PERFORMANCE NUTRITION
for Team Sports

MONIQUE RYAN, MS, RD, LDN

PEAK
SPORTSpress®

Performance Nutrition for Team Sports
© 2005 Monique Ryan

Printed in the United States of America.

10 9 8 7 6 5 4 3 2 1

Distributed in the United States and Canada by Publishers Group West.

Library of Congress Cataloging-in-Publication Data

Ryan, Monique, 1962-
   Performance nutrition for team sports / Monique Ryan.
      p. cm.
   Includes bibliographical references and index.
   ISBN 1-9746254-4-2 (pbk. : alk. paper)
  1. Athletes—Nutrition. 2. Physical fitness—Nutritional aspects. I. Title.

   TX361.A8R93 2005
   613.2'024'796—dc22   2004023040

Peak Sports Press®, an imprint of VeloPress®
1830 North 55th Street
Boulder, Colorado 80301–2700 USA
303/440-0601 • Fax 303/444-6788 • E-mail velopress@insideinc.com

To purchase additional copies of this book or other VeloPress® books, call 800/234-8356 or visit us on the Web at velopress.com.

Cover images by Thad Allender Photography
Interior photos by Eric Lars Bakke
Cover and interior design by Amber Salt
Interior production by Ronnie Moore

For Jack and James

CONTENTS

PERFORMANCE NUTRITION FOR TEAM SPORTS

A GUIDE TO USING THIS BOOK

Never has participation in team sports been so popular. Males and females alike at the junior high school, high school, college, and adult levels now regularly participate in basketball, soccer, baseball and softball, football, and hockey—the sports detailed in this book. Chances are that you are reading this book because you or a family member derives great satisfaction from participating, training, and competing in a team sport and appreciates that the proper fuel can greatly enhance your athletic accomplishments. Focused athletes realize that the daily food choices they make are highly interconnected with how they train, recover, and compete. Ultimately, consuming a quality training diet allows you to make the most of each training session and subsequently leaves you best prepared for competition.

Performance Nutrition for Team Sports is designed for the athlete interested in the everyday application of respected, cutting-edge sports nutrition science. Whether you are a basketball, soccer, hockey, football, or baseball player, providing your body with the proper food choices, consumed in the right amounts at the right times, lays a solid nutrition foundation for your chosen playing level, sport and competition goals, and optimum health. The high-quality training diet outlined in this book is designed to optimize your recovery, assist you in building muscle and strength, and sustain your energy during practice and competition.

Performance Nutrition for Team Sports has several unique features. First, it is designed to be a practical book and provides a bridge between sports nutrition science and real-life application of practical sports nutrition and health-related guidelines. In addition to the chapters that outline nutrition choices for good health and optimal fueling, specific advice for popular team sports are included. To provide this information, this book has been divided into three parts.

Part I, The Daily Performance Diet, emphasizes that good training and performance begins with a solid nutrition foundation of quality food choices. A quality diet consisting of the highest nutrient and food choices on a daily basis provides fuel and hydration for both training and competition, and nutrients for optimal health. This section also addresses the unique considerations of the many age groups of athletes that may participate in team sports, from high school to the masters athlete playing at the club level.

Part II, Training Nutrition, addresses the diverse nutrition training concerns of athletes participating in team sports, including fueling before and during practice, optimal food and fluid choices for recovery, and nutritional strategies to optimize muscle building. A full chapter on meal planning is provided to assist the high school, collegiate, and adult athlete in putting together the sport diet suited to your sport, training and body composition goals, and lifestyle. Supplement use and the research behind many products marketed to athletes are also covered in this section.

Part III, Sport-Specific Nutrition Guidelines, outlines specific nutritional considerations for the power sports of baseball and football and the power, middle-distance endurance sports of basketball, soccer, and hockey. This chapter will address some nutritional strategies unique to training programs and competition for these sports.

I trust and hope that the information provided in this book will enhance your health, enjoyment of your sport, and athletic accomplishments.

Monique Ryan, MS, RD, LDN

The Daily Performance Diet
Building a Healthy Sports Nutrition Foundation

For many athletes participating in team sports, interest in nutrition centers around performance at practice, muscle building, and being prepared for competition. But clearly, the quality of the foods and fluids you choose can have a significant impact on your health. Your daily food choices also provide a solid foundation for your training diet and optimizing your nutrient intake.

Part I provides you with nutrition guidelines on which to build your training diet, promote optimal health, support growth for younger athletes, and maintain and promote good health for masters athletes. You will learn about quality food choices for carbohydrates, protein, and fat and practical suggestions for integrating these choices into your life. You will also be provided with the information necessary for meeting daily hydration needs and the vitamin and mineral intakes required to build a foundation for a cutting-edge training and competition diet.

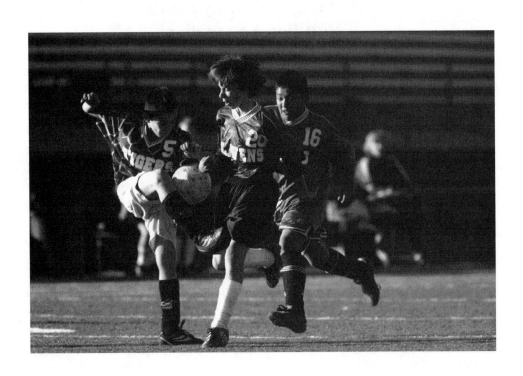

CHAPTER 1

THE DAILY PERFORMANCE DIET: YOUR KEY TO GOOD TRAINING AND GOOD HEALTH

Because you regularly put in hours of training for your chosen team sport or sports, your daily food intake has a significant effect on your recovery and your ability to build strength and muscle, and provide fuel during your daily workouts. In whatever sport you are involved at the high school, college, club, or professional level, the training sessions that you complete on a weekly basis require that you choose the right amounts and types of foods and fluids at the best times. Your nutrition efforts can maximize your various types of training efforts, whether during a team practice or when weight training, and replace fuel depleted during training. Optimal daily nutrition strategies and recovery means that you make the most of each training session and arrive to competition in the best form possible. You must meet the nutritional demands placed on your body in order to derive the maximum benefit from your training program.

Trained bodies also benefit from premium fuel by staying healthy. If you suffer from lackluster training days, injuries, and frequent infections such as colds, you may not be making the highest-quality fuel choices possible. Your body requires more than forty-five different nutrients for optimal functioning. Take a proactive and sensible approach to planning your diet by consuming a wide variety of wholesome foods in moderate amounts for the full spectrum of nutrients they provide. When it comes to nutrition, athletes participating in team sports should keep the big picture in mind when balancing their diet and appreciate that quality foods can taste good as well as fuel their active and well-trained bodies.

Variety, Balance, Moderation, and Quality

It takes planning, thought, and maybe some assistance to put together a diet balanced in nutrients. One clear way to regard and organize your diet is through food groups.

Often foods are grouped according to their carbohydrate, protein, and fat content, as the proper balance of these nutrients supports good health and gives an athlete training and competing in a team sport the proper ratio of nutrients and fuel for exercise and recovery. Foods may supply one of these three nutrients or a combination of two or three of these nutrients. For example, fruits are predominately a source of carbohydrate, while skim dairy milk is a source of both carbohydrate and protein.

You should also appreciate that foods are complex, providing nutrients beyond their basic carbohydrate, protein, and fat content and also containing important vitamins and minerals. While a morning glass of orange juice may be a good source of carbohydrate, it is also an excellent source of vitamin C and potassium. Vitamins and minerals are also essential to both your athletic performance and good health. Eating a variety of wholesome foods at meals and for snacks allows these nutrients to work together to improve the overall quality of your diet.

While a variety of foods are available in the North American diet, excessive amounts of highly processed foods are also available. Unprocessed and nutrient-dense foods should be emphasized in your diet as they provide a higher nutritional value than comparable processed foods in similar serving sizes. For lifelong good health and top performance, it is best if processed foods are not a mainstay in your diet. When you do choose a wholesome and varied diet the majority of the time, there is still some room for enjoyable foods that may not be as high in nutrients.

All nutrients are an important part of your diet. Whether you are weight training or practicing with your teammates, some carbohydrate is burned for energy. An adequate fluid intake supports delivery of nutrients to your body's cells when training. Healthy red blood cells are supported by an adequate intake of iron, vitamin B12, and folic acid. Healthy bones are also maintained when you consume not only enough calcium but also magnesium and vitamin D. Clearly, it is important to have the right balance of nutrients in your diet. Table 1.1 outlines the basic functions of the important nutrient classifications in your diet.

The optimal proportions of carbohydrate, protein, and fat for the athlete participating in team sports can vary somewhat from sport to sport, the position played in certain sports, and the type of training session in which you are participating. But because of the unique fuel requirements of weight training, stop-and-go training, power workouts, and two-a-day practices, it is generally recommended that your diet provide about 50 to 60 percent carbohydrate, 15 to 20 percent protein, and 20 to 30 percent fat. It is important to keep in mind that these percentages are all relative to the number of calories or the total amount of energy that your body requires to match up with your training needs that

TABLE 1.1 NUTRIENTS AND THEIR FUNCTIONS

Nutrient	Functions	Food Sources
Water	Carries oxygen and nutrients to cells Plays a role in digestion Cools the body through sweat production Important role in many cellular processes Important part of muscle tissue	Tap water Bottled water Fruit juices, dairy milk, soy milk Solid foods that contain water: fruits, vegetables, yogurt
Carbohydrate	Primary high-energy fuel source during exercise Replenishes body stores Provides dietary fiber	Grains, breads, cereals, rice, pasta Fruit and fruit juices Vegetables Dairy and soy milk, yogurt
Protein	Provide essential amino acids Required for maintaining and developing muscle and other body tissue Essential component of enzymes, hormones, and antibodies Needed for the formation of hemoglobin	Meat, poultry, fish, cheese, egg Soy, dried beans, lentils Dairy and soy milk, yogurt
Fat	Provides essential fatty acids Provides fat-soluble vitamins Adds flavor to foods Used as a fuel source Protects and insulates body organs Component of cell structures	Liquid oils Margarine and butter Nuts and seeds Avocado Fish
Vitamins	Enhance energy production Involved in tissue repair and protein synthesis Play a role in red blood cell formation Act as antioxidants	Fruits and vegetables Lean protein foods Whole grains Nuts and seeds
Minerals	Involved in energy production Play a role in building body tissue Play a role in muscle contraction Involved in oxygen transport	Fruits and vegetables Leans proteins Whole grains Nuts and seeds

day. Variations in these percentages can be adequate if that is what suits meeting the fuel demands of that day's training session. What is important is that you sufficiently replace the carbohydrate stores burned for fuel, consume enough protein for repair and rebuilding, and balance out your calorie needs with healthy fats. When the energy and fuel breakdown of your dietary intake matches and replaces what you burned and utilized that day, your recovery is enhanced and so is the quality of subsequent training sessions.

First, let's take a look at some of the food choices available from carbohydrates, proteins, and fats, so that you can appreciate which options are the most nutritious. How you portion and time these foods with your training is what distinguishes your sports nutrition diet from an ordinary healthy diet. More information on the timing and portioning of these fuels in relation to your training session, and how your diet replenishes your body stores on a daily and weekly basis, will be reviewed in Part II: Training Nutrition.

CARBOHYDRATES PROVIDE ENERGY
Classifying Carbohydrates—It's Not So Simple

Many athletes are familiar with the traditional classification of carbohydrates. Simple carbohydrates, often called "sugars," consist of one or two molecules, while complex carbohydrates or starches are composed of up to thousands of carbohydrate molecules joined together. What was long advised regarding these foods was that simple carbohydrates such as fructose and other sugars cause a rapid rise and subsequent fall in blood sugar that results in fatigue, and that these sugars are less nutritious. Conversely, it was maintained that complex carbohydrates resulted in a more gentle blood glucose rise and are more nutritious foods. In summary, simple carbohydrates were considered "bad" and complex carbohydrates were "good."

While this classification might seem logical, recent scientific data indicate that it is an outdated concept. What team sport athletes should truly be concerned about is the quality of the carbohydrate they consume, with an emphasis on wholesome versus refined sources. Wholesome carbohydrates provide vitamins, minerals, and fiber, while refined carbohydrates are processed foods with a much lower or poor nutrient content, providing little other than carbohydrate calories. What is important to appreciate is that wholesome carbohydrates are not always complex, and refined carbohydrates are not always simple. Fruit, a simple carbohydrate, is packed with nutrients, while products made from complex white flour such as white bread often have a much lower vitamin and mineral content. For optimal training and good health, wholesome carbohydrates are a very important component of your diet, because they are higher in nutritional value.

In addition to viewing carbohydrates as wholesome or refined, we can also categorize them according to how they affect blood sugar or blood glucose levels. The belief that simple carbohydrates cause a rapid rise in blood glucose and that complex carbohydrates cause a slower rise in blood glucose is outdated. Recent nutrition research has demonstrated that each carbohydrate food produces its own unique blood glucose profile that does not correlate with the simple-versus-complex classification.

The ranking system that describes the blood glucose profile of a food is referred to as the glycemic index. In this system, the blood glucose profile of 50 grams of pure glucose has been ascribed a glycemic index of 100. Other carbohydrates are tested in 50-gram doses and compared to glucose. High-glycemic foods are generally considered to have a glycemic index of greater than 70. Moderate-glycemic index foods are in the 55 to 70 range, and low-glycemic index foods have a score of less than 55.

Table 1.2 provides an abbreviated glycemic index ranking of high-carbohydrate foods (see Appendix A: Glycemic Index of Foods for a more complete listing). Interestingly fruits generally have a low glycemic index, despite being simple carbohydrates, while potatoes, a complex carbohydrate, have a high glycemic index. Many factors influence the glycemic index of a food, including the type of fiber in the food, how the glucose molecules in the food are connected, and the form of the food.

Currently, individuals with specific health concerns such as diabetes who need to control blood glucose and elevated blood lipids can manipulate their carbohydrate according to their benefit based on the glycemic index of the foods. The glycemic index can also play a role in treating individuals diagnosed with a condition referred to as *metabolic syndrome* that is characterized by a resistance to using the body's insulin appropriately. Ongoing research for individuals with these health concerns will fine-tune appropriate dietary recommendations.

Athletes may also be able to utilize the glycemic index to their performance advantage in regard to specific recommendations before, during, and after training. These sports nutrition applications of glycemic index will be reviewed in Part II. For their daily diet, athletes should try various nutrient-dense carbohydrate foods to determine what works best with their food preferences and schedules.

Go for the Grains

Wholesome grains are good sources of carbohydrate, fiber, and B vitamins. Because they are so concentrated in carbohydrate, they are excellent choices for replenishing your body's carbohydrate stores, namely muscle and liver glycogen, which become depleted from intense and demanding training sessions. Grains are easily obtained in the American diet, but unfortunately many of these choices are refined grains rather than whole grains.

For your health and your sports diet, choose whole grains whenever possible. Whole grains literally come from the entire grain, which includes the endosperm, germ, and bran portion of the grain, and retain all the desirable nutrients found in

TABLE 1.2 GLYCEMIC INDEX OF FOODS

Food, Portion	Grams Carbohydrate (CHO) per Serving	Glycemic Load per Portion	Glycemic Index for 50 g
High-Glycemic Foods (GI > 70)			
Potato, baked, 6.5 oz. (200 g)	29	27.3	94
Rice, instant, 5 oz. (200 g)	42	36.5	87
Corn Flakes, 1 oz. (30 g)	25	21.5	86
Rice Krispies, 1 oz. (30 g)	29	24.0	82
Total cereal, 1 oz. (30 g)	25	19.0	76
Waffle, 2 oz. (60 g)	25	19.3	76
Cheerios, 1 oz. (30 g)	25	18.5	74
Watermelon, 8 oz. (240 g)	12	8.6	72
Bagel, white, 2.25 oz. (70 g)	35.5	25.5	72
Millet, 5 oz. (150 g)	34.8	24.7	71
Bread, white, 2 oz. (60 g)	26.8	18.8	70
Moderate-Glycemic Foods (GI 55–70)			
Shredded Wheat, 1 oz. (30 g)	21.7	14.6	67
Pineapple, 4 oz. (120 g)	9.6	6.3	66
Oat kernel bread, 2 oz. (60 g)	25.6	16.6	65
Raisins, 2 oz. (60 g)	42.7	27.3	64
Muffin, 1.9 oz. (57 g)	27.7	17.2	62
Couscous, 5 oz. (150 g)	14.3	8.7	61
Spaghetti, white, durum wheat, 6 oz. (180 g)	44.3	25.6	58
Muesli, 2 oz. (60 g)	32	17.9	56
Oat Bran, raw, 2 oz. (60 g)	30	16.5	55
Low-Glycemic Foods (GI <55)			
Buckwheat, 5 oz. (150 g)	28.8	14.6	51
Bread, whole-grain, 2 oz. (30 g)	23.0	12.0	51
Banana, ripe, 4 oz. (120 g)	23.9	12.1	50
All-Bran, 2 oz. (60 g)	36.8	18.4	50
Rice, brown, 5 oz. (150 g)	47.7	23.9	49
Porridge oatmeal, 8 oz. (250 g)	20.3	9.9	48
Sweet potato, 5 oz. (150 g)	26	12.5	48
Grapefruit juice, 8 oz. (260 g)	15.7	7.5	41
Pear, Bartlett, 4 oz. (120 g)	11.3	4.6	40
Apple, 4 oz. (120 g)	14.6	5.9	33
Yogurt, fruited, 6.5 oz. (200 g)	33	10.9	32
Milk, skim, 8 oz. (259 g)	13	4.1	32
Spaghetti, whole-meal, 4 oz. (120 g)	30	9.6	28
Peach, 8 oz. (240 g)	15	4.2	28
Lentils, 5 oz. (150 g)	14.9	4.1	28
Kidney beans, 5 oz. (150 g)	24	5.5	23

Values are based on a glucose rating of 100. Source: *The GI Factor,* Dr. Jennie Brand-Miller, and www.glycemicindex.com

Consider the Glycemic Load

While the glycemic index (GI) is a ranking of carbohydrates based on their immediate blood glucose effect, the glycemic load (GL) builds on the GI to provide a measure of the total glycemic response of a food. Glycemic load takes into consideration the portion of the food consumed. It is the glycemic index of a food multiplied by the total grams of carbohydrate in the portion of the food. This number is then divided by 100. One GL unit is approximately equal to the glycemic effect of 1 gram glucose. The GL of all carbohydrate foods can be added up for the day. The total GL range for the day is typically 60 to 180. A low-GL day is less than 80, while a high-GL day is greater than 120.

GL = GI × grams of carbohydrate per serving divided by 100

Let's compare the GL of carrots to corn. Carrots have a glycemic index of 92 and corn a glycemic index of 60. Let's assume that one-half cup cooked of each is consumed, which is a reasonable portion.

1. Carrots have a GI of 92, and you eat one-half cup cooked, which has 6 grams of carbohydrate.

92 × 6 = 552 divided by 100 = a glycemic load of 5.52

2. Corn has a GI of 60, and you eat one-half cup cooked, which has 20 grams of carbohydrate.

60 × 20 = 1,200 divided by 100 = a glycemic load of 12

Although carrots have a higher glycemic index than that of corn, because of the portion consumed, the glycemic load of carrots is lower than a similar portion of corn. This example illustrates that many moderate- to high-GI carbohydrate foods may not be consumed in the 50-gram portion test dose and could potentially have a low GL. A low GL for a carbohydrate serving is 10 or less, moderate GL is 11 to 19, and high GL is 20 or more.

whole grains. For refined grains, the bran and germ are separated from the starchy endosperm. The endosperm is then ground into flour.

Whole grains are packed with vitamins and minerals and phytochemicals that have powerful antioxidant and disease-fighting properties that you won't obtain from white bread, processed cereals, white rice, and even many "enriched" multigrain breads. Some of the phytochemicals found in whole grains include oligosaccharides, flavinoids, lignans, phytates, and saponins, many of which have powerful antioxidant properties. Whole grains also provide vitamin E and selenium. Studies have shown that regular consumption of whole grains is linked to prevention of heart disease, diabetes, and certain cancers. Surveys indicate that most Americans consume less than one serving of whole grains daily. Consuming grains such as whole oats, barley, and bran can also reduce the glycemic load of your diet. High-fiber whole-grain bread that contains whole seeds will also have a lower glycemic index.

A variety of whole grains can be included in your diet. Even just making simple changes such as having brown rice instead of white rice and whole-wheat pasta rather than semolina pasta is beneficial. Buy 100 percent whole-grain breads and look for "whole grain" on the health claim packages, which indicates that more than half of the weight of the product comes from whole grains.

Athletes who are tired of the same wheat- and rice-based grain choices also have a few more adventuresome options. There are many whole-grain alternatives, including amaranth, kasha (buckwheat), quinoa, spelt, teff, triticale, bulgur, barley, brown rice, and millet. Table 1.3 provides a list of some top grain alternatives. They may take a bit more cooking time than pasta, rice, and potatoes, but they are nutritious and add variety to the diet. Experiment with various seasonings to further flavor these wholesome grains.

Whole grains should be an important part of your diet for the nutrients and carbohydrates that they provide. But you should also place a strong emphasis on fruits and vegetables, not only for their carbohydrate content but also the great health benefits that they offer. In fact, some health organizations and health researchers believe that fruits and vegetables should comprise the majority of our carbohydrate intake. Studies have shown that eating more fruits and vegetables can reduce your risk of heart disease, stroke, and some types of cancer. How you put together your sports diet will ulti-

Getting in the Grains

Aim for three servings of whole grains each day. One slice or one ounce of bread equals a serving and one ounce of cereal equals a serving.

Find a whole-grain cereal that you enjoy. Good choices include oatmeal or bran flakes.

Buy breads that list 100% whole-grain flour as the first ingredient and for all other listed flours as well.

Use brown rice instead of white and whole-wheat pasta instead of semolina.

Add bran or wheat germ to your yogurt, in smoothies, or in other cereals.

Look for the "whole-grain" health claim on the package, which indicates that more than half the weight of the products comes from whole grains.

TABLE 1.3 WHOLE-GRAIN ALTERNATIVES

Grain	Description	Tips
Amaranth	High in protein and fiber. Good source of vitamin E.	Boil and eat as a cereal. Cook 1 cup grain in 3 cups water for 1/2 hour.
Spelt	A distant cousin to wheat. High in fiber and B vitamins.	Used to make breads and pastas. Can be used in pilafs. Cook 1 cup with 4 cups water 30–40 min.
Millet	A staple in Africa. High in minerals.	Cook 1 cup grain with 2.25 cups water 25–30 min. Serve with meat or cook as a cereal.
Kasha (buckwheat groats)	Excellent source of magnesium and high in fiber.	Serve as a cereal, pilaf, or make pancakes. Simmer 1 part groats to 2 parts water for 15 min.
Quinoa	Excellent source of B vitamins, copper, iron, and magnesium.	Can make an oatmeal-like cereal. Rinse before cooking to remove bitter coating. Cook 1 cup quinoa in 2 cups water for 20 min.
Teff	The world's smallest grain. Rich in protein and calcium.	Serve as a hot breakfast cereal or as part of a stew. Cook 1 cup of teff in 3 cups water for 15–20 min.

mately depend on your food preferences, convenience, and personal health considerations. But chances are that boosting your fruit and vegetable intake would be a step in the right direction, for any athlete interested in optimal performance on the playing field and in lifelong good health.

Plenty of Fruit

Fruits are not only excellent sources of carbohydrate but also provide a number of health-protecting nutrients such as fiber, potassium, vitamins A and C, carotenoids, and a variety of disease-fighting substances called *phytonutrients*. Because they are so packed with disease-fighting nutrients, a high number of daily fruit servings are strongly recommended by the American Heart Association and the American Cancer Society. Fresh fruits, dried fruit, and fruit juice can also provide the team sport athlete with a significant and concentrated source of carbohydrates.

While all fruits are nutritious, some choices are *extremely* nutritious. Tropical fruits such as papaya, mango, kiwifruit, and guava have wonderfully high levels of vitamin C and carotenoids, which are potent antioxidants. Carotenoids are also found in signifi-cant amounts in deep-colored fruits such as apricots, cantaloupe, and nectarines. Citrus fruits such as oranges and grapefruits are known for being great sources of vitamin C. Phytonutrients, which appear increasingly important to maintaining good health, such as catechins, falvonols, stilbenes, allicin, quercetin, ellagic acid, anthocyanins, limonin, zeathanthin, and leutin, are also found in fruits. The best way to obtain a variety of phy-tonutrients is to consume a variety of fruits. Dried fruits and real fruit juices will provide the most concentrated sources of carbohydrate for athletes with higher energy needs. Dried fruits, however, will not be as great a source of vitamin C, though they may pro-vide more minerals and fiber than fresh because they are so concentrated. Try to avoid dried fruits prepared with sulfites if you are sulfite-sensitive. Sulfites are preservatives that trigger allergic reactions in some individuals. Fresh fruits are also great sources of fiber and the highest in nutrients. Table 1.4 provides a list of some top fruit choices.

TABLE 1.4 TOP FRUIT AND VEGETABLE CHOICES

Good sources of vitamin C	Good sources of carotenoids and vitamin A	Good sources of phytonutrients
Oranges	Apricots	Grapes
Blackberries	Cantaloupe	Blueberries
Kiwifruit	Nectarine	Citrus fruits
Papaya	Mangoes	100% real fruit juice
Pineapple	Peaches	Apples
Grapefruit	Guava	Blackberries
Strawberries	Broccoli	Watermelon
Tangerines	Carrots	Cherries
Mangoes	Romaine lettuce	Kale
Artichoke	Sweet peppers	Beets
Broccoli	Kale	Asparagus
Brussels sprouts	Sweet potatoes	Onions
Cauliflower	Spinach	Tomatoes
Okra	Winter squash	Cabbage
Potatoes	Swiss chard	Cruciferous vegetables
Tomatoes		
Peas		

Plenty of Vegetables

Like fruits, vegetables provide a wide variety of vitamins, minerals, and phytonutri-ents, and fiber that maintain optimal health. All vegetables are good healthy choices, but some stand out nutritionally speaking and are even more concentrated in nutrients than fruit. Color is often a good indicator of a higher nutrient content. Some stellar options include carrots, sweet potatoes, and red peppers, which are high in carotenoids.

Spinach and Romaine lettuce are good leafy choices for their vitamin C, folate, and phytonutrient content. Another group of vegetables that not only contain beta-carotene and vitamin C but also the cancer-fighting phytonutrients indoles are broccoli, cauliflower, bok choy, collards, Brussels sprouts, and kale.

Each day try to consume a variety of colorful vegetables that are yellow, orange, red, and deep green. Choose large servings of vegetables when you eat at home, as it can be challenging to obtain quality vegetable choices when eating out. Buy fresh vegetables when you know you will consume them in a few days and store them in the refrigerator crisper drawer. Frozen vegetables are a good second choice. Avoid overcooking your vegetables in order to preserve all the wonderful nutrients they contain. Steaming is your best nutrient-preserving choice, and try to microwave vegetables with as little water as possible. Table 1.4 provides a list of some top vegetable choices.

Fiber

Another good reason for choosing unprocessed carbohydrate foods is for the fiber they provide. This important nutrient has been linked to a reduced risk of heart disease, diabetes, and obesity. Fiber may also protect you from heart disease, hypertension, and some forms of cancer as well as help prevent many conditions related to colon function, including constipation, hemorrhoids, and diverticulosis.

Fiber is actually a class of compounds that can be divided into two main categories, water-soluble and water-insoluble fiber. Insoluble fiber is the most familiar form and is found in wheat bran, whole-grain cereals, dried beans and peas, vegetables, and nuts. This type of fiber aids digestion and regulates colon function. Water-soluble fiber can help control blood glucose and blood cholesterol levels. Good sources of water-soluble fiber include whole oats, oat bran, some fruits, and dried beans. Fiber can also increase your feeling of fullness after consuming a meal, a useful tool for individuals trying to reduce their caloric intake and lose weight.

Nutrition experts recommend consuming between 20 to 30 grams of fiber daily. This amount can usually be reached by eating more than five servings of fruits and vegetables daily and several servings of whole grains. By consuming fiber from food sources, you obtain a mix of fibers and other healthy nutrients that these foods provide, and the quantity of fiber you consume is consistent with your energy intake and not excessive.

Generally excessive amounts of fiber and fiber supplements are not recommended. The result may be bloating and other unwanted gastrointestinal side effects. If you do need to increase the amount of fiber in your diet, do so gradually and drink plenty of water. Team sport athletes with very high caloric requirements may find that excessive fiber is too filling and replaces more concentrated and needed sources of calories. High-fiber foods may also not be the best choices close to training and competition as they may cause intestinal discomfort with exercise. For the athlete who benefits from a comfortable stomach and intestinal system during training, fiber intake is not only about health but also about consuming the correct amounts at the safest times.

Sugar

Sugar is the most prevalent simple carbohydrate in the North American diet and the common name for sucrose. Nutritionists often refer to foods high in sugar as "empty calories" because of their low nutritional value. Sugar and other related substances such as high-fructose corn syrup, glucose, and honey provide energy but not much else in the way of nutrients. Experts recommend that sugar comprise no more than 10 percent of our total energy intake, though many individuals consume greater than 20 percent of their total energy intake from sugar. Excess intake of refined sugar has been associated with high triglyceride levels, a type of blood fat, and with dental cavities. Excess sugar intake is also considered a contributor to weight management problems because of the concentrated calories these foods provide due to their highly processed nature and portioning. Scientists are also concerned that high-fructose corn syrup may contribute not only to empty calories in our diet but also to an increased risk of insulin resistance and the development of obesity and Type II diabetes. More research in this area is needed, but all health experts agree that high-fructose corn syrup has no nutritional value other than calories.

Sugar is one of the major additives in processed foods and is often associated with a low-fiber, high-fat diet. Try to limit products in which sugar is the first ingredient on labels, and also look for labeling terms such as *beet juice, brown rice syrup, cane syrup, corn syrup, corn sweetener, crystalline fructose, dextrose, evaporated cane juice, fructose, high-fructose corn syrup, invert sugar, malt syrup, maltodextrin,* and s*ucrose* that reflect a high sugar content. Naturally occurring sugars may work to satisfy a sweet tooth. Try sweet and dried fruits and jams to satisfy your sweet tooth. Of course, you are only human and may crave sugar at times. Just keep the sweet choices in perspective and have them as occasional treats in your daily training diet.

Sugar and some of its derivatives, however, can play a much different role for the athlete as they are a major component of many sports nutrition supplements designed for consumption during training and for recovery. They provide the required amounts of carbohydrate in easily digested forms and can be utilized appropriately for athletic performance at specific times in conjunction with certain types of training sessions and during competition. Appropriate use of these products for training and recovery is reviewed in more detail in Part II.

The Power of Protein

While wholesome carbohydrates are a staple, athletes interested in maximizing power and strength also need adequate amounts of protein foods to perform their best. Proteins play an important role in the growth, repair, and maintenance of muscles and other body tissues. It is also required to form hormones, enzymes, and neurotransmitters, and key components of the immune system. Protein is needed for hemoglobin formation, the substance that carries oxygen to the exercising muscles. Protein can also supply fuel for energy if your body's carbohydrate stores run low.

Proteins are composed of amino acids, which are the building units that create protein-based tissues. We obtain amino acids from the protein-containing foods we consume and from the breakdown of muscle tissue. Amino acids that can be manufactured in the body are considered nonessential, as it is not required that we consume them from food. Conversely, amino acids that we cannot manufacture in our body are considered essential and must be obtained in our diet for good health and optimal performance. Proteins that we consume are digested into amino acids and go to the amino acid pool in your body. These amino acids can then be drawn upon to synthesize protein-based tissues or to use as energy if carbohydrate stores run low.

Your sports diet protein intake can easily comprise 15 to 20 percent of your daily energy consumption with a well-balanced and even typical North American diet. Generally, many athletes exceed their protein intake, most likely due to large protein portions prevalent in the North American diet. But weight- or body fat–conscious athletes who restrict certain foods in attempts to limit or avoid fat intake could be at risk for consuming inadequate protein.

Animal protein in the form of lean meats, poultry, fish, and eggs is the most concentrated source of protein. Many of these animal proteins are also good sources of iron and zinc. High-quality plant sources of protein include soy products such as tofu and tempeh, dried peas and beans, and lentils. Low-fat dairy foods are also an excellent source of protein and the important mineral calcium. What is important for optimal health is to choose lean protein sources, as this will reduce your intake of saturated fat. Too high an intake of saturated fat is a risk factor for developing heart disease. Table 1.5 lists the protein content of certain foods per specified portion. Try to emphasize leaner choices of red meats to limit your intake of saturated fat. More discussion on choosing protein and protein requirements for specific types of training will be provided in Part II.

TABLE 1.5 PROTEIN CONTENT OF SELECTED FOODS	
Food and Portion	**Protein (g)**
Chicken, white, 3 oz. (100 g) cooked	25
Pork, lean, 3 oz. (100 g) cooked	23
Beef, lean, 3 oz. (100 g) cooked	21
White fish, 3 oz. (100 g) cooked	20
Tofu, firm, 4 oz. (120 g)	20
Lentils, cooked, 1 c. (240 ml)	18
Soy milk, 1 c. (240 ml)	10
Milk, 8 oz. (240 ml)	8
Peanut butter, 2 tbsp. (40 ml)	8
Cheese, 1 oz. (30 g)	7

Facts about Fat

Fat is an important part of an athlete's diet. While fat is somewhat renowned for being a concentrated source of calories, it plays several key roles in keeping you healthy. Most important, fat is a source of nutrients known as *essential fatty acids.* Just as you need to obtain vitamins and minerals in your diet, you also need to obtain the two essential fatty acids, linoleic acid and alpha-linolenic acid, from the foods you eat. Another important function of fat is its role in the transport and absorption of fat-soluble vitamins and carotenoids. Fat can also add a wonderful flavor to our meals and make meals more filling and satisfying.

It is easy to obtain too much fat in the North American diet. A high-fat content often characterizes many convenience, restaurant, and fast foods. Fats are a concentrated source of calories, and excess fat does not provide optimum fuel for your body and may crowd out valuable carbohydrate and proteins. While consumption of less fat may take planning and knowledge of hidden fats, many North Americans consume too much of the wrong types of fats.

Fat comes in several chemical forms, some healthier than others. Depending on their composition, fats are categorized as saturated or unsaturated. *Unsaturated* fats include both polyunsaturated and monounsaturated fats. Currently the American Heart Association sets the recommended range of fat intake from 15 to 30 percent of total calories. Exceeding this range may increase risk of heart disease, while going below this range could result in essential fatty acid insufficiency in some individuals. For team sport athletes, a diet in which 20 to 30 percent of the calories are supplied from fat should be appropriate. This provides adequate fat to replenish fuel stores after training and leaves room for adequate carbohydrate and protein in the diet.

Being a Vegetarian Athlete

In recent years, many nutritionally aware high school and collegiate athletes have decreased their intake of specific proteins, such as meats high in saturated fat. Some have gone a step further and replaced animal proteins with plant proteins. Vegetarians are individuals who have consciously made the choice to completely exclude or include only specific animal foods in their diet, such as dairy products, eggs, or fish and obtain a significant portion of their protein from plant foods. Whether these dietary modifications are for health, environmental, animal rights, or taste-related issues, you need to pay attention to your vegetarian nutrition program to ensure that your diet is adequate in protein, specific vitamins and minerals, and is well balanced for your training program.

Vegetarianism is a term that actually incorporates a range of dietary exclusions. A plant-based vegetarian diet may refer to one of the following descriptions:

Semi- or near-vegetarians—Eat small amounts of fish, poultry, eggs, and dairy, and avoid red meat

Pescovegetarians—Eat fish, dairy, and eggs

Lacto-ovo-vegetarians—Eat dairy foods and eggs

Ovovegetarians—Eat eggs

Vegans—Eat no animal foods whatsoever

Depending on what type of vegetarian diet you follow, you need to carefully choose foods that provide specific nutrients in your diet. These nutrients include protein, of course, but also iron and zinc, as well as, particularly if you exclude dairy products, vitamin B12, calcium, and vitamin D.

Throughout this book, the unique considerations of vegetarian athletes will be addressed in regard to specific nutrients. Of course, any athlete can choose to include more plant sources of specific nutrients in their diet. Plant foods are filled with health-promoting minerals. Vegetarians appear to have a lower risk of hypertension, certain cancers, and a decreased risk for developing heart disease and diabetes. A plant-based diet also supplies plenty of carbohydrates for replenishing body fuel stores after training. Filling up on whole grains, fruits, and vegetables as described are healthy sources of carbohydrate for any endurance athlete. Milk and yogurt, though sources of high-quality protein, add nice amounts of carbohydrate to your diet as well.

However, an athlete training for a team sport should pay close attention to their vegetarian diet. Like a diet containing meat and other animal protein, a vegetarian diet can be well planned and support your training efforts, or it can be overly restrictive and ill conceived and hamper your training efforts.

For prevention of heart disease, it is important to limit the amount of saturated fat that you consume. Saturated fats raise the harmful low-density lipoprotein (LDL) cholesterol. This undesirable fat is found mainly in fatty animal foods such as cheese and whole-milk products, fatty cuts of meat, highly processed lunch meats, butter, lard, and shortening. Palm, palm kernel, and coconut oil are three highly saturated plant oils, which can sometimes be found in processed foods and commercially baked goods.

Another group of fats that are of concern in the North American diet are trans-fatty acids. Trans fatty acids are created from liquid oils that are "partially hydrogenated." Hydrogenation turns liquid corn oil into margarine sticks and increases the shelf life of commercial products that contain these altered oils. Some common sources of trans fat include cookies, crackers, and snack chips. These fats can increase LDL cholesterol, just like saturated fat, and lower the protective high-density lipoprotein (HDL) cholesterol. Check labels to limit hydrogenated oils as much as possible, particularly if they are listed as one of the first several ingredients. Choose margarine that lists "liquid oil" as the first ingredient.

Unsaturated fats, both polyunsaturated and monounsaturated, can help lower LDL cholesterol when they replace saturated fat in your diet. Sources of polyunsaturated oil include corn, safflower, and sunflower oil and walnuts and sunflower seeds. These oils should comprise no more than one-third of your total fat intake as large amounts have been linked to cancer in animals. Most health care professionals advocate that monounsaturated fats comprise the majority of your fat intake. Good sources include olive oil, canola oil, avocados, almonds, and hazelnuts. Table 1.6 outlines the types of fats contained in various oils.

Unfortunately, what has gotten lost in some of this heart-healthy advice is recommendations regarding the types of polyunsaturated fats that you should emphasize in your diet. Linoleic and alpha-linolenic essential fatty acids are both polyunsaturated fats, but they differ greatly in how they affect our health. Linoleic acid is from a family of fats knows as *omega-6 fats*, while alpha-linolenic acid is from the *omega-3* family of fats. Two other omega-3 fats, docosahexaenoic (DHA) and eicosapentaenoic (EPA), are abundant in fish oils such as salmon and tuna. The body can convert alpha-linolenic acid to DHA and EPA, though the conversion is inefficient.

DHA and EPA are of great interest to health experts. Consuming these fats, as well as alpha-linolenic acid, are needed to produce hormone-like compounds that can reduce unnecessary blood clotting, boost immune function, and decrease the disease-promoting condition of inflammation. Conversely, excess linoleic acid can produce

TABLE 1.6 PERCENTAGES OF FAT OF VARIOUS OILS			
Oil	% Saturated	% Polyunsaturated	% Monounsaturated
Canola	6	32	62
Hazelnut	7	11	82
Flaxseed	7	75	18
Safflower	7	79	14
Almond	8	19	73
Walnut	9	67	24
Grapeseed	10	73	17
Sunflower	11	69	20
Corn	13	62	25
Olive	14	9	77
Pumpkin seed	15	53	15
Soybean	15	61	24
Sesame	15	44	41
Margarine (tub)*	17	34	24
Wheat germ	17	61	22
Peanut	18	34	48
Rice bran	26	28	46
Cottonseed	27	54	19
Lard	41	12	47
Palm kernel	85	2	11
Coconut	92	2	6

*Also contains some trans-fatty acids. Different brands of margarine contain varying levels of hydrogenated oils. Some labeled as trans fat–free are available.

hormones that lead to inflammation, promote blood clotting, and promote constriction of arteries. Because linoleic and alpha-linolenic acid compete in the body for the same physiological pathway, it is best not to consume an excess of linoleic acid.

Keep in mind that both of these essential fats are good for you. What is desirable is to obtain the proper balance of the two essential fatty acids in your diet. However, most North Americans consume an excess of linoleic fat and need to increase their intake of alpha-linoleic acid. Table 1.7 will guide you in choosing food sources of these fats. Try to emphasize fatty fish and use soy, walnut, almond, and canola oils. Olive oil supplies very little of these essential fats but it is an excellent source of the healthy monounsaturated fat. Other good sources of alpha-linolenic acid include leafy green vegetables, walnuts, and flaxseed. Several foods are listed under both of these fat sources, as they are rich in both essential fatty acids. While scientists are still formulating specific recommendations, aim for a minimum 2 grams of the alpha-linolenic acid daily.

To emphasize the best fat choices, you can balance your intake in the following way:

- Consume fish like salmon, light tuna, sole, and tilapia two times weekly or more.
- Emphasize soy and canola oils and related products, and use olive oil as well.
- Have green leafy vegetables, walnuts, and ground flaxseed in your diet.
- Choose the leanest cuts of red meat possible.
- Limit fatty cheeses.
- Emphasize poultry, beans, lentils, and soy protein in your diet.
- Control margarine intake, and choose products with liquid oil as the first ingredient.
- Avoid processed foods that contain partially hydrogenated oil and trans fat.

TABLE 1.7 FOOD SOURCES OF ESSENTIAL FATTY ACIDS

Food Rich in Alpha-Linoleic Acid	Alpha-Linoleic Acid Content (g)
Flax oil, 1 tbsp. (20 ml)	6.6
Canola oil, 1 tbsp. (20 ml)	1.6
Soybean oil, 1 tbsp. (20 ml)	1.0
Walnut oil, 1 tbsp. (20 ml)	1.4
Flaxseed, ground, 1 tbsp. (20 ml)	1.8
Soy nuts, roasted, 1/2 c. (120 ml)	1.8
Tofu, firm, 1/2 c. (120 ml)	0.7
Soy milk, 1 c. (240 ml)	0.4
Legumes, 1/2 c. (120 ml)	0.05
Oat germ, 2 tbsp. (40 ml)	0.2
Wheat germ, 2 tbsp. (40 ml)	0.1
Sardines, 2 oz. (60 g)	0.28
Spinach, cooked, 1 c. (240 ml)	0.15
Kale, cooked, 1 c. (240 ml)	0.13
Almond butter, 2 tbsp. (40 ml)	0.12

Foods Rich in Linoleic Acid	Linoleic Acid Content (g)
Safflower oil, 1 tbsp. (20 ml)	10.1
Sunflower oil, 1 tbsp. (20 ml)	9.2
Corn oil, 1 tbsp. (20 ml)	7.8
Soybean oil, 1 tbsp. (20 ml)	6.9
Walnuts, 1 oz. (30 g)	11.0
Soy nuts, roasted, 1/2 c. (120 ml)	9.0
Brazil nuts, 1 oz. (30 g)	7.0
Pecans, 1 oz. (30 g)	6.0
Tofu, firm, 4 oz. (120 g)	5.4
Peanuts, 1 oz. (30 g)	4.5
Peanut butter, 2 tbsp. (40 ml)	4.4
Almonds, 1 oz. (30 g)	3.0
Almond butter, 2 tbsp. (40 ml)	3.8
Wheat germ, 2 tbsp. (40 ml)	0.8
Flaxseed, ground, 1 tbsp. (20 ml)	0.5

Consuming Fish Oils Safely

Fish is good for you because it is a great source of omega-3 fatty acids, which can reduce disease risk and enhance health. But when you consume fish, it would be appropriate to take into consideration choices that will reduce your mercury intake. Mercury is present in our air and water and, when converted to methyl-mercury, can accumulate in fish and humans. Methyl-mercury is a known toxin to developing fetuses, small babies, and children and is now considered a potential threat to adults as well. Mercury can damage the brain and nervous system, and cause symptoms such as fatigue and hair loss.

The health benefits of eating fish do outweigh these risks, if you make good choices regarding the type and amount of fish consumed. Currently the American Heart Association recommends eating fish twice weekly. Generally you can keep your total fish portions to about 12 ounces weekly, though mercury's effects are somewhat dose related based on body weight.

Next, try to choose fish lower in mercury. Fish highest in mercury include shark, swordfish, king mackerel, and tilefish. Other high-mercury fish are fresh tuna, red snapper, orange roughy, and mar-lin. Some of the fish lower in mercury include shrimp, salmon, pollack, catfish, tilapia, sardines, and sole. Canned white albacore tuna contains more mercury than canned light tuna and should be limited. Tuna lovers can switch to the light tuna. Other fish fairly low in mercury include haddock, herring, and whitefish.

Many salmon lovers are also concerned about the cancer-causing polychlorinated biphenyls (PCBs) in fish. Testing indicates that both farmed and wild salmon are contaminated with PCBs, with the farmed varieties containing much higher amounts. Farmed varieties from both the United States and Canada contain lower amounts of PCBs than those from European countries, but all levels were much higher than wild varieties. When in season, choose wild Alaska salmon, which is lowest in PCBs. You can also choose canned salmon, which comes almost exclusively from the wild Alaskan variety. Since September 2004, all seafood has been labeled as farmed or wild, with country of origin noted, which should assist you in making decisions around fish choices. Recent lab testing of several dozen fish oil supplement products found that none of the supplements contained detectable levels of mercury.

DAILY HYDRATION ESSENTIALS

Fluid is the most essential nutrient for any athlete, including those participating in team sports. Dehydration quickly results in adverse performance effects that are readily apparent and easily measured. When watching top players perform on the field or court, you may have been struck by their obvious sweat losses. Studies demonstrate that team sport athletes routinely replace less fluid than is lost in sweat during training and especially during competition. That is why adequate hydration is crucial for both general well-being and athletic performance, and every athlete should arrive to practice and competition well hydrated. In fact, even though it deserves top priority, daily water intake is often a secondary nutrition consideration, and many athletes frequently fall short on daily consumption of the most important nutrient in our daily diet. Team sport athletes should not only pay attention to their fluid intake before, during, and after practice and games but also throughout the day. More on fluid intake strategies are covered in Part II, and specific strategies are covered for each team sport in Part III: Sport-Specific Nutrition Guidelines.

Much marketing fuss has been made about the optimal fluids that athletes require. But before the plethora of sports-related drinks arrived and flooded the market, there was simply water. Water is basic and unpretentious and flows naturally into your active sport life with no packaging or gimmicks attached. Don't take water for granted, as it is an essential part of your daily training diet. Just as you don't want to arrive to training and competition with a low "fuel tank," your fluid stores should be topped off as well.

Water is both a significant part of your body and plays an integral role in its optimal functioning, whether you are training or not. Anywhere from 60 to 70 percent of your total body weight is water. Hydrated muscle tissue is also high in fluid content, with about 70 to 75 percent of your muscle comprised of water. Fat tissue is low in water content at about 10 percent. Consequently, muscular athletes will have high body water content when adequately hydrated. Clearly water is stored in many body compartments and moves freely between these various spaces. About two-thirds of your body's water is stored inside your body cells, giving them their shape and form. The rest of the water in your body is around these cells and within your blood vessels. About 93 percent of your blood is water and even your relatively solid bones are about 32 percent water. Water plays a role in cooling the body and also provides structure to body parts, consequently protecting important tissues such as your brain and spinal cord, and lubricating your joints. When fluid becomes depleted through sweating, both your cells and blood decrease in volume.

Athletes should appreciate that fluid is also the main component of their blood. Blood carries oxygen, hormones, and nutrients such as glucose to your cells and is linked to important body fuel and nutrient stores such as protein, carbohydrates, and electrolytes. The protein content of blood, muscle, and other tissues also binds water in those tissues. Muscle glycogen holds a considerable amount of water, and water removes lactic acid from exercising muscles, which can be an advantage to athletes. Water is involved in digestion through saliva and stomach secretions and it eliminates waste products through urine and sweat. Water is essential for all your senses, such as hearing, sight, and sound, to function properly.

Clearly the role water plays in maintaining your overall health is extremely important. That's why you can't live without water for more than a few days. But the role that water plays in your performance is also essential. Being even slightly under-hydrated is unacceptable for top athletic performance. As the primary component of sweat, water plays a major role in body temperature regulation. You are able to maintain a constant body temperature under various environmental conditions by continually making adjustments to either gain or lose heat. Your fluid balance is the result of your intake versus output. Intake is the net result of the water and hydrating fluids we consume, water in some of the foods we eat, and the metabolic water produced by the body. At rest, urine output represents our greatest losses, while sweating during exercise can incur significant fluid losses, especially for athletes involved in intense practice in hot and humid weather conditions. Fluid is also lost in feces and the air you exhale.

Warm or humid weather, living in a dry climate, or living at altitude all increase fluid losses. Traveling, especially by plane, can boost water loss. In general, your body loses about 64 to 80 ounces or 8 to 10 cups (2 to 2.4 liters) of fluid daily through the urine, feces, skin, and lungs. Your daily water requirements are based on the amount of calories you consume. Team sport athletes can have very high nutritional requirements, especially during periods of growth, during intense practices, and when participating in two-a-day practices. At rest, your body water levels can be replaced slowly, requiring a conscious effort to drink every 1 to 2 hours to replace these fluid losses.

What about Sweat?

When you train, heat is a major by-product of your working muscles. As this heat builds up, your body temperature rises. Water then acts as a coolant to keep the body from overheating. During exercise, sweating is the body's primary mechanism for getting rid of excess heat. Sweat losses can easily reach anywhere from 16 to 32 ounces

(500 to 960 milliliters) and sometimes even 48 ounces (1.5 liters) per hour depending on environmental conditions and the sweat rate of the individual athlete.

One of water's functions in the body is to maintain adequate blood supply to the skin. This blood transfers heat to the environment through sweating. When sweat evaporates it cools the skin, blood, and your body's inner core. Athletes who are in top shape actually sweat more than their sedentary counterparts, rendering their fluid needs quite high. So while it may appear that your tolerance to training in the heat improves, your fluid requirements go up.

Though sweating does the important job of keeping your body cool, the resulting minor to large fluid losses can impair your athletic performance during both training and competition. Even losing as little as 2 percent of your body weight (about 2 to 3 pounds for a 130-pound athlete) through sweat can impair your ability to exercise. When you sweat, blood volume is decreased and greater demands are placed on your cardiovascular system, which reduces your ability to take in and utilize oxygen. Muscular endurance ability is also impaired with dehydration and your heart rate may increase at a given level of intensity. When fluid losses through sweat are not replaced, your body temperature rises further and exercise becomes harder. Clearly, not meeting your fluid needs hinders your athletic goals.

Unfortunately, thirst is not a very good indicator of the amount of fluid that your body requires, during exercise or at rest. Some early signs and symptoms of dehydration are light-headedness, headaches, decreased appetite, darkly colored urine, and fatigue. When you are thirsty, you have already lost 1 percent of your body weight through fluid loss. When fluid losses reach about 2 to 4 percent of your body weight, increased thirst and symptoms such as irritability and nausea may occur. At losses of 5 to 6 percent of body weight, there will be an increase in heart rate and breathing regulation, and body temperature regulation will be significantly impaired. Table 1.8 describes some of the physiological effects and symptoms of dehydration. Pay attention to how you feel during the day. An annoying headache may indicate the need to up your fluid intake.

Daily Hydration Essentials

Because dehydration during exercise can hurt your performance, it is essential that you stay on top of your fluid needs by drinking a minimum of 60 to 80 ounces (1.8 to 2.4 liters) of fluid daily for basic hydration requirements off the field and court. Try to drink on a schedule of 8 ounces (240 milliliters) every hour. Water should comprise about half of your daily fluid intake, but you can also receive hydration benefits from

TABLE 1.8 EFFECTS AND SYMPTOMS OF DEHYDRATION

Physiological Effects of Dehydration	Symptoms of Dehydration
Decreased:	**Mild dehydration:**
Blood volume	Dark urine
Cardiac output	Decreased appetite
Skin blood flow	Headache
Sweat rate	Fatigue
Urine output	Heat intolerance
	Light-headedness
	Small amount dark urine
	Nausea
Increased:	**Severe dehydration:**
Body temperature	High temperature
Heart rate	Delirium, disorientation, dizziness
	Difficulty swallowing
	Dry, shriveled skin
	Muscle spasms
	Sunken eyes

other fluids. Hydrating choices include juice, dairy milk, soy milk, and various sports nutrition supplements.

Team sport athletes with very high energy requirements can consume high-calorie drinks such as juices and smoothies to assist them in meeting their fluid, carbohydrate, and energy needs. Caffeinated beverages can be incorporated into your diet in reasonable amounts but should not be your first choice for hydration purposes. Overdoing the caffeine may interfere with your sleep patterns and make you nervous and jittery. Excess caffeine may also act as a mild diuretic shortly after you drink a caffeine-containing beverage. However, overall, newer research suggests that caffeine-containing beverages are not as dehydrating as they were once thought to be and can be included in moderate amounts with other fluids in the diet.

You can monitor your hydration status by checking the color and quantity of your urine. Clear urine reflects adequate fluid intake, while darker urine indicates that you need to step up your fluid intake. Urine tends to be more concentrated when you first wake up but should be clearer throughout the day. You should urinate at least four full bladders every day. Certain vitamin supplements can darken urine, so volume rather than color may be a better indicator of hydration status if you take these products. You can also consider regularly monitoring of your weight during heavy training periods. If you notice significant weight losses at a morning weigh-in, this may also be an indicator of chronic dehydration.

Daily Hydration Strategies

Start your day with hydration in mind. Consume liquids such as juice, dairy, or soy milk at breakfast. Drink 8 to 16 oz. (240 to 480 milliliters) of water or hydrating fluid when you start your day. Don't overdo caffeinated beverages in the morning.

Don't rely mainly or solely on caffeinated beverages for daily hydration needs. Younger athletes should avoid or limit caffeine.

Carry water with you at all times; when you drive or commute, at work or school, and wherever the opportunity to drink presents itself.

Fit juices, milk, soy milk, or water into meals or snacks.

Spruce up your water with lemon or lime, or a small amount of juice for flavor.

Adults should consume any serving of alcohol with a full 8 to 12 oz. (240 to 360 milliliters) of hydrating fluid.

Consider consuming foods high in fluid such as fruits and vegetables, cooked cereals, and yogurt.

Consume 24 oz. (720 milliliters) of fluid, two hours before exercise and eight to 16 oz. of fluid (240 to 480 milliliters) 30 minutes before exercise to ensure adequate hydration prior to exercise.

Besides meeting your daily hydration requirements, consuming a planned amount of fluids before, during, and after exercise can have a positive effect on your training and competition efforts. Sports drinks are also a very important fluid consideration for team sport athletes. These topics will be covered in Part II.

Focusing and practicing to improve your daily fluid intake is definitely worthwhile. Athletes who have developed techniques for increasing their fluid intake have consistently found that improved hydration resulted in enhanced recovery and higher energy levels. Improving your hydration levels is really very simple. Just plan ahead and make sure that water and other hydrating fluids are available for consumption throughout the day. This will ensure that you begin your training sessions with a well-hydrated body.

Electrolytes

Sodium is one of the major electrolytes in the body and the one of greatest interest to team sport athletes who may have high-sodium sweat losses and practice in hot and humid conditions. Sodium is found outside the body's cells and helps to regulate blood pressure and blood volume. The concentration of sodium in your body plays a role in regulating the distribution of fluids and nutrients between the inside and outside of the cells. Your body has a fairly complicated system of regulating your sodium and fluid balance between your fluid intake and fluid losses, and the balance of other electrolytes including potassium and chloride. Sodium is also critical for nerve impulse transmission and muscle contraction, and it is essential in maintaining normal blood pressure.

Most important for team sport athletes is the fact that sodium is lost in sweat. The body can conserve how much sodium is lost in sweat when sweat rates are high. Any sodium losses can then be replaced through your daily diet. However, some strategies are designed to optimize sodium levels during more extreme weather training conditions that some athletes may have to consider, as well as recovery strategies. These recommendations will be covered in Chapters 5 and 7.

While you may have unique sodium requirements for some training and competition conditions, your daily sodium requirements are more than adequately met by the typical North American diet. Sodium is found in small amounts in most natural foods, but the processing that is so prevalent in our diet has added significant amounts of sodium to our daily intake. Because of health concerns, many individuals in North America are advised to limit their sodium intake. Excess sodium may exacerbate high blood pressure and interfere with calcium balance. However, many athletes with significant sodium losses from training are not advised to limit their sodium intake.

Adults require a minimum of 500 milligrams of sodium in their daily diet, and the upper recommended intake is 2,400 milligrams per day. But it is not unusual for individuals to obtain several thousand milligrams of sodium in their everyday diet, mainly through consumption of processed foods and table salt or sodium chloride, of which 40 percent is sodium. Be reasonable with your sodium and salt intake to minimize any health risks if this is appropriate or advised by your physician. However, as will be covered in later chapters, there may be specific athletic situations in which increasing sodium intake may benefit your athletic performance and recovery.

Alcohol

It is very possible that alcohol is a moderate part of your current lifestyle if you are of legal age to drink. But it is important for an athlete to use alcohol sensibly, as alcohol does not play any important role in your recovery and could have detrimental effects on your performance. Obviously alcohol abuse can affect your health and that of others by contributing to liver cirrhosis and irresponsible and drunk driving. But let's take a look at the implications of alcohol in regard to your training diet and athletic performance.

While alcohol is a drug, it provides calories just as foods do and makes for fairly high-calorie beverages. As far as your body is concerned, alcohol is merely a bunch of empty calories as these calories are not used for energy in the same way as carbohydrates, proteins, and fats. Beer and wine contain only small amounts of carbohydrates and only trace amounts of protein, vitamins, and minerals. In fact, alcohol can interfere with how your body uses vitamins and minerals. One-half ounce of pure ethanol is the equivalent of one drink, which equals 12 ounces (240 milliliters) of beer (150 calories), 4 ounces (120 milliliters) of wine (100 calories), and 1.25 ounces (38 milliliters) of liquor (100 calories).

Despite originating from fermented carbohydrates, alcohol is metabolized in your body as fat. Alcohol by-products are converted into fatty acids, which are stored in your liver and sent to your bloodstream. Obviously alcohol is not the best nutrient choice if your goal is to be a lean athlete. Alcohol is also a widely abused drug in North America, with a significant number of problem drinkers or abusers. Of course, alcohol should never be consumed during pregnancy.

Much has been made of alcohol's protective effects against heart disease. But while moderate amounts may raise the desirable and protective high-density lipoprotein cholesterol (HDL), too much alcohol may actually increase your risk of heart disease. Too much alcohol can raise your blood pressure and increase the amount of harmful blood fats called *triglycerides*, which, when combined with a low amount of the "good" HDL cholesterol, makes for a health profile associated with an increased risk of heart disease. Consumed in excess over a long period, alcohol may not only elevate blood pressure but increase the risk of stroke and certain cancers, and of course result in liver damage. Alcohol also provides empty calories.

Too much alcohol too soon after training and racing can impede recovery. Though you may rehydrate well after training, alcohol is a diuretic that causes your body to

Filtered, Bottled, or Tap?

While the tap water in the United States is very safe, many American consumers have purchased home filtration systems and consumed more than 5 billion gallons of bottled water in the year 2000 alone. Currently, the Environmental Protection Agency (EPA) estimates that 90 percent of the country's drinking water is safe.

Tap water does contain substances other than water. Depending on where you live, it can provide varying levels of minerals such as calcium, sodium, magnesium, iron, zinc, lead, and mercury. While calcium may be a beneficial mineral obtained from water, lead and mercury are not. As a health-minded athlete and consumer, you may lose more fluid than it takes in. That's why you need to replace losses even after drinking moderate amounts of alcohol. Alcohol may also interfere with glycogen synthesis. Athletes with soft-tissue damage or bruising may also want to consider that alcohol is a blood vessel dilator. Consuming alcohol after exercise may aggravate swelling or bleeding and impair healing. These types of injuries are usually treated with ice, which is designed to constrict blood flow to the injured parts.

Excessive alcohol consumed the night before, or alcohol consumed shortly before training, can impair fine motor ability and coordination, increase risk of dehydration, and impair fuel stores. Reaction times are delayed, as your brain's ability to process information is hampered. Know your limits and how they change with your training and fitness level. How fast you metabolize alcohol varies with body size. Average-sized men metabolize slightly less than one drink per hour, while smaller men and women take longer to metabolize this amount.

Underage drinking is also a problem for today's teenager and may adversely affect the high school athlete participating in team sports. Besides the obvious short-term risks involved, parents should emphasize that there are long-term health risks involved with alcohol consumption, such as liver damage and developing certain types of cancers. But they should also understand that there are clear adverse performance effects with alcohol consumption and a subsequent hangover. Alcohol will disrupt fluid balance and temperature regulation, impact fine-motor skills, and can cause athletes to have a subpar practice or competition.

Alcohol can be a small part of a healthy sports diet for adults, but drink sensible amounts. Have a large glass of water with each drink. Consider that your top priority as an athlete is recovery. Too much alcohol can compromise how effectively you do recover.

---

also be concerned about microbial contamination and pesticide residues in water.

Tap water is regulated under the strict standards of the EPA. Your local water municipality is required to supply you with an annual report and tests for microbes several times daily. You can also contact your local water municipality to obtain the names and numbers of certified testing labs to have the water from your own tap checked. Levels of lead and copper in your water may be higher than official reports due to leaching from household plumbing and faucets.

If you prefer, filtered water may be a viable option. Many filters attach right

Filtered, Bottled, or Tap? (continued)

to the tap and filter lead and other contaminants. Another convenient filter method is a pour-through filter that can be placed in a special pitcher and kept in your refrigerator as needed. You may also determine that bottled water is a convenient option for reaching your recommended daily water intake, though there is no guarantee that it is microbe free. Bottled water can be spring water, mineral water, well water, or distilled water.

Both water filter systems and bottled water can be certified by an independent organization called the National Sanitation Foundation (NSF). The NSF sets standards for and certifies water filtration systems. Its Web site at www.nsf.org lists filters and the contaminants that the filter is certified to reduce in your water. Look for a filter with a pore size less than one micron in diameter. Be sure to follow the manufacturer's directions for replacement of the filter cartridge. The best and most expensive systems are reverse osmosis.

Bottled water is currently regulated by the Food and Drug Administration (FDA), but it receives less scrutiny than tap water, which is regulated under stricter standards by the EPA. Water testing is required once weekly for microbes. Testing for contaminants and chemicals is also done more frequently on tap water than bottled water. That's why it is also a good idea to look for brands of bottled water that maintain the NSF certification. In order to maintain this certification, water bottlers must send daily samples for microbial testing to an independent lab and maintain records of filter changes and other quality checks. You can also determine if your brand of water is NSF certified by visiting the Web site mentioned earlier.

New varieties of bottled water include fortified waters, fitness water, waters supplemented with vitamins and herbs, and oxygen-enriched water. Some of these waters simply provide flavor for individuals who do not want to drink plain water. Some contain only a small number of calories, while others may provide more calories than consumers realize. Some of the new designer waters may contain artificial sweeteners. Herbal and vitamin-enhanced waters may not provide significant amounts of these nutrients per serving; however, you may consume enough servings in a day and take in too much of some of these substances. Currently there is no scientific backing to consuming oxygen-enriched water, which claims to boost energy by increasing the oxygen content of red blood cells.

CHAPTER 2

NUTRIENTS FOR OPTIMAL PERFORMANCE

As an athlete, you are understandably interested in consuming an optimal amount of vitamins and minerals in your diet for both maximum performance and good health. You may find yourself questioning just how your training program may alter or increase your requirements of these important nutrients. And, as an athlete, you also have a highly vested interest in keeping your immune system healthy so that illness does not put a halt to training. While athletes have long been advised by sports nutritionists to consume high-quality foods for an optimal nutrient intake, advertising targeting active individuals would suggest they require a daily vitamin and mineral supplement. Which is correct?

Of course, choosing foods that provide you with adequate amounts of vitamins and minerals is necessary for optimal performance. Correcting any dietary inadequacies could even improve your performance. However, research has not conclusively proven that taking "extra" amounts of vitamins and minerals when no deficiency is present will enable you to train harder and longer. While all vitamins and minerals are important, it would benefit you to be aware of nutrients that are especially important to an athlete. Certain groups of athletes may also benefit from nutrient supplementation beyond the basic assurance of a daily multivitamin and mineral supplement.

BALANCED EATING

As Table 2.1 indicates, balanced eating clearly provides variety and ample amounts of vitamins, minerals, phytochemicals, and quality carbohydrates, particularly in view of an athlete's higher energy needs for training. You should also keep in mind that nutrients exist together in foods in the proper balance.

VITAMIN BASICS

Vitamins consist of thirteen organic compounds found in small amounts in most foods. They play important roles in many physiological processes, many of which are greatly enhanced during exercise. Therefore, it is wise to ensure that you have high levels of

Optimal Health and Dietary Reference Intakes

In the early 1990s, the Food and Nutrition Board of the National Academy of Sciences revised the guidelines for the Recommended Dietary Allowances (RDAs), and subsequently a new family of nutrient reference values known as the Dietary Reference Intakes (DRIs) was born. For the past decades, these values more accurately reflect the health goals of the twenty-first century. Rather than merely preventing nutrient deficiencies, the new guidelines are set with the goal of optimizing health by reducing risk of chronic diseases such as heart disease, cancer, and osteoporosis.

Each updated nutrient has acquired a number of terms under the umbrella heading of DRI. The DRI values are provided in reports published over several years' time offering new guidelines on similarly grouped nutrients. Instead of a single category, the DRI include the four following classifications:

Recommended Daily Allowance (RDA): The RDA is the amount of a nutrient that should decrease the risk of chronic disease for most healthy individuals in a specified age group and gender. It is based on estimating the average requirement plus an increase to account for individual variation. It is to serve as a goal for individuals only.

The RDA is a good starting point for athletes to determine the nutritional adequacy of their diet. Athletes of all ages are likely to have energy requirements higher than the average person, and some vitamins and minerals are required to process this energy. Athletes may also have a body reserves of these nutrients in order for these processes to function optimally. While it is true that inadequate intake of vitamins may result in deficiencies, whether or not it will adversely impact your performance depends on the extent of that deficiency. Extreme deficiencies are not very commonplace in North America, and many dietary inadequacies can be corrected by making the proper food choices.

Athletes most likely to have problems with an inadequate vitamin intake are those following a restricted calorie diet for weight loss, athletes who have adopted an extreme or fad diet, and perhaps those on a very restrictive vegetarian diet. But overall, athletes training and competing in team sports can greatly minimize their risk of vitamin deficiency by consuming a wide variety of nutrient-dense foods and adequate calories to match their training needs.

higher nutrient intake than the average person, simply because of their high energy needs and quality food choices.

Adequate Intake (AI): The AI is used when there is not enough scientific evidence to set an RDA. It is a recommended daily intake based on observed or experimentally determined approximations of nutrient intake by a group of healthy people. The AI can be used as a goal for individual intake when an RDA does not exist.

Estimated Average Requirement (EAR): The EAR is the nutrient value estimated to meet the requirements of half the healthy individuals in a group. The EAR represents the average nutrient intake required to maintain a specific body function. For example, the EAR for vitamin C is set at a level that prevents scurvy, a deficiency disease. The EAR is used to develop the RDA, assess adequacy of intakes, and plan diets for population groups.

Tolerable Upper Intake Level (UL): The UL is the highest level of a daily nutrient intake recommended, from both food and supplements, which should not be exceeded or individuals may experience adverse or toxic health effects. This is not a recommended amount but rather an upper limit. For most nutrients, the UL refers to the total amount obtained from the total food intake, fortified foods, and supplements. This number may be of interest to athletes who consume a number of such fortified foods, take various vitamin and mineral supplements, and frequently use sports nutrition products that are supplemented with nutrients as well.

Vitamins play a major role in catalyzing energy production reactions from body fuel stores. For instance, a number of B vitamins are essential to converting carbohydrate into energy for muscular contraction. Vitamins themselves do not directly provide energy, which must be obtained from consuming carbohydrates, protein, and fat. The vitamins B12, B6, and folic acid also play an important role in the development of red blood cells that deliver oxygen to the exercising muscles. Vitamins are also involved in tissue repair and protein synthesis. Several vitamins such as E and C are antioxidants that protect cells from potentially toxic free radicals. *Free radicals* are unstable molecules produced by oxygen-related reactions in the body and have been implicated in contributing to a number of diseases. Each vitamin is unique in the functions it performs in the body and in how it interacts with other dietary nutrients.

TABLE 2.1 BALANCED FOODS FOR ATHLETES

Food Group	Serving Sizes	Number Servings	Nutrients Provided
Fruits	1 c. fruit (240 ml) 1 medium piece	3 daily	Carotenoids Vitamin A Vitamin C Phytonutrients
Vegetables	1 c. cooked (240 ml) 2 c. raw (480 ml)	2–3 daily	Carotenoids Vitamin A Vitamin C Phytonutrients Calcium
Dairy milk, yogurt fortified soy milk	8 oz. milk (240 ml) 6–8 oz. yogurt (200–240 ml)	2–3 daily	Calcium Riboflavin Vitamin A Vitamin D
Poultry, fish, lean red meat	3–4 oz. (100–120 g)	2–4 daily	Thiamin Niacin Iron Zinc
Whole grains and starch	2 oz. bread (60 g) 1-1/2 c. cereal (360 ml) 1 c. cooked (240 ml)	6–12 daily	Thiamin Niacin Iron Riboflavin
Fats and oils	1 tsp. to 1 tbsp. (7–20 ml)	4–6 daily	Vitamin A Vitamin D Vitamin E

Vitamins are separated into two classifications: fat-soluble and water-soluble. Your body may contain large stores of the fat-soluble variety—A, D, E, and K. Deficiencies of these nutrients are rare, though excessive intakes may have toxic effects. The water-soluble variety—which include vitamin C and the eight B vitamins: thiamin (B1), riboflavin (B2), pyridoxine (B6), niacin, B12, folacin, biotin, and pantothenic acid—are not stored in your body in significant amounts. Harmful effects of excessive intakes of these water-soluble vitamins are not as likely, though there are exceptions. Appendix B provides a list of vitamins, their functions, DRIs, and food sources.

IMPORTANT MINERALS
B Vitamins
Due to their role in processing energy from the metabolism of carbohydrate, B vitamins have received much attention from athletes. However, several of these vitamins are easily obtained from a variety of carbohydrate-rich foods such as breads and whole

grains and other foods that are found in relatively high amounts in the high-energy athlete's diet. Often intake of the nutrients exceeds the RDAs when an athlete consumes the calories required for training and competing.

Thiamin and Riboflavin

Thiamin or vitamin B1 is present in a wide variety of food sources besides whole grains, including nuts, dried peas and beans, and pork. It plays an important role in deriving energy from carbohydrates. A thiamin deficiency is unlikely to occur in athletes. Many athletes with high energy needs likely consume thiamin above the current RDA of 1.2 milligrams daily.

Riboflavin is also involved in energy production from carbohydrates, proteins, and fat. Vegetarians should pay attention to their riboflavin intake, as milk, meat, and eggs are good sources. Some plant sources include brewer's yeast, wheat germ, soybeans, avocados, green leafy vegetables, and enriched bread and cereals. Training for your sport may slightly increase your riboflavin requirements, but the higher amounts are easily met in a well-balanced diet.

Pyridoxine and Niacin

Pyridoxine or vitamin B6 is found mainly in whole-grain cereals, brown rice, wheat germ, bananas, legumes, fish, and poultry. This vitamin is closely linked to protein metabolism, the manufacture of muscle and hemoglobin, and the breakdown of muscle glycogen. Athletes who consume adequate calories should get plenty of vitamin B6 in their diet. Though most water-soluble vitamins are easily excreted, excess supplementation of B6 can present a problem. Doses of more than 1 gram daily over several months may cause numbness and even paralysis. Symptoms have also been experienced with chronic doses as low as 200 milligrams.

Another B vitamin, niacin, is involved not only in carbohydrate, protein, and fat metabolism but also in glycogen synthesis and cellular metabolism. Good food sources of niacin are meat, whole or enriched grains, nuts, seeds, and dried beans. Because it is in such a wide variety of foods, it is relatively easy to obtain enough niacin in your diet. In fact, excess niacin from oversupplementation can block the release of free fatty acids, resulting in greater use of muscle glycogen and thereby depleting a limited energy source for exercise. Large doses may actually reduce performance.

Vitamin B12

Vitamin B12 plays a major role in red blood cell development, among other important functions. Vegetarian athletes who are strict vegans should pay close attention to their

B12 intake. Your vitamin B12 needs are easily met by consuming animal foods, so if you consume eggs and dairy foods, your intake should be fine. But the only plant foods that can be counted on for their B12 content are those that have been fortified with this vitamin. Some reliable fortified food sources are soy milk, soy burgers, and some breakfast cereals. Plant proteins such as tempeh and miso may not contain the active form of vitamin B12. The human intestinal tract does make some vitamin B12, but this is generally not well absorbed. While requirements of this vitamin are relatively low, deficiencies can have serious implications and even lead to irreversible nerve damage. Vegans who do not regularly consume fortified foods should take a vitamin B12 supplement.

Folacin

Folacin is a B vitamin that has deservedly received much increased attention from health professionals over the past several years. *Folacin* is the collective term for folate, folic acid, and other forms of the vitamin. Folate is the form found naturally in foods, and folic acid is the form of the vitamin found most often in your body and added to foods and supplements. Folic acid is actually absorbed twice as well as the folate that occurs naturally in foods.

Since January 1998, manufacturers were required to add folic acid to all enriched products including flour, bread, rolls, grits, cornmeal, rice, pasta, and noodles. There is good reason for this fortification. Obtaining enough folic acid in the early weeks of pregnancy can significantly reduce the risk of neural tube defects such as spina bifida in newborns. Prior to fortification, most Americans consumed only about 200 micrograms of folic acid daily, falling short of the recommended 400 micrograms. Fortification will continue to prevent a significant number of all neural tube defects, but this fortification may benefit others as well as pregnant women and newborns.

Evidence is building that folic acid may reduce the risk of heart disease, stroke, and certain cancers. Folic acid helps reduce blood levels of the amino acid homocysteine. High levels of homocysteine appear to be a strong predictor for heart disease and stroke. Keeping homocysteine low also requires adequate intake of the vitamins B6 and B12. At least 30 percent of all older Americans don't produce enough stomach acid to absorb the B12 found in foods. Synthetic B12, however, doesn't have this stomach acid dependency. Connections between folic acid and the prevention of certain cancers, through prevention of damage to DNA, have also been suggested.

Many researchers suggest that individuals over the age of 50 take a supplement providing the RDA (high doses are not advised) of folic acid, B12, and B6. Older individuals are also more likely to take medications that interfere with folic acid absorption.

Of course, every active individual should increase the intake of folate-rich foods because of folate's relationship to maintaining red blood cells. Folate is easily destroyed by long storage times and common cooking techniques. Try to obtain folate from fresh foods (see Table 2.2).

Vitamin C

Another water-soluble vitamin of interest to and heavily marketed to athletes is vitamin C. Several important functions of this vitamin impact athletes. It is necessary for the formation of connective tissue, scar tissue, certain hormones, and neurotransmitters that are secreted during exercise. Vitamin C plays a role in iron absorption and in the formation of red blood cells. This vitamin is also strongly promoted because of its role as a powerful antioxidant. Symptoms of vitamin C deficiency could impair athletic performance.

Despite being a water-soluble vitamin that is easily excreted, the human body actually has a pool of vitamin C ranging from 1.5 to 3.0 grams. Serious vitamin C deficiencies are rare because fresh or frozen fruits and vegetables are so abundant in our food supply. Though vitamin C is readily available from food, athletes often consume vitamin C supplements. Correcting a deficiency clearly improves performance, but research does not demonstrate that vitamin C supplements enhance performance when a vitamin C deficiency is not present.

TABLE 2.2 FOLATE-RICH FOODS

Food	Portion	Folate content (mcg)
Lentils, cooked	1 c. (240 ml)	358
Brewer's yeast	1 tbsp. (20 ml)	312
Liver, beef	3 oz. (100 g)	285
Garbanzo beans, cooked	1 c. (240 ml)	282
Kidney beans, cooked	1 c. (240 ml)	229
Turnip greens, cooked	1 c. (240 ml)	171
Asparagus, boiled	6 spears	131
Beans, white, baked	1 c. (240 ml)	122
Orange juice	1 c. (240 ml)	110
Spinach, raw, chopped	1 c. (240 ml)	108
Mustard greens, cooked	1 c. (240 ml)	103
Broccoli, cooked	1 c. (240 ml)	78
Romaine lettuce	1 c. (240 ml)	76
Endive	1 c. (240 ml)	72
Wheat germ, raw	1/4 c. (60 ml)	70

On the other hand, because exercise places stress on the body, moderate amounts of vitamin C, above the Recommended Daily Allowance of 75 to 90 milligrams, may be appropriate for athletes. Some scientists have recommended 200 to 300 milligrams daily, which can be obtained from a diet abundant in fruits and vegetables. Research indicates that 200 milligrams daily of vitamin C leads to full saturation of plasma and white blood cells, which supports optimal immune function. Vitamin C supplements may also reduce the symptoms and duration of upper respiratory tract infections often seen after strenuous physical efforts. Vitamin C is also an important part of the healing process when there is injury or muscle soreness. Despite popular perceptions, however, most studies have not found vitamin C supplementation to prevent the common cold.

A diet rich in fruits and vegetables provides ample amounts of vitamin C and other healthful substances found in those foods. Table 2.3 lists the vitamin C content of some top sources of this nutrient. Avoid excessive intakes of vitamin C supplements reaching 1,000 to 3,000 milligrams daily, which can cause side effects such as diarrhea and kidney stones.

Vitamin E

Vitamin E also receives much attention from athletes because of its major role as an antioxidant. This vitamin prevents the oxidation of unsaturated fatty acids in cell membranes and protects the cell from damage. Vitamin E is widely distributed in foods and stored in the body, so vitamin E deficiencies are rare. The current RDA is 22 international units (IU). Polyunsaturated oils such as soybean, corn, and safflower are the most common sources of vitamin E. Other good sources are fortified grain products and wheat germ.

TABLE 2.3 VITAMIN C CONTENT OF FOODS		
Food	**Portion**	**Vitamin C (mg)**
Pepper, green	1 large	130
Orange juice	1 c. (240 ml)	124
Cranberry juice	1 c. (240 ml)	108
Grapefruit juice	1 c. (240 ml)	94
Broccoli, cooked	2/3 c. (200 ml)	90
Brussels sprouts, cooked	7	85
Strawberries, raw	1 c. (240 ml)	85
Orange, navel	1	80
Kiwi	1 medium	75
Cantaloupe, pieces	1 c. (240 ml)	70
Cauliflower, cooked	1 c. (240 ml)	65

Experiments on vitamin E supplementation at altitude have produced some interesting results, but more research is required, especially to determine if there is any real performance benefits. Vitamin E may also be beneficial to athletes training in high-pollution areas due to its antioxidant effects. Though no performance benefits have been established, vitamin E supplements may be recommended for possible prevention of chronic diseases, especially heart disease. Some researchers currently feel that a daily supplement dose of 100 to 200 IU is safe, though the upper limits of safety for long-term vitamin E intake have not been firmly established. People with a bleeding disorder or who are on anticoagulant medication or statin medications designed to lower elevated blood lipids should be cautious and first check with their physician before taking vitamin E. If you do take a vitamin E supplement, choose one that provides the natural source of the vitamin. See Table 2.4 for good sources of vitamin E.

Carotenoids

Beta-carotene is just one of 600 carotenoid pigments that give fruits and vegetables their yellow, orange, and red colors. Carotenoids are also abundant in green vegetables. While carotenoids are not vitamins, many act as antioxidants and also protect cells from free radicals.

Carotenoids most commonly found in blood and tissues are alpha-carotene, beta-carotene, beta-cryptoxanthin, lycopene, lutein, and zeaxanthin. Only alpha-carotene, beta-carotene, and beta-cryptoxanthin can be converted to vitamin A in the body. Research is just beginning to determine how specific carotenoids can boost immunity and protect the heart and eyes from chronic disease.

To obtain a variety of carotenoids in your diet, aim for at least five servings combined of fruits and vegetables daily, focusing mainly on yellow-orange, red, or dark green choices. You can easily obtain ample amounts in your diet.

TABLE 2.4 VITAMIN E CONTENT OF FOODS		
Food	**Portion**	**Vitamin E (IU)**
Wheat germ oil	1 tbsp. (20 ml)	25
Sunflower seeds	1 oz. (30 g)	21
Almonds	1 oz. (30 g)	11
Sunflower oil	1 tbsp. (20 ml)	10
Wheat germ	1 oz. (30 g)	5
Margarine, soft	1 tbsp. (20 ml)	3
Mayonnaise	1 tbsp. (20 ml)	3
Brown rice	1 c. (240 ml)	3
Mango	1 medium	3
Asparagus	4 spears	2

Super Sources of Carotenoids

Apricot halves, 6 dried	Orange, 1 medium
Broccoli, 1/2 c. cooked (120 ml)	Papaya, 1/2 medium
Cantaloupe, 1 c. chunks (240 ml)	Pepper, red, 1/2 raw
Carrot, 1 medium raw	Pumpkin, 1/2 c. cooked or canned
Collard greens, 1/2 c. cooked (120 ml)	(120 ml)
Grapefruit, 1/2 medium	Spinach, 1/2 c. raw (120 ml)
Kale, 1/2 c. cooked (120 ml)	Sweet potato, 1/2 c. mashed (120 ml)
Mango, 1 medium	Tangerine, 1 medium
Mustard greens, 1/2 c. cooked (120 ml)	Tomato sauce, 1/2 c. (120 ml)

Taking a supplement with carotenoids requires some caution, particularly in the case of beta-carotene supplements, which were found to increase cancer in smokers. It is advised not to supplement but to stay under 3 milligrams daily if you do take a supplement. In addition, carotenoids interact with one another. Supplementing with one carotenoid may impair the absorption of others. Carotenoids are converted to vitamin A as the body requires. But vitamin A supplements can be highly toxic at greater than the daily RDA of 5,000 IU. Besides, foods high in carotenoids may provide health-promoting substances not found in supplements. It's quite possible that these protective nutrients work best when they are packaged together, as in food.

Phytochemicals

While vitamin A can be formed from some carotenoids, this group of nutrients is actually one of many that fall under the broader classification of phytochemicals. Many important disease-fighting properties have been attributed to these plant chemicals. Unlike vitamins and minerals, phytochemicals are not nutrients. Most phytochemicals are found in carbohydrate-containing foods such as fruits, vegetables, and grains. Some phytochemicals you may have heard about include allylic sulfides found in garlic, flavonoids found in citrus fruits, genistein found in soybeans, indoles in broccoli and cauliflower, and phytoestrogens in soy products, to name a few. To take advantage of these phytochemicals, eat plenty of fruits and vegetables, dried peas and beans, and soy products. In the future, probably even more phytochemicals will be discovered.

MINERAL BASICS

Like vitamins, minerals are involved in energy metabolism and play important roles in building body tissue, forming the base of the strength and structure of the skeleton, in muscle contraction and oxygen transport, in maintaining acid–base balance of the blood, and in regulating normal heart rhythm. All of these functions are important for top athletic performance. Weak bones can contribute to the development of stress fractures, acid-base imbalance and muscle contraction affect endurance, and energy metabolism impacts fuel utilization when training. Minerals are involved in metabolizing carbohydrates, proteins, and fats and in obtaining energy from an important fuel source, phosphocreatine.

There are two classes of minerals, both important to optimal body functioning. The *macrominerals* are present in relatively large amounts in the body and include calcium, phosphorus, and magnesium. *Trace* or *microminerals* include iron, zinc, chromium, copper, and selenium. All together there are 25 essential minerals, all with their own unique functions.

Minerals are obtained in our diet from the water we drink and both plant and animal foods. Training-induced mineral losses can occur through urine, sweat, and gastrointestinal losses. Two very important minerals to the athlete are calcium, because of its essential role in maintaining healthy bone structure, and iron, which plays a crucial role in oxygen transport.

IMPORTANT MINERALS

Calcium

Calcium is the most abundant mineral in the body. Ninety-eight percent of calcium is found in bone, a dynamic tissue that is constantly being broken down and rebuilt. The remaining 2 percent of calcium in your body is in your teeth and circulates in your bloodstream.

This circulating calcium has a significant effect on metabolism and physiological functions. It is involved in all types of muscle contraction, including the heart muscle, skeletal muscle, and smooth muscle found in blood vessels. By activating a number of enzymes, calcium also plays a role in both the synthesis and breakdown of muscle and liver glycogen. Calcium is also involved in nerve impulse transmission, blood clotting, and secretion of hormones. These physiological functions of calcium take precedence over formation of bone tissue. If the diet is low in calcium, calcium can be pulled from the bone for these functions.

Calcium deficiency can develop from inadequate intake or increased calcium excretion. Strenuous exercise increases sweat loss of calcium. One of the major health concerns associated with inadequate intake of calcium is osteoporosis, a disorder in which bone mass decreases and susceptibility to fracture increases. Optimal bone building takes place until age 25, but you can continue to build some bone until 35 years of age. After this age, your efforts should focus on maintaining your current level of bone mass.

Hormonal status, more specifically estrogen loss, also contributes significantly to the development of osteoporosis, making women more susceptible to this disease after menopause occurs, though men may also develop osteoporosis. Hormonal status in younger female athletes also plays an important role in bone health. Extra calcium is recommended for female athletes with absent or irregular menstruation and for post-menopausal female athletes. Weight-bearing exercise such as running and weight training enhances calcium skeletal absorption, increases bone mass, and can help prevent bone loss at any age. Calcium recommendations for various ages are cited in Table 2.5. Vitamin D recommendations are also provided, as this vitamin is essential for adequate calcium absorption. As we age, our bodies become less efficient at converting sunlight to vitamin D.

Dairy products are very concentrated sources of calcium and for many individuals provide about three-fourths of their total calcium intake. Athletes who do not have a high intake of dairy products and vegan athletes need to focus on alternative plant sources of calcium intake and increase their intake of calcium-fortified foods. Try to choose low-fat options as much as possible. Some good plant sources of calcium include dark leafy greens, broccoli, bok choy, dried beans, and dried figs. Some good fortified sources (check labels) are soy and rice milk, orange juice, cereals, tofu processed with calcium sulfate, and various energy bars. Look for products marked as "high" or "rich in" or an "excellent" source of calcium. They contain over 200 milligrams per serving. Some good calcium sources are listed in Table 2.6.

Individuals who are lactose-intolerant can buy specially formulated lactose-free milks, or take lactase supplement enzymes before consuming milk products. Yogurt

TABLE 2.5 CALCIUM AND VITAMIN D REQUIREMENTS		
Requirements	**Calcium (mg)**	**Vitamin D (IU)**
Ages 19–50 years	1,000	200
Ages 51–70	1,200 (on hormone replacement therapy [HRT])	400
Greater than 70 years	1,500 (not on HRT)	600
	1,200 (on HRT)	
	1,500 (not on HRT)	

TABLE 2.6 FOOD SOURCES OF CALCIUM

Great Sources, 300-mg Serving	Good Sources, 200-mg Serving	Fair Sources, 100-mg Serving
1% milk, 8 oz. (240 ml)	Cheddar cheese, 1 oz. (30 g)	Skim milk, dry, 1 tbsp. (20 ml)
Skim milk, 8 oz. (240 ml)	Brick cheese, 1 oz. (30 g)	Cottage cheese, 1%, 1 c.
Yogurt, 6 to 8 oz. (200–	Colby cheese, 1 oz. (30 g)	(240 ml)
240 ml)	Edam cheese, 1 oz. (30 g)	Parmesan, grated, 1-1/2 tbsp.
Swiss cheese, 1 oz. (30 g)	Mozzarella cheese, 1 oz. (30 g)	(30 ml)
Mackerel, canned, 3 oz.	Instant breakfast, 1 packet	Frozen yogurt, 1/2 c. (120 ml)
(100 g)	Broccoli, cooked, 1 c. (240 ml)	Pudding, 1/2 c. (120 ml)
Sardines, canned, w/bones,	Kale, cooked, 1 c. (240 ml)	Shrimp, cooked, 6 oz (200 g)
3 oz. (100 g)	Turnip greens, cooked, 1 c.	Lobster, cooked, 6 oz (200 g)
Salmon, canned, w/bones,	(240 ml)	Tofu, 1/2 c. (120 ml)
3 oz. (100 g)	Mustard greens, cooked, 1 c.	Navy beans, cooked, 1 c.
Rhubarb, cooked, 1 c.	(240 ml)	(240 ml)
(240 ml)	Bok choy, fresh, 1 c. (240 ml)	Pinto beans, 1 c. (240 ml)
Collard greens, cooked,	Sesame seeds, 2 tbsp. (40 ml)	Orange, 1 large
1 c. (240 ml)	Soybeans, cooked, 1 c.	Tempeh, cooked, 1 c. (240 ml)
Blackstrap molasses,	(240 ml)	Swiss chard, cooked, 1 c.
2 tbsp. (40 ml)		(240 ml)
Orange juice, calcium		Figs, dried or fresh, 5 medium
fortified, 1 c. (240 ml)		

and cheese have lower lactose levels than milk and may be well tolerated. You may also be able to tolerate small amounts of lactose-containing foods.

A well-balanced training diet should provide many of the essential nutrients needed to build and maintain healthy bones; however, a calcium supplement may also be indicated if your food intake is not adequate. If you do take a calcium supplement, find one that provides more than 500 milligrams per pill and take one pill at a time. Amounts greater than 500 to 600 milligrams will not be fully absorbed. Calcium carbonate should be taken with meals to increase absorption, while the calcium citrate form can be taken at any time. Avoid calcium made from oyster shells, bone meal, or dolomite as it may contain lead, though major brand-name products of these sources should be safely consumed. Look for calcium supplements that contain "USP" on the label, which indicates that it meets the standards of the United States Pharmacopia.

Good food sources of vitamin D are relatively limited. They include fatty fish and egg yolks. Fortified sources include milk, soy milk, butter, margarine, and cereals. Some athletes may spend a considerable amount of time outdoors during certain times of the year, and your bodies can make enough vitamin D when your skin is exposed to sunlight. However, sun exposure may not be adequate from October to April in the northern parts of the United States and in Canada. Our ability to make vitamin D from sunlight also decreases as we age. Older athletes, those living in northern climates, and vegetarians may want to consider taking a vitamin D supplement. Use of sunscreen products can also decrease our ability to form vitamin D from sunlight. Vitamin D is often conveniently combined with calcium in supplement form, and can also be obtained from a multivitamin.

Other nutrients are also an important part of building healthy bones:

Vitamin C—Plays a role in collagen production that helps hold bone together. A diet with plenty of fresh fruits and vegetables provides ample amounts.

Vitamin K—Activates osteocalcin, which is needed for optimal bone strength. Good sources are dark leafy green vegetables.

Magnesium—Another important mineral for bone formation. Good sources are almonds, bananas, avocados, dried beans, lentils, nuts, tofu, wheat germ, and whole grains.

In contrast, some dietary factors are actually harmful to calcium absorption. Excess sodium, protein, and caffeine increase calcium excretion. Alcohol can also be damaging to bone cells. Try not to consume excessive sources of caffeine. Excessive intakes of phosphorus, namely from carbonated beverages, should also be limited, as too much of this mineral can upset calcium balance in the body. Keep your protein intake at an appropriate level for training, but do not consume excessive and unneeded amounts from supplements.

Obtaining adequate calcium in your diet takes planning. Here are some tips for maximizing your calcium intake:

- Have a breakfast every day that includes high-calcium milk, yogurt, or a calcium-fortified soy product.
- Plan a high-calcium food into three meals or snacks daily.
- Prepare or order low-fat milk and soy milk smoothies whenever possible.
- Make some great stir-fried vegetables for dinners that include one of the following: bok choy, kale, broccoli, and leafy greens.
- Add reduced-fat cheeses to sandwiches.
- Drink a glass of calcium-fortified orange juice on a regular basis.
- Buy tofu high in calcium for stir-fries and other recipes.

Iron

Many athletes are aware of the important role that iron plays in exercise metabolism. Hemoglobin transports oxygen in the blood, and myoglobin transports oxygen in the muscle. Both of these oxygen-carrying molecules require iron for optimal formation. Many muscle enzymes involved in metabolism require iron. Other iron compounds facilitate oxygen use at the cellular level. The body storage form of iron, ferritin, is used as an indicator of iron stores, as are transferrin and hemoglobin. About 70 percent of the iron in your body is involved in oxygen transport, while the other 30 percent is stored in the body. It makes sense that poor iron status could impair these functions and exercise performance. This has been demonstrated when an athlete has iron deficiency that has progressed to anemia. Anemia causes fatigue and intolerance to exercise.

Iron deficiency is the most common nutrient deficiency in the United States. It is estimated that 22 to 25 percent of female athletes are iron deficient, with 6 percent having full-blown anemia. When iron stores are low, total hemoglobin drops, and the muscles do not receive as much oxygen. Normal hemoglobin levels for males are 14 to 16 grams per deciliter (g/dl), with anemia classified as less than 13 g/dl. The normal range for women is 12 to 14 g/dl, with anemia diagnosed at less than 12 g/dl. Blood work can be interpreted to determine if you have early iron deficiency or full iron deficiency anemia. However, endurance training can affect your blood measurements of iron. Training produces an increased blood volume, which dilutes hemoglobin, making it appear low in some athletes when iron stores are adequate. This increased blood volume often occurs at the start of a training program and has no harmful effect on performance. In fact, this increased blood volume means that your heart can pump more blood to your working muscles, enhancing oxygen delivery.

Data clearly indicate that true iron deficiency anemia will impair exercise performance. While there is less data regarding the performance effects of a low ferritin level, athletes may experience symptoms of fatigue and poor recovery with this condition. Of course, it makes sense to treat low ferritin levels so that full-blown iron deficiency anemia does not develop and to improve any reoccurring symptoms. Your blood work should be monitored by a physician and treated as appropriate. Inadequate dietary intake of iron is the most common cause of iron deficiency or anemia.

Women with heavy menstrual blood loss may also experience iron deficiency. Strenuous exercise can also increase iron sweat loss, precipitate gastrointestinal bleeding, and decrease iron absorption. Strenuous training may also accelerate red blood cell destruction from mechanical trauma, such as during running. Training at altitude can also place you at risk for developing iron deficiency. Development of iron deficiency is also associated with low-calorie diets, vegetarian diets, very high-carbohydrate diets containing only small amounts of animal protein, and various fad and unbalanced diets.

Iron is obtained from food in two forms. Heme iron is found in animal foods—good sources are lean meat and dark poultry. About 10 to 30 percent of heme iron is absorbed from the intestines. Nonheme iron is found in plant foods—dried peas and beans, whole-grain products, apricots, and raisins are good sources. About 2 to 10 percent of nonheme iron is absorbed. Nonheme iron absorption is compromised by the phytates that are found in many vegetables and whole grains.

Consuming meats and plant iron sources together can enhance iron absorption from plant foods. Small amounts of red meat in bean chili, spinach with chicken, and turkey with lentil soup combine heme and nonheme iron. Vitamin C–containing foods also enhance plant iron absorption. Try having orange juice or strawberries with fortified cereal. Table 2.7 lists good sources of iron.

TABLE 2.7 IRON CONTENT OF SELECTED FOODS

Sources of Heme Iron	Portion	Amount (mg)
Liver, beef, cooked	3 oz. (90 g)	6.0
Beef, cooked	3 oz. (90 g)	3.5
Pork, cooked	3 oz. (90 g)	3.4
Shrimp, cooked	3 oz. (90 g)	2.6
Turkey, dark, cooked	3 oz. (90 g)	2.0
Chicken, breast, cooked	3 oz. (90 g)	1.0
Tuna, light	3 oz. (90 g)	1.0
Flounder, sole, salmon	3 oz. (90 g)	1.0

Sources of Plant Iron	Portion	Amount (mg)
Cereal, iron-fortified	1/2 cup (120 ml)	2–18
Cream of wheat	3/4 cup (180 ml)	9
Lentils	1 cup (240 ml)	6
Instant breakfast	1 envelope	4.5
Kidney beans, canned	1 cup (240 ml)	3.2
Baked potato, with skin	1	3.0
Prune juice	8 oz. (240 ml)	3.0
Wheat germ	1/4 cup (60 ml)	2.6
Apricots, dried	10 halves	1.7
Spaghetti, enriched, cooked	1/2 cup (120 ml)	1.4
Bread, enriched	1 slice	1.0

To boost iron intake, you can take the following measures:

- Incorporate lean meat regularly into your diet. Have small amounts several times weekly.
- Try adding small amounts of red meats to your favorite recipes like stir-fry, soups, pasta sauces, and casseroles.
- Mix heme-iron foods with nonheme choices, such as bean chili with dark turkey meat.
- Incorporate iron-fortified cereals into your diet.
- Consider increasing fish and shellfish in your diet for their iron content.
- Increase your intake of plant irons such as whole-grain cereals, legumes, and green leafy vegetables. Have them with a vitamin C–containing food to improve iron absorption.

Athletes training at altitude and female athletes may want to supplement with the RDA of iron. Many multivitamins contain this amount of iron, so check labels. You should also have your hemoglobin, hematocrit, and ferritin stores monitored regularly. Taking excess iron from supplements, however, does carry some risk.

Iron and Zinc Supplements

Zinc is another important mineral for athletes who train hard. An adequate amount of zinc keeps your immune system strong and promotes healing of wounds and injuries. Zinc is also a component of several enzymes involved in energy metabolism and is involved in protein synthesis. Good sources of zinc include red meat, turkey, milk, yogurt, and seafood—especially oysters. The zinc from animal foods is better absorbed than that found in plant foods. Plant sources of zinc include garbanzo beans, lentils, lima beans, brown rice, and wheat germ.

It is important that you do not self-diagnose low iron stores but rather have your blood work evaluated by a physician. If you take a supplement providing greater than 100 percent of the RDA for iron and zinc, your hemoglobin, hematocrit, and ferritin should be monitored regularly. Higher doses of iron, even as little as 25 milligrams, can inhibit absorption of zinc and another mineral, copper. Oversupplementing with zinc can also interfere with absorption of other minerals.

Excess iron supplementation may also adversely affect individuals who have a genetic predisposition to iron overload. Iron overload, a condition known as *hemochromatosis*, is a genetic disorder that affects one in every 200 people. This condition can result in excess iron deposits in the heart, liver, joints, and various body tissues, with the potential for damaging these tissues. High levels of iron supplements can also lead to gastrointestinal intolerance and constipation. Vegetarians can consider a supplement that provides 100 percent of the Daily Values (DV) for iron and other trace minerals, such as zinc and copper to ensure that they obtain adequate amounts of these nutrients.

Multivitamin and Mineral Supplements

Athletes training in team sports have the distinct advantage of being able to eat more than their sedentary counterparts. With a focus on quality food choices, this generally means a diet filled with variety and nutrients. While a multivitamin and mineral supplement does guarantee that you will obtain all the Daily Values for vitamins and minerals, it is not the same as eating food. Nutrients from foods tend to be optimally absorbed and will provide you with all the phytochemicals, undiscovered or otherwise, that are not in your supplement. However, a broad-range, reasonable dose supplement may just be that little extra insurance that athletes who care about their health often seek. However, some active individuals may want to seriously consider taking a vitamin and mineral supplement. This would be the case for athletes who consume fewer than 1,500 calories daily (not a recommended calorie level for team sport athletes); have food allergies that restrict a significant number of choices from one food group; travel frequently; have disordered eating and erratic diets (which should be corrected with proper food plans and strategies); are vegans or vegetarians who may need additional vitamin D, zinc, iron, B12, and riboflavin; are picky eaters who may restrict many foods; are at risk for osteoporosis; or are pregnant or planning a pregnancy.

If you decide to take a multivitamin and mineral supplement, try to stick to the following guidelines:

- Choose a broad-range, balanced supplement of vitamins and minerals that provides 100 percent of the Daily Values. These doses are known to be safe.
- Avoid supplements that contain an excess of minerals or any one mineral, as these nutrients compete with one another for absorption.
- Choose a supplement with the USP stamp of approval on the label to guarantee that it dissolves properly in your body.
- Choose a supplement in which the majority of vitamin A is actually beta-carotene, the precursor to vitamin A.

- A blend of natural and synthetic supplements is fine. Don't pay more for "timed-release" or "chelated" products.
- Calcium and magnesium may need to be purchased separately as they are too bulky for a regular multivitamin pill.
- If you take antioxidant supplements, keep doses to 100 to 200 IU vitamin E and 250 milligrams vitamin C.
- Take your multivitamin with a meal or snack and plenty of water.
- Don't double up on one-a-day vitamins. You may get too much of certain nutrients.
- Avoid megadoses, and be sure to account for any vitamins and minerals you may be taking from sports nutrition supplements.
- Individuals over 50 years of age can opt for iron-free formulas; look for B6 and B12 content in the higher range.

Antioxidant supplements are strongly marketed to athletes, but it is actually diets abundant in foods that contain antioxidant nutrients that have been shown to prevent cancer and other diseases. So don't discount the importance of increasing food sources of these nutrients. You may also wonder if training increases the effects of free radicals or if athletes learn to cope with these negative by-products. Probably both situations occur. It is impossible to directly measure free radical production in humans. Free radical by-products do increase with exercise, but trained athletes may dispose of them more effectively.

Moderate doses of vitamin C, beta-carotene, and other carotenoids are easily obtained with educated food choices. However, one nutrient that may be difficult to obtain at antioxidant levels on a diet of under 30 percent fat is vitamin E. Good sources are high in fat, and you would need to consume large amounts of them to reach even the low antioxidant dose of 100 IU. Researchers still need to determine the optimal doses of antioxidant supplements needed for preventing heart disease and cancer, and that can be safely supplemented.

If you do supplement, do so wisely. A multivitamin and mineral supplement providing 100 percent of the DV should be safe, though not always necessary. But keep in mind that the hazards of vitamin and mineral overdosing are real and can be subtle. If you do take a supplement, understand the good reasons for taking it, consume appropriate doses, and discontinue its use when it is no longer needed.

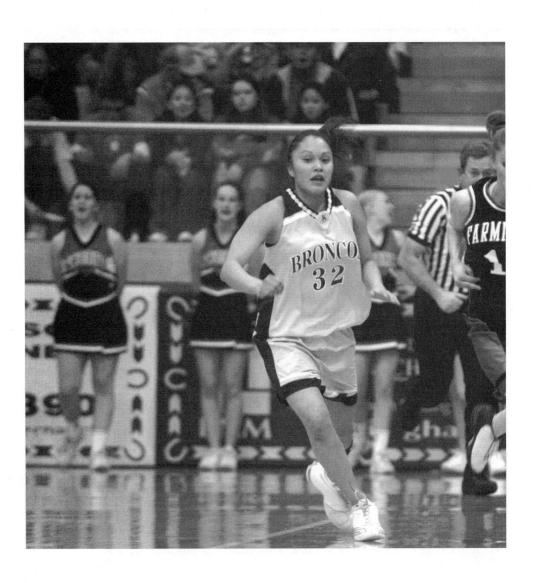

CHAPTER 3

PERFORMANCE NUTRITION FOR ALL AGES

Athletes of all ages participate in team sports, from grade school, to high school, through college, and later as a masters athlete who wants to enjoy club sports after college. Many professional team sport athletes now continue playing at a high level in their sports well into their thirties. It is important to appreciate some of the differences in nutrition that exist for athletes of all ages to support growth, increased strength, optimal recovery, specific nutrient requirements, and optimal health, and provide a sound nutritional framework to support and enhance the athlete's enjoyment of their sport and competitive endeavors.

FUEL FOR THE PREADOLESCENT ATHLETE

Many children develop an appreciation and enjoyment of their sport at an early age. It is important that these active children be well nourished and properly fueled for their activity and competition. Athletes aged 5 to 12 years must consume a diet designed to support both growth and development, and training and performance.

When feeding these athletes, it is important to appreciate that they are not mini-versions of adolescent or adult athletes. The preadolescent athlete's nutritional needs cannot be easily quantified as one diet fits all because of the wide variation in growth rates among children, variety in training programs, and the lack of scientific data on child athletes. Parents and coaches need to be sensitive to these children's nutritional needs and provide the food choices and direction required by their young bodies.

Calories

Children involved in team sports should be observed in regard to their growth and energy levels to effectively determine if they are consuming adequate calories or energy. Chronic poor calorie intake can result in many health concerns such as short stature, delayed puberty, poor bone health, menstrual irregularities, increased susceptibility to injury, fatigue and poor performance, and higher risk of developing an eating disorder. Energy requirements in children are not only affected by growth and training. Their energy needs are also increased due to the fact that they are not as metabolically efficient and also waste calories by being more mechanically inefficient due to relative lack of coordination.

Children often do the best job of determining their caloric intake simply by choosing foods and eating in accordance with their hunger and fullness levels. Calorie intake is affected by the training program, as well as other lifestyle issues, and may vary throughout the season as sport involvement changes from club to school involvement or off-season. The parents' role is to provide three regular, structured meals and healthy between-meal snacks and foods and fluid around practice times. Children involved in sports may be unaware of the important role nutrition plays in the enhancement of their athletic performance. Children can also be encouraged to take some responsibility for their own food and fluid choices. Education in this area may benefit both the parent and child, as it is easier to adopt healthy eating practices earlier in life.

The child athlete's growth should be monitored at regular intervals and can include height, weight, skinfold, and circumference measurements. If children are growing appropriately for their own specific growth curve, their energy needs are likely being met. Any substantial deviation from this growth curve should be investigated. Growth may be affected by an increase or decrease in training intensity, and various medical or psychological problems can affect food intake.

Protein

Child athletes have higher protein requirements than adults because of the extra amounts required for growth. The younger the child, the more protein required per pound of body weight. However, these higher protein amounts are easily met with good food choices and a well-balanced diet. The child athlete who consumes enough calories will also use the protein provided in the diet more efficiently and for important, unique protein functions.

Children may often gravitate toward lower-quality protein sources such as hot dogs, fatty luncheon meats, and fast-food fare. Adding choices such as nonhydrogenated peanut butter, lean poultry meat, and yogurt or milk to meals and snacks can contribute to their total protein intake and lay the foundation for good eating habits early in life.

Fluid

Younger children are more likely than older children to become dehydrated, and consequently active children need to consume plenty of fluids. Because children don't sweat as easily as adults, their bodies do not cool as efficiently. Children should arrive for practices fully hydrated and drink at regular pauses during the training session. Cooled beverages are more appealing and accepted by children, and they are absorbed more quickly. Children are less likely to drink than adults, even when pushed to do so at practice. Checking weight before and after practice can also provide information on how well children are meeting their fluid needs. Any weight loss can completely be attributed to fluid loss. Young children also need more time than adults do to acclimatize to hot weather. When children start practice in hotter weather, they should be given time to adjust and adequate fluid intake is imperative.

While water is adequate for rehydration, children are more likely to drink adequate amounts when provided flavored drinks. Real fruit juice, dairy and soy milk, and foods that are high in water such as oranges, watermelon, and apples can also be used to rehydrate the body. Some of the fluid and high-water food choices cannot only replace lost fluid but provide carbohydrates for replenishment as well. Fluids consumed during exercise that provide carbohydrate and sodium, such as sports drinks, are also appealing to children.

Minerals

Calcium is a very important mineral for the child athlete because of its role in developing strong, hard bones and teeth properly. Adequate calcium also reduces the risk of fractures and is essential to the healing of broken bones. Calcium requirements are very high during childhood, and many young athletes have an inadequate calcium intake, perhaps as consumption of milk has decreased in favor of less nutritious fluids. Children need at least three servings of calcium-rich foods daily. (Good sources of calcium have been presented earlier, in Table 2.6.)

Iron is also an essential mineral for the child athlete, as iron requirements are extremely high at this stage of life, mainly because of its role in the formation of hemoglobin. (A list of iron-rich foods was provided in Table 2.7.) Children should be encouraged to consume low-sugar, iron-fortified cereals and other high-iron foods such as raisins, iron-enriched grains, and protein sources such as lean beef and poultry.

Many school-age children skip breakfast, an important meal that helps them perform better in school and perform during practice. Breakfast fills up carbohydrate stores in the liver, an important fuel source that becomes depleted overnight when sleeping. Maintaining this fuel source with a steady supply of fuel from breakfast, lunch, and an afternoon snack ensures adequate stores for afternoon training.

A balanced school lunch is also important. Parents should consider the choices offered at school or pack a lunch as appropriate. The child's friends can often influence food choices. Parents should ask children what they eat at school, if they eat the entire lunch packed, and find out what snacks are consumed away from home. Many child athletes practice after school, making an afternoon snack appropriate and well timed. This snack provides fuel for training and can prevent extreme hunger during practice. This is also a convenient time for the athlete to hydrate prior to practice.

Vitamin and mineral needs of young athletes are easily met through a well-balanced diet. Achieving nutrient balance over the week is what is important. If a child athlete is provided with a basic multivitamin and mineral supplement, it should not provide children with a false sense of security, and nutritious foods should still be encouraged and consumed. Ergogenic aids such as creatine are not suitable for child athletes for a number of reasons, but particularly for the potential short-term and long-term harmful effects.

Prepubescent athletes can be sensitive to the normal body changes that occur with growth and development. Young athletes may be skilled at their sport before going through puberty. As the body starts changing, some athletes may attempt to control food intake and maintain their current "competitive" weight. Even young children can experiment with fad diets and disordered eating behavior. Coaches and parents can help by appreciating the normal growth stages of the prepubescent athlete and by being prepared to help children cope with normal body changes.

Weight Control

Unhealthy weight management strategies should not be practiced when trying to achieve top athletic performance. A diet that is restricted in calories and nutrients and that may compromise the health of a child should not be promoted. Parents should not inappropriately eliminate food groups or over-restrict foods in an attempt to control weight or prevent disease later in life. Parents can encourage long-term healthy eating habits that support growth, provide fuel for sport, and reduce unnecessary amounts of saturated fat, hydrogenated fat, and sugars in the diet.

Children with very high energy needs may find it difficult to consume adequate calories and may require concentrated food sources. Smoothies, low-fat milk shakes, concentrated starches, and dried fruits may help them consume adequate calories. These children should consume three meals and at least two snacks daily to stay in calorie balance.

Conversely, child athletes should not be encouraged to eat excessively in the belief that they will build strength and endurance more quickly. Inappropriate calorie consumption can lead to the start of a lifelong struggle of being overweight. Parents who require some nutritional guidance for their child athlete can consult a qualified sports nutritionist.

Children can be encouraged in taking some responsibility for their own food intake and developing their own nutritional strategies. Children should not be dictated what they are allowed to eat and not eat but rather be offered a variety of healthy choices.

FUEL FOR THE HIGH SCHOOL ATHLETE

The adolescent or high school athlete will experience a significant growth spurt and body changes that may concern or even frustrate them. Every high school athlete will develop and grow at their own pace. In any one high school grade, you will see a wide variety of normal body shapes and sizes.

Teenagers can be very sensitive about their changing bodies. Girls may desire to be both lean and fast, while boys may focus on being stronger and bigger for increased strength. This may conflict with the fact that acquiring increased body fat is normal for a developing female athlete, and that some boys may develop later than their classmates. It is important that high school athletes appreciate good nutrition practices, the physical demands of their sport, and how nutritional decisions affect both their short-term and long-term health.

Calories

The energy requirements of the high school athlete depend on the basic (basal) energy expenditure for adolescence, growth requirements, daily activities, and of course the energy burned when training and competing for their sport. Many teenage athletes have high calorie needs, and eating enough to support all their activities is important.

Table 3.1 reviews daily calorie intake for preadolescents and teenagers. These caloric intakes do not include calories that need to be consumed for exercise. The longer and harder these young athletes train, the more food they should consume. (Estimation of

TABLE 3.1 DAILY CALORIE INTAKES FOR TEENAGERS	
Males age 11 to 14 years	**Females age 11 to 14 years**
2,500 calories/day	2,200 calories/day
Males age 15 to 18 years	**Females age 15 to 18 years**
3,000 calories/day	2,200 calories/day

energy needs is described in Chapter 5, Eating for Training and Recovery, with the energy expenditures for various sports listed in Table 5.1.)

An ideal calorie level for growing teen athletes will reflect all of their energy expenditure, but it should be interpreted with caution as these numbers are only an estimate. Calorie needs vary greatly from teenage athlete to athlete depending on their growth, age, and type of training. The athlete's energy level, recovery, body weight, growth, and general health should all determine if adequate calories are being consumed. When an athlete does not eat enough food, her metabolism slows down, resulting in fewer calories being burned. This in turn means that an athlete requires less food for the same amount of activity, which could lead to future eating and weight control problems. Athletes with a slowed metabolism may also feel tired, underperform in their sport, and not grow to their full potential.

Estimates of energy requirements for adolescent athletes range from 2,200 to 4,000 calories per day for females and 3,000 to 6,000 daily for males in high school, depending on their total energy expenditure. Let's say we have a 16-year-old male basketball player who trains 90 minutes daily. His weight is 170 pounds (77 kilograms). He burns 11.2 calories per minute, for 90 minutes of practice, for a total of 1,008 calories. Add this to the basic energy expenditure of 3,000 calories, and his energy needs for a heavy practice day are over 4,000 calories. Now consider a 14-year-old female soccer player who also practices 90 minutes daily. At a weight of 130 pounds (59 kilograms), she burns 702 calories during practice. Added to 2,200 calories daily, her total calorie needs are approximately 2,900 daily.

Protein

Healthy teenagers require about 0.4 to 0.45 grams of protein per pound of body weight (0.8 to 1.0 gram/kilogram body weight) daily. No scientific data are available to indicate if teenage athletes require additional protein. Team sport athletes who may require additional protein include athletes who are just starting a training program and athletes who are actively weight training as part of their overall program. As for most North Americans, the protein intake of teenagers usually exceeds the recommended amounts. While exceeding their protein requirements does not build more muscle in teenagers, consuming adequate calories ensures that protein is used for unique protein functions and will not be wasted as a fuel source during exercise. High-quality protein sources should be emphasized, such as lean meats, fish, poultry, eggs, and dairy products. Vegetarian teenage athletes need to emphasize soy and dairy protein sources, and consume plenty of dried peas and beans.

Iron and Calcium

Even teenagers not involved in sports have a high risk of developing low iron stores, but athletes are at risk due to increased demands of growth, sports-related blood loss, poor iron absorption, menstruation in female athletes, and possibly poor nutritional intake and unbalanced eating. Good sources of iron should be emphasized.

Calcium is also a very important mineral for the teenage athlete, as this is one of the most critical times for building bone. It is not usual for teenagers to consume inadequate amounts of calcium. Female athletes who restrict calories often restrict more concentrated food sources of calcium such as dairy products. Dairy products are usually the main source of calcium in the adolescent's diet.

Poor calcium intake may not be apparent until the athlete experiences a stress fracture, and it is often not apparent until identified with laboratory or bone density tests. Female athletes with irregular periods, and amenorrhea or cessation of menstruation are at great risk for poor bone status. Amenorrhea is often related to inadequate calorie intake for growth and training needs, and it may also reflect disordered eating. The recommended daily calcium intake for adolescents is 1,300 milligrams, and high school age

Iron Tips for the High School Athlete

- Teenagers who do not have a variety of foods in their diet such as meat, fish, and poultry may be at greater risk for developing poor iron status.
- Restrictive eating, fad diets, and poorly balanced vegetarian diets can significantly decrease iron intake.
- Full-blown iron deficiency in adolescents will impair athletic performance. While iron deficiency without anemia may not have the same effect, it should be treated with appropriate food intake and supplementation as the more serious condition of anemia can develop.
- Nutritional intake of iron must be adequate to meet needs for training, support growth and development, and produce adequate hemoglobin and ferritin to maintain iron status.
- Teenage athletes should appreciate that poor iron status can result in symptoms such as fatigue when training, breathlessness, paleness, slightly elevated heart rate, and inability to keep warm.
- Iron deficiency is more common in female athletes because of menstrual losses, rapid growth in the early high school years, and inadequate dietary iron intake.
- Iron loss can also be associated with weight-bearing exercise as seen in team sports, gastrointestinal losses, and losses from excessive sweating.

females may consume 400 to 700 milligrams daily. Males may consume half to all of their calcium needs of 1,300 milligrams daily. High school athletes should be educated on good sources of calcium, ways to increase calcium absorption, and the number of food servings required for meeting their calcium needs. Teenagers may respond better to the more immediate concerns of poor calcium intake such as stress fractures, as well as the long-term concern of osteoporosis.

Other Supplement Use

High school athletes may take a daily multivitamin and mineral supplement for a variety of reasons, including the desire to improve athletic performance. Supplements can offset any uneven eating habits, though good food choices should be encouraged whenever possible. Supplements themselves will not improve athletic performance, though they can correct marginal deficiencies that may impact exercise performance. Adolescent athletes who may benefit from a vitamin and mineral supplement include vegetarians, girls who are iron-deficient, and those who are amenorrheic. Misuse and overuse of supplements is possible and could have adverse effects on health. These supplements should be taken as directed.

Young athletes participating in team sports should also be advised that athletic performance is dependent on a number of important factors, such as years of good training, sound nutrition practices, skill acquisition, and growth stages, and they should be advised to not place unrealistic and high expectations on the use of nutritional supplements. Supplements designed to specifically enhance performance such as ergogenic aids, as described in Chapter 6, are often supported by flashy advertising and anecdotal success stories. Many of these ergogenic aids are frequently used by male adolescent athletes interested in building muscle or female athletes interested in losing body fat. These products may include protein powder, creatine, and hydroxyl-methyl butyrate or HMB, with the short- and long-term effects of these on adolescents not known. These products may often contain banned ingredients due to poor product purity and quality control and could have harmful side effects, as well as result in a positive drug test. Many of these products are often not backed by scientific testing and appropriate safety data and have not been tested on young athletes. It has been suggested that athletes under 18 years of age do not consume ergogenic aids.

Fluid and Hydration

Adolescents training in the heat should be monitored closely for signs of heat stress and dehydration. Younger bodies and smaller bodies are at greater risk for developing dehydration due to greater heat production. Athletes with higher levels of body fat and heavier builds are more susceptible to heat stress as they are less efficient in dissipating heat when exercising. Adequate fluid consumption during exercise is essential to preventing heat-related problems. Athletes should start training in a well-hydrated state, as even training situations that make room for ideal fluid consumption during exercise may not allow them to keep up with their fluid losses. Starting the training session well hydrated can lessen the degree of dehydration that can develop during training. Dehydration in adolescents will result in a greater increase in core body temperature than in adults. (Guidelines for fluid intake during training will be covered in Chapter 5.)

Developing Good Eating Habits

Adolescents often have distinct eating habits from both younger children and adults. Older adolescents, particularly girls, may become regular breakfast skippers and not rely as much on snacking to meet their daily nutrient intake. Older adolescents are also more likely to obtain and consume food away from home. A number of factors influence the food choices of adolescent athletes, including convenience and time considerations around busy school and training schedules, both hunger and cravings, food appeal and appearance, peer and parental influences, beliefs about health often influenced by the media, moods and feelings, body image, and cost. Girls are more likely to obtain their nutrition and weight loss information from magazines that may not be accurate and factual. Other major sources of nutrition information include physicians, the school environment, and coaches. Adolescent athletes may have exposure to accurate information from sports nutritionists, usually as a result of parental initiation, though some schools may include this service in their programming for athletes.

Body Image Concerns

Body image is an important issue for many adolescents as this is a period of quick and often unpredictable growth, as well as significant emotional changes. Becoming self-conscious about the body starts at an early age as many males strive for a muscular physique, while females attempt to be small, lean, and thin.

These body image concerns can sometimes translate into poor nutrition practices. Males may consume large and unnecessary amounts of protein in the belief that this will build more muscle, while females may develop restrictive eating patterns in hopes of losing weight and body fat. Disordered eating patterns can also occur in hopes of enhancing performance, attempting to change body type to reach an ideal for their chosen sports, and attaining the physique idealized in society. Athletes who are at a healthy weight and attempt to lose or drastically decrease body fat can resort to weight loss techniques that have negative effects on nutrient intake and balance in the diet, as well as harmful effects on physical and psychological health. Some ill-advised and unhealthy techniques can be skipping meals, decreasing meals, eliminating food groups, use of laxatives, purging after meals, and using over-the-counter weight loss supplements.

Nutrition Education

Adolescent athletes can benefit from repeated and regular sound nutrition advice. Support in preparing or purchasing healthy school lunches, consuming healthy snacks, and taking responsibility for meal preparation should be encouraged. Adolescents can become quite independent in meeting their nutritional needs, and this practice is often essential due to demanding school and training schedules, and conflicting schedules for various family members. Education of other family members, particularly the person responsible for food shopping and meal preparation, is also indicated.

Specific strategies may be required for athletes with high energy requirements, such as nutrient-dense food choices in the form of smoothies, low-fat shakes, and concentrated carbohydrate choices. These athletes may need to base most meals and snacks on carbohydrate-rich foods, pack foods for school, and make good use of high carbohydrate liquids. Filling foods that are low in nutrients and calories should be kept to appropriate levels.

Athletes identified as having weight management concerns should be referred to a sports dietitian who can provide healthy nutrition guidelines so that restrictive eating and disordered eating behaviors are prevented. Rapid weight loss is not recommended; when indicated, gradual weight loss is recommended. Regular monitoring is also essential. Vegetarian adolescent athletes and their families could also benefit from qualified nutritional guidance.

FUEL FOR THE COLLEGIATE ATHLETE

In the United States, hundreds of thousands of male and female collegiate athletes participate in all sports, with team sports being some of the most popular. College athletes often appreciate the importance of nutrition in athletic performance but may have had limited exposure to sound sports nutrition advice. Many of these athletes may have gone though high school sports thriving on convenience items and fast food and have not developed the sports nutrition practices required for optimal performance. Moving to the school's dining hall, which provides a variety of food choices, may or may not support a positive change in nutrition habits. These athletes may not always like college dorm food choices or may have trouble adapting a vegetarian diet to college life. Class schedules often require that some meals be eaten on campus, where a variety of food choices may be offered, including fast food. Athletes may opt to consume some meals in their room, or on their dorm floors, with options limited to microwaving and other simple food preparation techniques. Most college athletes are not proficient cooks and may lack some of the equipment and facilities previously utilized at home.

Even for collegiate athletes motivated to shop for healthy foods and comfortable with meal planning and cooking, time may be a great limitation in achieving these tasks. Frequently, these athletes have very busy schedules with little free time for off-campus activities such as food shopping. Between training, class time and studying requirements, and participation in other hobbies and interests, they have heavy demands on their time. Collegiate athletes may train more than once daily and take demanding academic classes.

Nutrition Assessment Education

Nutrition education and support programs can vary widely among locations, with some of the larger universities more likely to offer comprehensive programming. Ideally a sports nutritionist is available to offer a variety of services and is part of a comprehensive program that works closely with the athletic department and the food service offerings available to student athletes. Collegiate athletes are also exposed to a variety of nutrition information sources, both accurate and healthy, and inaccurate and perhaps risky. Student athletes have exposure to the Internet and advertising for supplement use, as well as weight loss products.

In addition to the risk of nutrition misinformation, research indicates that collegiate athletes may experience other health risks. These athletes may be focused on an ideal weight that may conflict with good health and appropriate nutrition habits. Males in team sports may be preoccupied with building muscle and may be exposed to and use anabolic steroids. They are also more likely to consume alcohol and even engage in binge drinking, and be a passenger in a vehicle driven by a driver under the influence of alcohol. Female athletes can also be at risk. Preoccupation with weight and disordered eating habits can result in a higher rate of irregular and absent menstruation and a higher incidence of stress fractures.

Sports nutrition evaluation and services that the collegiate athlete can be offered include the following:

- Assessment of body composition and evaluation to determine weight and body fat goals. This can include body fat loss and ongoing monitoring of a strength and conditioning program designed to build muscle mass.

- Evaluation of blood chemistry and lipid profiles. These tests can be part of the yearly physical conducted on athletes.
- Screening of iron deficiency and iron deficiency anemia
- Nutrition education at the training table/food hall that provides nutrition examples and food strategies
- Nutritional information on the dishes and meals offered at the training table
- Diet and nutritional analysis
- Team seminars
- Individual nutritional counseling to provide meal plans for training, during the training season, for competition, and off-season
- Assistance with on-campus meal choices and strategies at various venues frequented by the athlete
- Nutritional counseling for health-related concerns that can be integrated with the sports nutrition meal plan
- Team seminars on various sports nutrition topics such as fluids and hydration, nutritional recovery strategies, and sports nutrition supplements
- Nutritional protocols for providing foods and fluid for pregame ingestion
- Nutritional protocols for fluids and sports supplement availability at games

Unfortunately, not all of these services and follow-up are available to the collegiate athletes, with the athletic trainer often fielding sports nutrition concerns. If on-campus sports nutrition services are not available, off-campus qualified sports nutritionists can be contacted to provide various services.

Energy and Protein Requirements

Fuel needs of many collegiate team sport athletes can be high, though this can vary depending on the sport and the position played within the sport. For example, soccer players may actually run several miles in one practice session, whereas a football player playing a linebacker position may not expend as many calories as a running back. Energy needs of various sports are outlined in Table 5.1. As indicated, the energy burned per hour can vary with body weight and sport.

Protein requirements need to be calculated to encompass the strength-training program of the athlete and the number of hours spent training. As with younger athletes, the protein needs of collegiate athletes are easily met with an appropriately chosen diet, and expensive protein supplements are not needed. For serious weight training, timing of protein intake around the training sessions may significantly enhance muscle building. (More of these strategies are covered in Chapter 6.) Lean protein sources low in saturated fat and prepared with less fat should be emphasized. Adequate caloric consumption also ensures that the protein consumed is used for important protein functions.

Fluids and Hydration

College athletes also need to have workable strategies for maintaining daily hydration. They can carry water bottles and consume other hydrating fluids such as milk and juice to maintain hydration levels. Caffeine intake should be kept to moderate levels. Fluids should also be easily available during practice sessions. (More on fluid intake before, during, and after practice is covered in Chapters 5 and 7.) Players should be educated on how to monitor fluid status. For example, pale urine reflects adequate hydration, as does four full bladders of urine daily.

Supplements

Athletes should be aware of supplements that are banned by the National Collegiate Athletic Association (NCAA). Over-the-counter nutritional supplements may also contain banned substances due to poor quality control at the time of production of raw materials and product manufacture. Many schools may have a dietary supplement policy designed to prevent ingestion of banned substances, prevent harmful effects of products, keep the athlete from spending money on unnecessary products, and take legal supplements appropriately.

Collegiate athletes may benefit from a daily multivitamin and mineral supplement providing 100 percent of the DVs, to augment any marginal intakes of nutrients. Iron supplementation to treat or prevent anemia should be monitored with regular blood work. Any other vitamin and mineral supplement recommendations should be provided under the recommendations of a sports nutritionist.

Food Service

A sports nutritionist can work directly with the food service program and chef to make menu recommendations and suggest recipe modifications. Athletes can be offered a wide variety of menu items and also be educated on appropriate choices and portions to consume for their nutritional plan. Some healthy offerings may include a nutrient-dense salad bar, pasta and potato bars, whole-grain choices, and fresh fruits.

Both high school and collegiate athletes may frequent fast-food establishments. It is important that they make the best choices possible at these establishments not only for performance but also for lifelong good health. (Chapter 8 outlines some fast-food options.)

Team personnel, with the assistance of the sports nutritionist, can also set up healthy meals for the team when traveling for away games. Restaurants can be contacted ahead of time to set up team meals. Athletes should be educated on healthy food choices when eating out for fast food, in airports, and at various types of restaurants and ethnic cuisine.

FUEL FOR THE MASTERS ATHLETE

With baby boomers now well into their forties, it is not unusual to see many masters athletes participating in team sports. They may have participated in the sport in college and have found a club or league that allows them to participate in their chosen sport for part of the year. Besides training and competing for the love of their sport, they also receive the added bonus of staying fit and healthy. Masters athletes often also participate in a weight-training or resistance-training program to maintain lean body mass and strength.

Plenty of data indicate that these older athletes enjoy better health than nonathletes, as many of the supposed normal age-related health changes could actually result from a sedentary lifestyle. However, masters athletes will experience some physiological changes with aging, such as decreases in heart function, muscle mass, and aerobic capacity. These changes are not as pronounced in masters athletes as they are in their sedentary peers. Masters athletes are also more likely to experience sports-related injuries, and adjust to training at a slower rate. They also recover from training more slowly than their athletic younger counterparts.

Nutritional considerations for masters athletes focus both on these physiological changes as well as on the nutritional demands of the training program for their team sport. Masters participation varies from sport to sport, with playing time often limited to two or fewer practices per week. The age at which an athlete is defined as being a master can vary from sport to sport.

Performances of world-class athletes tend to decline after ages 30 to 35 years due to a number of physiological age-related factors. Muscle strength peaks at around 25 years of age, levels off from 30 to 35 years, and then declines after ages 35 to 40. This decrease is related to reduced muscle mass, rather than an actual decrease in the capacity of muscle fibers. Training programs that incorporate muscle building can offset some of this muscle loss and help maintain strength. Specific nutrition strategies can also maximize your muscle-building efforts. These guidelines are covered in Chapter 6. Aerobic capacity decreases each decade beginning at about 25 years. This age-related rate of decrease is slightly slower in athletes than their sedentary counterparts. However, it is clear that masters athletes benefit from a health perspective and likely have a lower risk of chronic diseases such as cardiovascular disease, hypertension, and diabetes.

Energy and Protein Requirements

There is a decline in basal metabolic rate with aging, and there may also be a decrease in calories burned with exercise, depending on the intensity and duration of the training program. While the energy or calorie needs of masters athletes may decline over the course of their athletic career, they can still consume more than their sedentary counterparts. Adjustments in food intake may be required to prevent unwanted weight gain. Resistance training also increases calorie needs. Masters athletes should continue to consume more protein than their sedentary counterparts, and they likely require the same amounts as younger athletes. Their total protein needs are easily met by making the proper food choices and do not demand any specific protein supplements.

Carbohydrate should continue to be the major source of energy in the masters athlete's diet, though the amount required can vary depending on the training program, specific training session, and time of the season. Fat intake can make up the remainder of the calories consumed, with the emphasis being placed on healthy types of fats (reviewed in Chapter 2).

Vitamins and Minerals

Both male and female masters athletes should pay close attention to optimal bone health and the nutrients that support this important body tissue, particularly calcium and vitamin D. It is important that you meet your calcium needs on a daily basis. From ages 30 to 50, men should obtain at least 1,000 milligrams of calcium daily and supplement as needed if this is not provided in the diet. Calcium needs increase further beyond these ages, with 1,200 milligrams being the recommended amount for men aged 50 to 70. Many experts believe that women should consume at least 1,200 milligrams of calcium daily from ages 30 to 50 and 1,500 milligrams after menopause.

Vitamin D is also crucial for healthy bones, aiding in the optimal absorption of calcium. Aging decreases the capacity to synthesize vitamin D from sunlight, and less vitamin D is absorbed with age. For these reasons, vitamin D requirements double from 200 to 400 IU daily at age 50, for both men and women. A standard multivitamin can supplement your food intake of this nutrient, and many formulations for individuals over 50 provide the full daily requirement.

There are several other important nutrients that the masters athlete should consider increasing in their diet by choosing good food sources. Vitamin B6, vitamin E, and zinc are important to maintaining optimal immune function, which can decline with age. Folate, vitamin B6, and vitamin B12 are important nutrients that keep levels of homocysteine in the blood down to acceptable levels. High levels of homocysteine are associated with increased risk of developing heart disease. Absorption of B12 also decreases with age due to decreased gastric acid levels. Increasing food sources of these nutrients is one important strategy, but you can also consider a standard-dose multivitamin mineral supplement that provides 100 percent of the daily values. Formulations for older individuals that specifically provide higher amounts of these nutrients are also available.

Fluid and Hydration

Masters athletes should pay extra attention to daily fluid intake for a number of reasons related to aging. As we age, thirst sensation decreases, affecting regulation of hydration status. Body water also declines in older persons. After age 40, the kidneys require more water to remove waste products from the body.

Not keeping up with sweat losses can impair training, particularly when exercising in the heat. Masters athletes may be more susceptible to overheating and should consume as much fluid as possible before and after training. They should give themselves more time to acclimate to hot weather and pay attention to warning signs of dehydration and heat exhaustion. They should also be aware of how any prescription drug they take can affect body temperature regulation in a hot environment, discussing this with their physician as needed. More specific guidelines on hydration strategies before, during, and after exercise are outlined in Chapter 5.

SPECIAL CONSIDERATION FOR FEMALE ATHLETES

Female athletes may need to pay special attention to specific nutrients at various stages in their training and in their lives. Bone health is a special concern in females, as they are at greater risk for osteoporosis, and those who develop menstrual irregularities are at even greater risk. Because our society places such value on thinness in women, they are highly susceptible to developing eating disorders.

Body Weight, Amenorrhea, and Bone Density

Bone health is an issue that has received heightened attention over the past two decades due to the increasing rate of osteoporotic fractures and a focus on stress fractures. The athlete at risk for development of compromised bone health should appreciate the influence of exercise, hormone balance, and nutritional factors such as calcium intake on maintaining appropriate levels of this important body tissue.

Bone is a dynamic tissue that is constantly being broken down and rebuilt under the regulation of your body's hormones. When the process of bone breakdown or bone resorption exceeds bone formation, bone loss occurs. If this bone loss is prolonged, osteoporosis, a condition in which low bone mass has developed and bone is fragile, can result, and there is greater risk for fracture. Calcium balance is maintained by the amount of calcium you both consume and absorb, and how much calcium you lose in your urine. The hormone estrogen plays a crucial role in maintaining bone in women. When estrogen levels are low, the bone serves as a source of calcium to maintain normal levels of calcium in the blood and perform important physiological functions in the body. Even if physical activity is high, low estrogen levels, as seen in amenorrhea and after menopause, can result in bone loss. Female athletes seem to have a higher incidence of menstrual irregularities than the general population. Genetics also has a large influence on your bone density.

The hormone estrogen plays a crucial role in maintaining bone in women. When estrogen levels are low, the bone serves as a source of calcium to maintain normal levels of calcium in the blood and perform important physiological functions in the body. Even if physical activity is high, low estrogen levels as seen in amenorrhea and after menopause can result in bone loss. Female athletes seem to have a higher incidence of menstrual irregularities than the general population.

The term *athletic amenorrhea* has been used to describe menstrual imbalances in female athletes. A variety of factors have been implicated in the development of amenorrhea in athletes. It appears that the predominant factor in development of amenorrhea is inadequate energy intake. An excessive training load or increase in training that is not matched with proper food intake creates a caloric deficiency that can result in amenorrhea. Of course, disordered eating and a full-blown eating disorder can also result in chronically low intake of calories. Amenorrhea may also be more common in certain sports such as running, gymnastics, and dance, rather than team sports, but can occur in any sports under the proper precipitating conditions.

What has been determined is that female athletes with amenorrhea have lower bone mass than athletes who menstruate regularly. Greater incidence of stress fractures has also been reported in athletes with current or past menstrual disturbances. Athletes

TABLE 3.2 NUTRITIONAL CONSIDERATIONS FOR SPECIFIC POPULATION GROUPS

Athlete	Nutritional Considerations
Children	• Monitor growth curve to assess nutritional adequacy • Quality protein sources to meet high requirements • Higher risk of overheating and becoming dehydrated • Good calcium and iron intake • Teach sound eating habits
Adolescents	• Significant growth spurt and varying rates of growth affects body image in boys and girls • Protein needs met in well-balanced diet • Calcium and iron intake very important • May want to try various sports supplements for muscle building and decreasing body fat • Often eat on the run and are involved in own meal preparation • Sound nutrition education very beneficial
Collegiate	• May bring fast-food eating habits to college • Benefit from nutritional assessment and monitoring • Supported by healthy training table programs • Benefit from nutrition team seminars and individual counseling • Require healthy guidelines for eating on campus and eating out • Benefits from education on proper food and fluid intake before, during, and after practice/games
Masters	• Changes in physiology that affect performance • Often include strength training in their program • May have decreased energy needs • Have higher protein needs than sedentary counterparts • Require higher amounts of calcium and iron • Require higher amounts of vitamins B6 and B12 • Should pay close attention to adequate daily and training hydration
Females	• At higher risk for developing disordered eating • At higher risk of anemia • Need to pay careful attention to adequate calcium intake • May require special nutrition considerations during pregnancy and lactation

with health concerns should see a sports medicine physician for assessment of bone mass, hormonal status, and appropriate medical treatment. This may include hormone replacement, weight gain recommendations, and modifications in training. These female athletes can benefit greatly from guidance from a sports nutritionist regarding appropriate calorie intake and the balance of other nutrients in their diet.

Athletes being treated for amenorrhea should increase their calcium intake to 1,500 milligrams daily. Refer back to Table 2.6 for a list of foods high in calcium. If this amount cannot be achieved through diet, calcium supplements can make up the difference. Doses of 500 milligrams of calcium carbonate or calcium citrate can be taken one to two times daily. Excessive intake protein when combined with inadequate calcium intake and high intakes of caffeine and sodium can also aggravate calcium absorption. Overall balance in the diet, especially adequate calorie intake, should also be restored. Weight-bearing exercise may also be continued, though not at excessive levels.

The Spectrum of Disordered Eating

For many female athletes, team sports competition involves moving your body quickly over short or longer distance, often at top speeds, and requires the need to reaccelerate several times during practice or competition. Because of the desire to be quick, having a lower level of body fat is considered to be a mechanical advantage. However, many female athletes do become overly focused on their weight and body fat levels. Because athletes may be obsessive by nature, as well as perfectionistic and very competitive, some of these qualities may manifest in unrealistic weight and body fat goals, placing a high degree of importance on losing a few pounds. Pressure to lose this weight may come from a number of outside sources, including trainers, coaches, and athletic peers. Chapter 6 discusses issues pertinent to the team sports athlete interested in changing body composition. An overview of eating disorders in athletes is also provided. Table 3.2 summarizes the nutritional concerns of specific athletic population groups.

Nutrition for Pregnancy and Exercise

Many pregnant female athletes desire to maintain a high degree of fitness during pregnancy and often return to training and competition as quickly as possible. It is no longer unusual for Olympic or professional athletes to have a child and resume training at a high level. While these athletes may be most concerned about consuming an adequate number of calories for a healthy and appropriate weight gain, the nutrients consumed while planning a pregnancy are also very important.

Often women plan to see their physician before trying to conceive and take a prenatal multivitamin mineral supplement in order to obtain folic acid and other important nutrients. Folate (found from food sources) and folic acid (from supplement sources) deserve serious attention from women athlete's even contemplating pregnancy. An adequate intake of folate, both prior to conception and during the first several weeks of pregnancy, can help prevent birth defects such as spina bifida. Folate is used for the synthesis of DNA, the building block of all cells. During the first twenty-eight days of pregnancy, cells divide rapidly and form the neural tubes

Nutrition for Pregnancy and Exercise (continued)

that become the baby's brain and spine. Many Americans fall short of the recommended 400 micrograms of folate.

Good food sources include asparagus, lentils, spinach and other leafy green vegetables, dried beans such as kidney beans, and orange juice. Grain products such as bread, pasta, rice, and enriched flour have been fortified with folic acid for several years, and a decrease in these types of birth defects has been the result. Many health experts also recommend that any woman who may become pregnant take a multivitamin providing 400 micrograms of folate.

During the first 3 months of pregnancy, it is normal to have no weight gain or up to a 5-pound weight gain. After the first trimester, a weight gain of up to 1 pound weekly is normal. Generally a total weight gain of 25 to 35 pounds is recommended. Underweight or lean women may be advised to gain more weight, at about 28 to 40 pounds. Adequate weight gain comes down to finding the right balance of calories to build your own tissue during pregnancy, to support the growth of the baby, and to meet your energy needs from exercise in order to prevent having a low-birthweight baby or a premature delivery. Starting in the second trimester, pregnancy requires only an additional 300 calories daily above your usual energy needs and another 10 to 12 grams

of protein. These additional nutrient amounts are easily met with an increased food intake—for example, 8 ounces of milk and a small turkey sandwich.

The expectant mother's weight gain comes from growth in her own body tissues, the baby's body weight, and tissues that support the baby's growth. It includes an increased blood volume, body fluid, breast tissue, and weight gain from the placenta, umbilical cord, and amniotic fluid. Body fat stores increase in anticipation of lactation, which requires at least an additional 500 calories or more daily, above normal nonpregnancy requirements. The physician will monitor not only your total weight gain but also the pattern of weight gain to make sure that it is appropriate.

Fluid requirements also increase during pregnancy, and it is critical to maintain proper hydration during exercise and training. Basic fluid requirements are about 2.5 to 3 quarts daily, plus sweat losses during exercise. It is essential that exercise begin in the well-hydrated state. Overheating could have serious negative effects on the unborn baby. Plenty of fluids should be consumed several hours before exercise and at least 4 to 8 ounces of fluid consumed every 15 to 20 minutes. Carbohydrates can be consumed several hours before exercise to prevent hypoglycemia. Sports drinks, carbohydrate gels, and energy bars that have no extra vitamin, mineral, or herbal additives can be consumed during exercise to maintain blood glucose levels. Food choices and prenatal vitamin and mineral supplements should be more than adequate to meet these nutrient requirements, and they should not be overconsumed. Herbal products have not been tested in pregnancy and should be avoided.

Other important nutrients to include in the diet during pregnancy are iron and calcium. Iron requirements double due to a pregnant woman's expanded blood volume. Most pregnant women receive adequate iron in their prenatal vitamin and mineral supplement, but some require an additional iron supplement in order to prevent anemia. Anemia can result in fatigue, shortness of breath, and increased delivery risks. The baby also runs the risk of developing anemia if iron stores run too low, and athletes may already have low iron stores. Iron levels should be checked early in pregnancy and at regular intervals afterward. Concentrate on including plenty of high-iron foods in your diet as listed in Table 2.7.

Calcium plays an important role in every woman's health and deserves extra attention during pregnancy. Calcium requirements increase to 1,200 milligrams daily. As the baby builds bone, the mother's bones serve as a calcium source. If her diet is inadequate to replenish this calcium reservoir, the risk of developing osteoporosis later in life increases. High calcium food sources are listed in Table 2.6. You can also consider taking a separate calcium supplement during pregnancy to meet your elevated requirements.

Certain nutrients and foods should be limited during pregnancy. Excess vitamin A intake from supplementation can increase the risk of birth defects. Intake from a supplement should not exceed 5,000 IU of vitamin A daily. There is also no room for alcohol in the diet as it can produce severe negative effects on the baby, such as fetal alcohol syndrome. Caffeine should be restricted to no more than 300 milligrams daily or avoided altogether. Avoid saccharin and limit other artificial sweeteners as much as possible. Limit soft cheese such as Brie, Camembert, blue cheese, and feta cheese because they can increase the risk of bacterial contamination. In general, pregnant women should be careful with food safety, never eat raw fish, and make sure that all meats are well cooked. Avoid any unpasteurized milk products and raw eggs.

Fish can also be contaminated with mercury, which can have adverse effects

Nutrition for Pregnancy and Exercise (continued)

on the developing baby. Fatty fish such as swordfish, mackerel, shark, bluefish, tilefish, and striped bass should be avoided completely. Other high-mercury fish to avoid include lobster, marlin, red snapper, trout, fresh tuna, and white canned albacore tuna. Canned light tuna should be limited to less than 6 ounces weekly, and keep your total fish intake to 9 to 12 ounces weekly. Lower-mercury fish include sole, tilapia, scallops, shrimp, canned salmon (wild Alaskan), and catfish. Eat low-fat fish and trim excess fat as much as possible. Avoid all herbal supplements and herbal products such as teas, as they have not been tested in pregnancy.

Lactation or breast-feeding increases daily energy requirements 500 calories or more above nonpregnancy requirements.

Fat stores accumulated during pregnancy also serve as an important energy source for lactation. Fluid needs are also high during this time. Weight loss can occur gradually with lactation, but it is best to try not to lose more than one pound weekly, as an overly restrictive diet will decrease the quantity of milk that you produce. High calcium and iron intakes from pregnancy should be maintained, and the prenatal multivitamin mineral supplement can be continued. Limit alcohol and caffeine as they can enter breast milk. It may be best to nurse before exercise due to transient changes that occur in breast milk with exercise. When women train at very high intensities or complete interval training, higher levels of lactic acid in the breast milk may result.

PART II

Training Nutrition
Fine-Tuning Your Diet for
Top Performance, Maximum Strength,
and Optimal Recovery

While the optimal training diet is based on a solid foundation of wholesome food choices, specific nutritional strategies distinguish a top training and competition diet from a healthy diet. Training for your sport often places high energy demands on your body, and optimal recovery is essential for quality training. Not only do your specific food choices make an impact on your health and performance, but how you portion and time your intake of foods and fluids before, during, and after training is also essential to optimizing your energy levels and recovery, as well as performance during practice and competition.

Maximizing your body fuel stores leading up to challenging training sessions supports your hard efforts and results in high-quality training. Fine-tuning your nutrition practices during training also replaces fuel and minimizes fluid losses that can slow down your athletic efforts. Fine-tuning your nutrition practices before, during, and after training gives you the opportunity to identify the nutrition techniques that will work best for you on competition day.

Part II provides specific nutrition guidelines for increasing muscle mass and the strategies for making the most of your weight-training sessions. Ergogenic aids or nutritional supplements marketed to build muscle, burn fat, and improve performance are also reviewed. To bring all this important information together, a very practical chapter describes concrete strategies for planning and consuming an optimal training diet. Guidelines for eating out, food shopping, and meal planning are provided, along with sample menus.

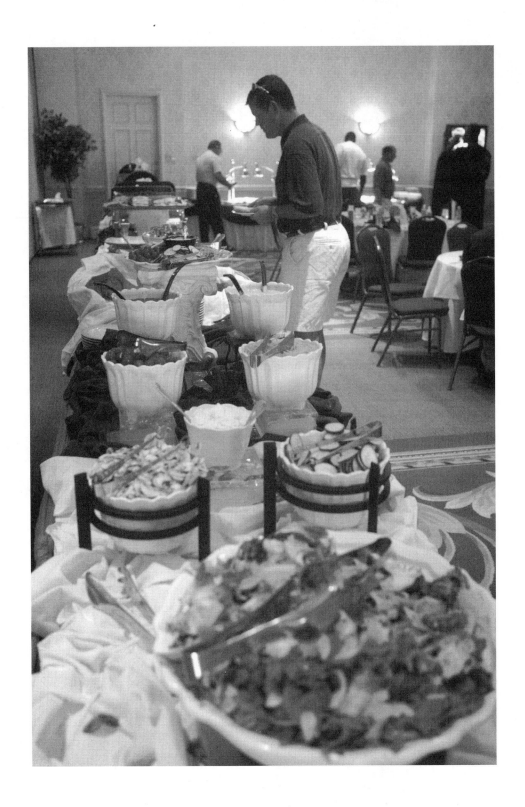

CHAPTER 4
BODY FUEL: POWER FOR TRAINING

For athletes participating in team sports, energy is everything. At times, training and competing in your chosen sport require tremendous amounts of effort. One very important performance-determining factor is optimal energy production or power output over a designated amount of time or distance, while performing the skills specific to your sport. Hockey players must be able to skate explosively while handling the puck. Players running up and down the basketball court must use the highest dexterity when handling the ball. Soccer players who can repeatedly perform short bursts of high-intensity efforts on the field will contribute to a winning match. Sports such as baseball and football rely heavily on short bursts of power, though being able to run at top speed is an essential component of the game, especially for key playing positions.

You may wonder what fuel sources your body uses for exercise, how your training session affects energy use and fuel depletion, and how you can best refuel your body to replenish your stores. Because the way your body uses energy during training directly impacts the nutritional requirements of your sport, team sport athletes can benefit from a basic review and understanding of energy production and the fuel demands placed on the muscles. Specific nutritional strategies can enhance your body's energy systems and muscle-building efforts, and affect your athletic performance. This chapter provides a brief overview of these energy systems and how they each contribute to meet fuel demands for the different types of exercise sessions that you complete and that are unique to your training program for your sport.

All of these energy systems utilize different metabolic pathways to produce energy. How significantly each system will contribute to the energy required for exercise depends on the type of activity performed, which is determined by how intensely you train or the speed at which you train and how long you train. Obviously, your training sessions can vary in intensity and makeup depending on whether you are building your aerobic system, endurance, or speed, and whether you are training on the field, ice, or court or in the weight room. Some training sessions require quick bursts of activity, some may require steady activity with some periods of faster movement or specific interval training, and other types of training sessions require that your muscles work slow and continuously.

Several team sports—namely, soccer, hockey, and basketball—require players to sustain at least an hour of on-and-off high-intensity activity during training and perhaps competition depending on the amount of playing time for each athlete. Often much of this activity is at the very least at moderate speed and may increase to close to maximal speed. Players may have varying playing times and be in and out of the game, but significant fuel depletion can still occur, particularly for the sports of basketball, hockey, and soccer, which are power sports that also incorporate varying amounts of middle-distance and endurance work in the training and competition mix. But all team sport athletes need to be aware of their potential level of fuel depletion and adequately replace this fuel with optimal food choices. Although skill and tactics are an important component of any team sport, having a high level of overall fitness can still be an advantage over the opposing team. To prepare effectively for competition, the team sport athlete incorporates a variety of training sessions and fitness strategies into a weekly program, during the preseason, regular playing season, postseason, and off-season.

Although a variety of nutritional strategies are specific to each of the five team sports outlined in Part III, there are important sports nutrition principles for each team sport athlete to consider. During games, the power sports football and baseball are characterized by short bursts of high-intensity activity with significant periods of rest. The power, middle-distance, endurance sports of basketball, soccer, and hockey are different in that they are characterized by periods of high-intensity activity, often with periods of active or very short rest during which athletes are still moving. Of course, athletes rest more when they are on the sidelines and not on the playing field or court, or when on the bench or sidelines during competition.

The energy to power the intense activity is referred to as *anaerobic*, while the energy that powers the recovery process is mainly *aerobic*. For the team sport athlete, being able to recovery quickly from the last all-out burst of activity is essential to prepare for the next similar burst of speed.

Your muscles have three energy systems from which to obtain fuel:

- The phosphagen (creatine phosphate) system
- The anaerobic glycolysis (lactic acid) system
- The aerobic system

High-speed activity such as football line play demands the all-out effort of the anaerobic phosphagen system, which may provide energy for up to 10 seconds. While this fuel is quickly depleted, muscles can also use stored carbohydrate or glycogen for fuel, also without oxygen or anaerobically and at high intensities. There are still limits to this fuel supply, which lasts about 90 seconds or slightly longer. Obviously, soccer, basketball, and hockey players will need to go longer and then rely on the aerobic system for fuel, which can burn oxygen for a much longer time. The aerobic system only predominates as a fuel source when you are working at low to moderate intensities. Once the pace picks up and your muscles start working faster, oxygen cannot be supplied quickly enough, and it is back to the anaerobic system that predominates. Eventually the anaerobic system runs low on fuel and the athlete becomes fatigued.

Well-trained athletes are able to provide plenty of oxygen to the muscles when needed and limit their reliance on the anaerobic system, delaying fatigue. All of these systems, whether aerobic or anaerobic, work best when they have the right fuels available. Some of these fuels are easier to supply than other fuel sources. Fat is in abundant supply, even in the leanest athletes. Carbohydrates are in more limited supply, and are needed not only as a direct fuel supply but also to allow fat to be burned effectively as a fuel.

ATP: THE ULTIMATE ENERGY SOURCE

Although your muscles contain three different power systems that supply your body with energy for training, ultimately, only one source of fuel can be used for muscle contraction: adenosine triphosphate (ATP). You are constantly using ATP for both daily living and training, whether simply to breathe, go to school or work, run drills, or practice your skills. ATP is a high-energy chemical compound found in all muscle cells. When ATP is broken down, the energy released is used for muscle contraction. Because your muscles contain only a small amount of ATP, it must be steadily recharged for training to continue. The rate at which ATP is recharged in your body must meet the demands of the exercise you are performing. Slower-intensity exercise requires a steady supply of ATP, while higher-intensity exercise requires a more rapid supply of ATP.

Because your body stores ATP in only small amounts, you require plenty of stored energy to recharge ATP and keep the energy flowing while you train. Body stores of carbohydrate, protein, and fat release varying amounts of ATP at varying rates when they are burned for fuel. Carbohydrate is stored in limited amounts in your blood as glucose and in your muscles and liver as glycogen. Blood glucose is your brain's sole source of energy at rest and during exercise. A steady supply of blood glucose keeps you focused while you skate across the ice, for example, or refine your puck-handling skills.

However, your blood glucose levels can quickly run low to meet the energy demands of training. When this occurs, the liver breaks down its supply of glycogen into glucose and releases it directly into the bloodstream to maintain your blood glucose levels. A well-fed liver can store up to 400 calories worth of glycogen. But liver glycogen is a relatively short-lived fuel supply that fills up and empties depending on the timing and composition of your last meal. Depending on what you ate and how much you ate, liver glycogen stores generally last from 3 to 5 hours. You have likely experienced hunger and some of the symptoms that come with low blood glucose levels when you have not eaten for several hours. This hunger, which signals the need for fuel, can occur 3 hours after breakfast, in the afternoon before an evening training session, or anytime that your liver stores run low.

Your liver glycogen and blood glucose levels clearly are a relatively limited supply of fuel. In fact, they can both become depleted relatively quickly during certain types of practice training sessions and during competition. In contrast to your liver glycogen stores, your muscle glycogen is a much larger storage supply of energy, providing anywhere from 1,400 to 1,800 calories, depending on your body weight and the makeup of your diet. When you train at any intensity from easy to hard, steady or stop-and-go exercise, this glycogen is converted into glucose and used by the muscle fibers for energy. However, when your muscle glycogen stores run low, as can occur during long practices or hard interval training sessions, your muscles can also utilize the glucose in your bloodstream for fuel. You are constantly using your glycogen stores when training at most intensity levels, but how much carbohydrate you actually need, or the rate at which you burn carbohydrate (fast, medium, or slow), depends on how hard and how long you train that day.

Team sport athletes benefit greatly from ensuring that their muscle glycogen stores are refueled after training sessions that significantly deplete these stores. Even if your training session does not fully deplete muscle glycogen stores, constant partial replacement of stores can drain your performance efforts. Several days of successive training, without adequate glycogen replacement, could ultimately result in poor energy levels and poor training.

Table 4.1 clearly indicates that your body's supply of carbohydrate is relatively limited. These carbohydrate stores are easily depleted during very high-intensity exercise. You have probably experienced the symptoms of low body carbohydrate stores during one training session or another. When your blood glucose levels hit bottom, you may have felt dizzy and been unable to focus and concentrate. You may have had to stop exercise altogether or slowed down considerably while consuming carbohydrate to get your blood glucose levels back up. Many team sport athletes have probably also experienced muscle glycogen depletion during which their legs felt heavy and sluggish and normal training seemed harder. Team sport athletes can avoid these energy-draining training experiences by starting exercise properly fueled and by consuming enough carbohydrate during exercise to offset body fuel losses. More information on the proper nutrition techniques used specifically for training will be covered in Chapter 7.

A quick look at Table 4.1 reveals that fat is the body's greatest supply of energy even in the leanest athletes, providing over 50,000 stored calories depending on the athlete's body composition. During exercise, when your muscles require fat for fuel, the fat stored within your muscle cells, known as *intramuscular triglycerides,* is used for energy. Just like your muscle glycogen stores, intramuscular triglycerides must be replenished after training, though this fuel is not likely as easily depleted as muscle glycogen. Depending on the intensity and duration of the training session, you will also tap into the fat stored in adipose tissue and convert this fat into fatty acids that are transported to your muscles. It is these more visible body fat stores that provide a relatively unlimited supply of fat for fuel and that are often a focus of the weight management efforts of some team sport athletes, who may include specific training sessions into their program in order to decrease body fat levels.

Muscle protein stores can also potentially supply several thousand calories worth of energy. However, breaking down your muscle protein for fuel is not ideal for both your recovery and health, and it could be detrimental to your performance. Muscle tissue

TABLE 4.1 CALORIES PROVIDED BY BODY FUEL STORES	
Carbohydrate Stores	
Blood glucose	80
Liver glycogen	400
Muscle glycogen	1,400–1,800
Fat Stores	
Blood fatty acids	7
Serum triglycerides	75
Muscle triglycerides	2,700
Adipose tissue triglycerides	80,000
Protein Stores	
Muscle protein	30,000

maintains strength, and constant excess breakdown of this tissue places undue stress on your body and immune system. Preventing muscle tissue breakdown can best be prevented by maintaining optimal carbohydrate and calorie consumption.

Essentially, fat and glycogen are the major fuels that the body uses for energy during training. Exercise intensity, which can be measured as a percentage of your heart rate or VO$_2$max, is particularly important in determining which of these two fuels your body prefers. Generally, the harder you train, the more carbohydrate you burn. Interval training or intermittent high-intensity training, in which you take your heart rate to higher intensities repeatedly, burns a significant amount of carbohydrate. Training simply activates the energy system that can best meet the fuel demands of your training session. It is your job to ensure that this energy system is well supplied.

The three energy systems in your body are activated to supply the most appropriate type and amount of fuel that can best meet the energy demands of your training session. If your body needs carbohydrate quickly, then the lactic acid system is activated. If your body requires a steady supply of fat, the aerobic system is activated. The ATP-CP system can be activated for an all-out sprint effort. Table 4.2 summarizes the characteristics of these energy systems.

TABLE 4.2 THE BODY'S ENERGY SYSTEMS

Anaerobic System

ATP-CP System
- Highest rate of ATP production
- Very limited supply of ATP lasting 6–8 seconds
- Highest power output and intensity level
- Uses ATP and creatine phosphate stored in body
- Development explosive power

Anaerobic Glycolysis (Lactic Acid System)
- High rate ATP production
- Limited supply ATP lasting 1.5–2 minutes
- High power output and intensity level
- Uses ATP, creatine phosphate, and muscle glycogen for fuel
- Development of lactate tolerance

Aerobic System

Glycolytic (Aerobic Glycolysis)
15–90 minutes of exercise
- Low rate of ATP production
- High supply ATP
- Low power production
- Lower intensity
- 15–30 minutes of exercise: use muscle glycogen and blood glucose for energy
- 60–90 minutes of exercise: use muscle glycogen, blood glucose, and intramuscular fat for energy

Glycolytic and Lipolytic
Greater than 90 minutes of exercise
- Lowest rate of ATP production
- High supply ATP
- Lowest power output
- Lowest intensity level
- Longer than 90 minutes of exercise: use muscle glycogen, blood glucose, intramuscular fat, and adipose tissue fat for energy

It's also important for you to realize that although you may specifically train a selected energy system, sometimes neither aerobic nor anaerobic metabolism works exclusively to provide energy during practice and competition, though one energy system may predominate during various types of play. While one system may predominate during a training session, these two metabolic pathways can work together and complement one another to meet the body's energy demands.

The Phosphagen System (The ATP-CP System)

As its name indicates, the ATP-CP system consists of both ATP and another high-energy compound called *creatine phosphate*, or CP. Because ATP is in such short supply, it must be continuously and rapidly resynthesized to provide energy. Like ATP, CP is an energy-rich compound. When it is broken down, it, too, supplies energy. However, CP's released energy does not directly fuel muscle contraction. Rather, the energy released by CP resynthesizes ATP. Like ATP and the energy released from it, CP is in short supply. Energy from the ATP-CP system can fuel high-intensity efforts for only 6 to 8 seconds. Even at 6 seconds' duration, only half of your energy needs come from ATP-CP. Fast-twitch muscle fibers use the ATP-PC system rapidly. This system fuels the initial seconds of sprint events and other events where maximal force is required. It is an important fuel source for baseball and football players who experience single bursts of high-intensity activity. For soccer, hockey, and basketball, any type of workout that involves successive bursts of high-intensity activity intermingled with lower-intensity activity will also rely on the phosphagen system for fuel.

The team sport athlete who has the ability to store more creatine would have an advantage during this type of training. With enhanced storage of this important fuel, you can maintain a higher power output on the successive bouts of very high-intensity activity. To improve the storage of creatine in your muscles, you must do activities that focus on this energy system by performing high-intensity movements that are repeated multiple times during an exercise session. Also, consuming enough calories and protein for recovery improves your short-duration, high-intensity performance.

Anaerobic Glycolysis

Glycolysis is the second metabolic pathway within your muscle cells that is capable of rapidly producing ATP. As its name indicates, glycolysis occurs through the breakdown of glycogen or carbohydrate, without oxygen being present. A single glucose molecule is broken down from muscle glycogen to produce ATP. Anaerobic glycolysis provides energy for short-duration, high-intensity exercise, lasting 10 seconds to several minutes.

As exercise continues beyond 1 to 2 minutes, this system provides less than half of your energy needs. Anaerobic glycolysis fuels activities such as sprinting down a basketball court or training at high-intensity intervals. At the onset of intense exercise when oxygen cannot be delivered to your muscles quickly enough, this energy system is rapidly ignited to supply ATP.

The predominant source of energy during this type of activity is stored muscle glycogen. When this fuel runs out, your muscle cannot continue to perform at the same intensity, and you become fatigued. This anaerobic energy source runs out quickly (about 1.5 minutes) and must be followed by a period of rest, about 3 to 5 minutes, for your muscles to become replenished with energy. This rest and recovery time is just as important as the high-intensity training time. For basketball players going at full efforts at various moments in a game, this anaerobic pathway is crucial.

For the power sports of baseball and football, fat is less likely to be metabolized as a fuel, whereas creatine phosphate and muscle glycogen are mainly utilized for energy. Because of this low reliance on fat for fuel and the lower amount of calories burned during training, baseball players and football players have a higher potential for gaining too much weight and body fat. Another important aspect of these two sports is that they have an off-season during which the athlete's training program may change dramatically. Often weight and body fat can be gained during the off-season. However, due to heavy training schedules and weight-training programs, many team sport athletes may actually have fairly high energy needs due to their large level of muscle mass and the high amount of energy required for training, which can include several practices a day and often weight training. Nutrition programs need to be adjusted for various times of the season to prevent extremes in weight gain or weight cycling. Since weight training is often a large part of the team sport athlete's diet, Chapter 6 is devoted to nutritional strategies for maximizing muscle building.

Aerobic Metabolism

The aerobic pathway is the primary energy source for lower-intensity, prolonged exercise. This system is glycolytic and lipolytic as it derives energy from both carbohydrates and fat, respectively. This pathway provides half of the energy for exercise lasting longer than 1 minute and the majority of the energy for exercise lasting longer than 2 minutes. When you begin exercise, you initially use the anaerobic pathways for energy but then switch to a predominantly aerobic pathway. An adequate supply of oxygen must be delivered to the muscles in order for the oxygen system to release the energy stored in carbohydrates and fats. Protein is not normally used for energy production, but under certain conditions it may become a significant source of energy for the oxygen system.

Although the aerobic system cannot produce ATP as rapidly as the two anaerobic systems, it can produce much greater quantities at a slower rate. The rate at which the oxygen system produces ATP also depends on whether aerobic glycolysis (carbohydrate) or aerobic lipolysis (fat) is burned for fuel. Carbohydrate is a more efficient fuel than fat and is the predominant fuel for steady exercise lasting over 2 minutes and up to 3 hours. But your storage capacity for carbohydrates in the muscles and liver is inadequate for certain endurance events, whereas fat stores are extensive. For the team sport athlete, however, glycogen depletion can occur when combining aerobic training with anaerobic training, eventually depleting muscle glycogen stores. For longer and lower-intensity ultraendurance events, lasting 4 to 6 hours, fat is primarily burned for energy, though this aspect of fuel burning is less applicable to the team sport athlete than to the long-distance cyclist or long-distance runner.

The endurance, middle-distance power sports of hockey, basketball, and soccer do utilize the aerobic system as training combines periods of steady, continuous movement with occasional fast bursts of movement. Having adequate fuel stores for this type of training is crucial, and running low on fuel leads to fatigue and poor-quality training sessions. These types of training sessions benefit not only from the right nutrient mix in the daily diet but also proper nutrient intake immediately before, during, and after training.

Although team sports have distinct differences in terms of their physiological profiles (see Table 4.3), training programs, and ultimately nutritional requirements (see Table 4.4), one basic nutrition profile describes them. The unique nutritional demands for each sport will be addressed in Part III, but we can summarize the following about team sports:

- They all rely heavily on the short-lived phosphagen with ATP and creatine phosphate as fuel sources, and the anaerobic glycolytic systems with muscle glycogen as a fuel source.
- They rely to varying degrees on the aerobic system, but mainly through carbohydrate as a fuel source, with limited use of intramuscular fat as a fuel source.
- The majority of fuel that supplies energy for athletes participating in team sports is stored within the muscle.

TABLE 4.3 PHYSIOLOGICAL PROFILE OF TEAM SPORTS

Team Sport	Characteristics
Baseball	• Mainly power sport • Relies heavily on phosphagen system • Also utilizes anaerobic glycolysis system • Requires explosive bursts of speed and strength • Requires flexibility and agility • Requires running speed and quickness
Football	• Mainly power • Somewhat middle-distance sport depending on position played • Relies heavily on phosphagen system • Also utilizes anaerobic glycolysis system • Requires explosive bursts of speed and strength • Requires high level anaerobic strength and endurance • Requires flexibility and agility
Hockey	• Power sport • Middle-distance sport depending on practice and playing time • Heavy reliance on phosphagen system, moderate reliance on anaerobic glycolysis and somewhat on aerobic • Trained aerobic system improves recovery • Requires variety of skills including skating at high speeds, turning and maneuvering, and racing for the puck • Requires strength, endurance, agility, and balance
Soccer	• Power to middle-distance sport • Develops aerobic endurance • Uses phosphagen system, especially goalies and fullbacks • Utilizes anaerobic glycolysis system for all positions, especially forwards, halfbacks, and wings • Uses aerobic system for stamina and recovery between high-intensity efforts for forwards, halfbacks, and wings • Requires a variety of skills including jumping and sprinting ability, ball control, quick changes in direction, and endurance
Basketball	• Power to middle-distance to endurance sport • Relies on all three energy systems, phosphagen, anaerobic glycolysis, and aerobic endurance • Similar energy needs for different positions • Requires variety of skills including jumping, sprinting, agility, ball control, and endurance

TABLE 4.4 NUTRITIONAL PROFILE OF TEAM SPORTS

Team Sport	Characteristics
Baseball	• Meeting fluid needs most important • Good pretraining and precompetition meal • Generally do not have high energy demands • Calories adjusted for strength-training phase of program • Carbohydrate intake to maintain muscle and liver glycogen stores • Adequate protein for strength training • Avoid excess fat and choose healthy fats • Focus on healthy eating on the road
Football	• Adequate fluid and electrolyte replacement to protect from heat illness, particularly preseason • Calorie intake to match energy needs of position played • Calorie intake adjusted for heavy weight-training phase • Calorie adjustment for body composition goals • Calorie adjustment for time of season and off-season training • Proper balance of carbohydrate, protein, and fat for training and not to exceed protein and fat requirements • Require safe and legal nutritional methods for increasing lean body mass
Hockey	• High energy needs for training • Carbohydrates are the preferred fuel to replace muscle glycogen stores • Higher protein needs for building strength easily met by balanced diet • Require safe and legal nutritional methods for increasing lean body mass • Replace high sweat losses during practice and games • Need to replace carbohydrates during practice and games • High-carbohydrate, moderate-protein precompetition meal • Practice appropriate postgame recovery nutrition • Optimal nutrition plan to meet body composition goals
Soccer	• High energy requirements based on needs of individual player and position • Carbohydrate important fuel source to maintain/replace muscle glycogen • Prehydrate before practice and games • Replace fluids and carbohydrates at halftime and during game • Increased protein requirements easily met by diet • Recovery nutrition after practice and games • Include reasonable amount of healthy fat in diet
Basketball	• High energy needs based on high body weight and training demands • Higher amount of carbohydrates to replace muscle glycogen • Higher protein requirements for strength and cross-training • Reasonable amount of healthy fats in diet • Replacement of fluid losses during practice and prehydrate • Intake of fluid and carbohydrates at breaks, halftime, and time-outs • Recovery nutrition to speed recovery for the next game or practice • Carbohydrate-rich, moderate protein pregame meal

- These sports benefit from the development of moderate to high aerobic power for moderate-intensity activity and improved recovery.
- Team sports all require a high level of skill and technique development unique to that particular sport.
- The proper nutrient diet mix and energy intake maximize recovery of fuel stores and support the development of optimal body composition.
- Adequate amounts of carbohydrate are required to replenish muscle glycogen stores (discussed in Chapter 5).
- Team sport athletes frequently include resistance training in their program to varying degrees during the season and require the proper nutritional program to support these efforts (outlined in Chapter 6).
- Timing of nutrient intake before, during, and after practice can improve the quality of training.
- Optimal fluid, electrolyte, and carbohydrate intake during practice and competition can improve performance (outlined in Chapter 7).

CHAPTER 5

EATING FOR TRAINING AND RECOVERY

Several essential nutrition practices transform a healthy, well-balanced diet to a scientifically sound, cutting-edge sports nutrition plan designed to support your training and recovery for your team sport:

- Consuming optimal energy or balance of calories for recovery from training, muscle building, and growth if appropriate
- Consuming enough grams of carbohydrate to match that day's training depletion and to prepare for the next training session
- Timing your intake of carbohydrate to expedite the process of muscle glycogen resynthesis
- Eating adequate amounts of protein for recovery, muscle tissue repair, and maintenance of a strong immune system
- Consuming fat to balance out the diet and provide essential fatty acids
- Consuming adequate amounts of fluid and electrolytes, particularly sodium, for specific training situations and environmental conditions for optimal recovery
- Timing your nutritional intake properly to optimize recovery until the next training session, particularly immediate postexercise nutrition recovery guidelines and the meal and snacks in the several hours after training

Recovery for athletes starts when training finishes and takes place until the next training session begins. Depending on your training schedule and training cycle, you may have 24, 12, 8, or 4 hours of recovery time to restore body fuel and begin exercise again. Your daily diet is really your recovery diet, and you must understand the amount and types of fuels burned during training in order to time your meals and snacks properly.

First, as a team sport athlete, you must consume the right amount of energy or calories. Your training can be tough and tiring, and eating enough food is essential to completing demanding training programs that test your power, endurance, skill, and ability to exercise at high intensities. Even with the intermittent activity seen in team sports training, the demand for glycogen as a fuel source can be high, particularly for hockey, basketball, and soccer. Team sport players in football and baseball may also have high energy requirements, particularly during a weight-training cycle, but also need to balance calories for optimal body composition depending on the time of season and position played. But because of their integral role in fueling exercise and the limitations of your body's fuel stores, carbohydrates are the foundation of your training diet for any team sport, with protein also playing an all-important supporting role, and fat rounding out the remainder of your calorie intake. Recovery is the process of eating properly, which provides you with the fuel to go from one training session to the next with the fuel stores required. Begin by choosing high-quality foods for your sports diet as outlined in Part I to lay the foundation for your diet. Consuming the optimal fuel for recovery and your training program and putting in your best performance on game day comes down to consuming these foods in the right amounts, at the right times.

ENERGY FOR TRAINING

This chapter will outline your total carbohydrate, protein, and fat requirements for various levels of training, but it is also important to appreciate how your daily training affects your energy requirements. Determining energy needs is not a precise science, but there are some general indicators that can give you an appreciation of just how low, moderate, or high your calorie needs may be for daily recovery from one training session to the next. You should also consider the proper level of calories to maintain your optimal body weight. This may include efforts to maintain muscle mass you have acquired through resistance training and proper diet in anticipation of the upcoming season (more on nutrition for building muscle mass appears in Chapter 6).

Energy needs are presented as the amount of calories required per pound of weight. Your energy requirements can vary daily as your sport and current training program dictates. When in serious training mode and preparing for the competitive season, it is best not to fall short on your calorie requirements. Several days in a row of not recharging your batteries fully or too low a calorie level may result in some needed unplanned rest days and days off or poor-quality training sessions, all of which can hamper your competition goals and tire you even further.

Training calories can be estimated as a function of how hard and how long you train. The descriptions listed here explain how your activity can affect your calorie needs. For adult team sport athletes training more than 90 minutes daily, 18 to 24 calories per pound of body weight can meet your training needs, while high-intensity multiple workouts of more than 3 hours daily may require 24 to 29 calories per pound of body weight.

- For mild activity with no purposeful exercise or training: 12 to 14 calories per pound
- For moderate activity with up to 1 hour daily of moderate intensity exercise: 15 to 17 calories per pound
- For high activity of 1 to 2 hours daily of moderate intensity: 18 to 24 calories per pound
- For very high activity of several hours training daily: 24 to 29 calories per pound

Calories burned during training can also be estimated based on current body weight and the amount of energy expended for each individual sport. As Table 5.1 indicates, the amount of calories expended can vary from sport to sport. While the energy expenditures of the power sports of baseball and football are described as lower per pound of body weight and minutes of activity than for the power, middle-distance endurance sports of basketball, hockey, and soccer, calorie needs can be significantly affected by the position played, efforts to increase muscle mass, and overall body composition goals of an athlete. Let's take a look at general energy requirements of the various team sports.

TABLE 5.1 AVERAGE CALORIE EXPENDITURE FOR TEAM SPORTS (PER MINUTE OF ACTIVITY)

Weight in Pounds (kilograms)

Activity	100 (45)	110 (50)	120 (55)	130 (59)	140 (64)	150 (68)	160 (73)	170 (77)	180 (82)	190 (86)	200 (91)
Hockey	6.6	7.3	8	8.7	9.4	10	10.7	11.4	12.1	12.7	13.4
Basketball	6.5	7.2	7.8	8.5	9.2	9.9	10.5	11.2	11.9	12.5	13.2
Soccer	5.9	6.6	7.2	7.8	8.4	9	9.6	10.2	10.8	11.4	12
Baseball	3.1	3.4	3.8	3.9	4.2	4.5	4.8	5.1	5.4	5.7	6
Softball	3.3	3.5	3.8	4.1	4.4	4.7	5	5.3	5.6	5.9	6.2
Football	3.3	3.6	4	4.3	4.6	5	5.3	5.7	6	6.3	6.7
Weight training	5.2	5.7	6.2	6.8	7.3	7.8	8.3	8.9	9.4	9.9	10.5

Baseball

Baseball places a high emphasis on skill and requires quick reaction time, coordination, and fine-motor control. It is clearly not a game of continuous activity but does require general aerobic conditioning for basic fitness (and good health) and clearly anaerobic power, such as when running the bases or batting a ball. Baseball does not have significantly high demands for calories and consequently carbohydrates, though pitchers have higher energy needs than fielders.

Football

Overall calorie needs for football players can vary depending on the position played and whether the athlete is involved in a serious resistance-training program. However, football players may have total high-calorie needs due to their actual weight, often over 200 pounds for a lineman. Many high school and collegiate football players are highly focused on building muscle mass and gaining weight, which requires a significant amount of calories.

Basketball

Energy needs of basketball players can vary depending on the athlete's age, competition level, and training program. A high school basketball player may expend half the calories of a professional player. Generally, basketball players have the high-energy needs exhibited by many hard-training athletes. Basketball players often include aerobic conditioning and resistance training into their programs, which increase their calorie requirements. Calories burned can fluctuate daily depending on how long and intense the training sessions are and whether resistance training is part of the program that day. Professional players typically practice twice daily, up to 5 hours daily.

Soccer

One of the most widely played sports in the world today, soccer requires running, walking, and jogging on the field, in addition to jumping, accelerating, and turning. Much of this distance covered by a player in practice may be at slower speeds, but periods of very high intensity are not uncommon. Midfielders tend to cover the most distance in a game, compared to defenders or attackers. Goalies expend the least amount of energy. Adequate energy intake is important to support the training needs of soccer players.

Hockey

Hockey players generally have high-energy needs due to both their aerobic and anaerobic conditioning. Resistance training is often part of the overall program, as they require muscular strength needed for fast acceleration, quick stopping, direction change, and physical contact. In addition to their usual daily energy needs, a 180-pound hockey player may burn 720 calories in an hour of intense practice. It is very important that hockey players meet their energy needs for full recovery.

Carbohydrate: The Recovery Fuel

While you may not have experienced the symptoms of glycogen depletion during a single training session, the symptoms of gradual glycogen depletion due to inadequate carbohydrate recovery can occur over successive days of training and be much more subtle. Symptoms of glycogen depletion can creep up over a week's time or longer, producing feelings of sluggishness or heaviness. Besides general lethargy, you may put out an increased or even normal effort during training and find it difficult to maintain your usual intensity and stamina. The more muscle glycogen stores in your body, the faster you can run up and down the field or court or the faster you can skate across the ice.

Numerous scientific studies have measured that a diet adequate in carbohydrate is superior in building, maintaining, and replenishing muscle glycogen stores. The amount of carbohydrate you consume in your diet directly affects the amount of glycogen you store in your muscles and liver. Inadequate intakes of carbohydrate will only lead to partial replenishment of muscle glycogen stores. If this incomplete replenishment occurs from one day to the next, glycogen stores are gradually depleted over a week's time or more, and your training will suffer. Adequate recovery allows you to start the next training session, whether it is 4, 8, 12, or 24 hours away, with optimal fuel to complete the exercise at the desired duration and intensity spelled out in your training program.

Carbohydrate Requirements: Matching Intake to Training

Carbohydrate recommendations are often expressed as a percentage of total calories. This is appropriate for general recommendations for the community, when the goal is to decrease unwanted fat intake and to increase wholesome carbohydrates from whole grains and fruits and vegetables. However, for team sport athletes, it is more appropriate to express carbohydrate needs as grams per pound of weight based on the intensity and duration of your training session or sessions for that day. Regardless of the type of training session, your muscles require an absolute amount of carbohydrate to recover sufficiently, particularly after intense training sessions with plenty of high-intensity efforts that can quickly deplete carbohydrate stores.

The ceiling for daily carbohydrate consumption, at which point your muscle storage capacity has been reached, is 4.5 to 5.5 grams of carbohydrate for every pound of weight. Depending on the size of the athlete, this translates to anywhere from 500 to 700 grams of carbohydrate daily, and higher levels than these absolute amounts may not resynthesize muscle glycogen stores faster. Most team sport athletes who meet both their energy and carbohydrate needs can average about 50 to 60 percent carbohydrate calories in their training diet. But depending on whether you are restricting calories for weight management or have very high-energy needs, the percentage of carbohydrate consumed may vary. Typically, as an athlete, you will have to consume greater quantities of carbohydrate than most people, including athletes participating in sports that do not have as high a fuel demand. Table 5.2 outlines your daily carbohydrate requirements.

Practical Carbohydrate Issues

As an athlete, you must make a concerted effort to obtain adequate amounts of carbohydrate at specific times in portions that allow you to prepare for training, recover from training, and get ready for competition. Some team sport athletes can meet their carbohydrate requirements on specific training days with plenty of well-chosen wholesome carbohydrates. However, on specific training days for many team sport athletes, the amounts required for fuel may exceed appetite and hunger levels and exceed the portions that are typically provided in the North American diet. Although wholesome carbohydrates provide nutritional content and health benefits, for specific times around training, you may need to focus on carbohydrate-rich foods that are appealing, convenient, and carbohydrate-dense for a given serving in order to maximize your nutritional recovery.

Food tables listing carbohydrate portions for 30-gram servings are provided in Chapter 8, which covers meal planning and provides practical guidelines for putting together a top team sport diet. You can match up these carbohydrate amounts to provide you with the total grams of carbohydrate required for training on a given day. A

TABLE 5.2 DAILY CARBOHYDRATE REQUIREMENTS	
Grams per Pound of Weight	**Training Regimen**
4.5–5.5	Duration 3–4 hours daily Moderate/high intensity
3.0–4.5	Duration 90 minutes to 3 hours daily Moderate/high intensity
2.25–3.0	Moderate intensity under 1 hour daily Low intensity for several hours daily

180-pound basketball player training three hours daily may require a full 700 grams of carbohydrate, while a baseball player of the same weight practicing skills may require only 400 grams of carbohydrate daily. Consuming 400 grams of carbohydrate in a given training day is much simpler than consuming 700 grams, as attaining the higher carbohydrate amount would likely require more structure and planning.

The food system outlined in Chapter 8 provides you with the flexibility to emphasize various carbohydrate sources from one day to the next, depending on your food preferences, fuel needs, training schedule, and training cycle. However, for those very high-carbohydrate days, you may want to consider the suggestions described in the following paragraphs.

Sports bars or energy bars are a concentrated and convenient source of carbohydrate, supplying up to 50 grams per serving. They travel well and can be consumed quickly between training sessions or on the way back to class or work. But do keep in mind that these bars are often vitamin and mineral fortified. Make sure that you do not consume too high doses of these nutrients simply by overconsuming sports bars. Energy bars should not replace fruits, vegetables, and whole grains in your diet.

Low-fiber carbohydrate foods may be more practical when carbohydrate needs to be consumed in very large amounts on hard and intense training days. They can be consumed in combination with higher-fiber items and still be part of a diet that is adequate in fiber, vitamins, and minerals. Choices include large bagels, calorically dense cereals, fruit juices, jams, honey, and syrup.

A well-timed snack of yogurt with fruit, a low-fat milk shake, or a fruit smoothie can up your carbohydrate intake considerably and provide needed fluid as well. They also taste good!

High-carbohydrate supplement drinks or meal replacements may also be a convenient source of carbohydrate and are easy to carry and quickly consumed. These products should not replace wholesome foods.

Desserts can be part of a nutritious diet in reasonable amounts. Some carbohydrate-dense choices include sherbet, sorbet, and frozen yogurt topped with fruit.

Meeting your daily carbohydrate intake often requires consuming between-meal snacks and "grazing" throughout the day. Carbohydrate-rich foods should comprise at least half of your meals and snacks. Low-fiber choices may be best tolerated when food is consumed close to the start of exercise.

Keep an eye out for carbohydrate foods that are also high in fat (often unhealthy fats), such as croissants, creamed or deep-fried vegetables, doughnuts, French toast, fried rice, muffins, pancakes, pastry, potato chips, snack crackers, and popcorn popped with oil.

Obtaining the total grams of carbohydrate that you require to match your training may be your biggest nutritional challenge of the day, particularly on hard training days. Although you want to emphasize fruits, vegetables, and whole grains, higher carbohydrate needs for more intense and longer training may require that you incorporate less filling but carbohydrate-dense foods into your diet. Meeting these higher carbohydrate amounts requires planning and a good appetite.

Protein and Your Recovery Requirements

While carbohydrate intake is clearly emphasized in your team sport diet, your training program and training for power and strength also increase your need for protein. Protein needs are higher in team sport athletes who incorporate resistance training into their program and who benefit from increased muscle mass for athletic performance. Team sports such as hockey can also have significant wear and tear on the muscles and ligaments, requiring protein for repair. Team sport players who engage in strength training can rely on glycogen for fuel during this mode of exercise and, most important, should consume enough adequate carbohydrate so that protein is not utilized for fuel during training.

You should appreciate, however, that your elevated protein requirements are easily met by choosing a well-balanced sports diet. Protein powder and special supplements usually are not necessary for your training program, though the proper use of supplements is discussed in Chapter 6. Table 5.3 outlines the protein requirements of team sport athletes.

What is most important for you to appreciate is that your elevated protein requirements are easily met by a well-planned sports diet. Often the higher calorie intake of

TABLE 5.3 DAILY PROTEIN REQUIREMENTS	
Exercise Type	Protein Requirements per Weight
Endurance and team sport training	Moderate training: 0.45 g/lb. (1 g/kg) Heavy training: 0.50–0.75 g/lb. (1.1–1.6 g/kg) Very intense training: 0.8–0.9 g/lb. (1.8–2.0 g/kg)
Growing teenage athlete	0.8–0.9 g/lb. (1.8–2.0 g/kg)
Athlete restricting calories	0.8–0.9 g/lb. (1.8–2.0 g/kg)
Strength-training phase of training	Experienced: 0.5–0.7 g/lb. (1–1.5 g/kg) Novice: 0.8 g/lb. (1.8 g/kg)
Maximum recommended amount for extreme exercise loads	1.0 g/lb. (2.2g/kg)

your sports nutrition plan simply results in more protein being consumed. Most North Americans consume a diet that easily meets the protein needs of an athlete participating in a demanding training program. Inadequate protein intake may only be a concern for a poorly planned vegetarian diet or athletes following calorie restriction.

Consider how easy it is to meet your daily protein requirements. Having some peanut butter and cereal with milk for breakfast, followed by a turkey sandwich for lunch and a stir-fry of lean red meat and rice for dinner, will supply about 90 grams of protein. You will obtain additional protein from between-meal snacks. Foods such as whole grains and vegetables, which are not as concentrated in protein, still contribute to your total protein intake, with moderate amounts over the course of a day supplementing your intake of more concentrated protein foods.

Healthy Proteins in the Right Amounts

A well-balanced diet with adequate calories and up to 15 to 20 percent or more of protein calories provides enough total grams of protein for the muscle growth and repair required for team sport athletes engaged in hard training who also strength train. Protein in excess of your requirements is simply excess calories that are either burned for energy or stored as fat. Converting protein to fuel for exercise is inefficient when compared to carbohydrates, which are much more easily burned for energy.

Consuming excess protein results in other negative effects. Protein from both food and supplements increases your need for fluid, because your kidneys require more water to eliminate the end products of protein metabolism. Individuals with liver or kidney problems are also susceptible to negative effects of excessive dietary protein. Excess dietary protein leads to a short-lived increased urinary excretion of calcium, an important mineral for building healthy bone tissue. Although food sources of protein are best, they can also contribute substantial amounts of fat and cholesterol to the diet. Consuming excess protein can mean taking in excess fat and cholesterol and raising your risk of heart disease and other health problems. You should be selective regarding the type of protein foods you eat. There are plenty of low-fat animal protein food sources to choose from and plenty of healthy plant proteins as well.

Your protein needs for your training program, and for muscle repair and other important protein functions, are easily met through a well-planned diet providing ample calories. The key is to obtain adequate amounts of quality lean or low-fat protein sources throughout the day and to consume enough calories so that protein is not burned for energy.

Fat Requirements

Team sport players have total fat requirements at about 0.5 gram per pound of body weight to obtain adequate amounts of essential fatty acids. Fat can provide from 15 to 30 percent of the day's calories depending on the carbohydrate, protein, and especially energy needs for that day's training. Once carbohydrate and protein requirements are met for your training program and recovery, fat can make up the remainder of the calories appropriate for your weight and body composition goals.

The most important strategy regarding fat intake is to consume enough healthy fats high in essential fatty acids, as outlined in Chapter 1. Athletes who may need to monitor their weight closely and prevent unwanted weight gain (e.g., baseball and football players) may have a problem of too much fat in their diet, especially when away at training camps or traveling for competition. Some athletes may be used to eating out and frequenting fast-food establishments. A high-fat diet is often very calorie-dense and leaves less room for quality carbohydrates. Weight-conscious athletes should keep fat calories to 20 to 25 percent of total intake. (More on body composition strategies will be covered in Chapter 6.)

Although several team sports have some component of aerobic activity in their training plan, having or not having adequate fat stores in the muscle should not be a limiting fuel source during hard training.

Daily Recovery

Overall, your daily recovery hinges on obtaining the appropriate amount of calories for your training, with the proper amounts of carbohydrate, protein, and fat in your diet to replace the fuels you burned in training and to maximize your strength- and power-building efforts. Because of the relatively limited supply of glycogen in the body and the integral role of glycogen in supplying some amount of fuel during all types of training, carbohydrate is an important nutrient for the team sport athlete. Carbohydrates are needed to synthesize glycogen, and you must consume enough total grams of carbohydrate to fully replenish stores, whatever the level of depletion, to continue to participate in high-quality training sessions. It is also important that the amount of carbohydrate you consume match your training specific for that day.

Protein is also needed for recovery to build and repair muscle tissue. Adequate protein in your diet will also maintain a strong immune system. Your higher protein requirements are easily met through a well-planned diet that is adequate in calories. Fat can provide the remainder of calories, and levels can be adjusted whether the athlete is trying to meet high energy needs or control calories.

Fine-Tuning the Recovery Process
Carbohydrate, Protein, Fluid, and Sodium Immediately after Exercise

While the most important factor affecting daily muscle glycogen recovery is the total amount of carbohydrate consumed, eating carbohydrate within 30 minutes to 2 hours after training can speed up the recovery process and provide you with a good jump-start toward total carbohydrate replenishment. Several scientific studies have resulted in the recommendation to consume anywhere from 0.5 to 0.7 gram of carbohydrate per pound of body weight (1 to 1.5 gram/kilogram) within 30 minutes after completing intense exercise—a time when a significant depletion of muscle glycogen stores occurs. One study demonstrated that subjects fed carbohydrate a full 2 hours after exercise synthesized the carbohydrate into glycogen 45 percent more slowly than subjects fed carbohydrate immediately after exercise. It appears that muscle glycogen storage is slightly enhanced 2 hours after exercise, during which time the muscle has a greater capacity to take up blood glucose.

Studies have shown that both liquid and solid carbohydrates are adequate in refueling the body after hard exercise. However, emphasizing higher-glycemic carbohydrates that elicit a higher insulin response, such as sports nutrition supplements and breads and cereals, may enhance glycogen resynthesis. A list of high-glycemic foods is provided in Appendix A.

For the rest of the day, carbohydrate can be consumed as a series of snacks or a few larger meals, depending on your training schedule, food preferences, and total daily carbohydrate requirements. Both eating styles will sufficiently promote glycogen recovery if the total amount of carbohydrate consumed is adequate. Eating a balanced mix of low-, moderate-, and high-glycemic carbohydrates throughout the day will support the glycogen recovery process. But consuming an adequate amount of total carbohydrate grams over the 24-hour period is a very important carbohydrate recovery strategy.

A fair amount of debate has focused on the benefits of adding protein to the recovery carbohydrate snack immediately after exercise. Study results have varied depending on whether the protein provided additional calories or whether researchers supplied the same amount of calories when comparing a carbohydrate-only dose to a carbohydrate-and-protein combination dose. What is certain is that having protein comprise about one-fourth of your recovery snack will not compromise your muscle glycogen recovery, and it could facilitate muscle glycogen recovery. Consuming some protein immediately after exercise may also speed up the repair of muscle tissue and provide important nutrients for your immune system. It will also send you on your way to optimizing your protein intake until the next training session when you have two-a-day or even three-a-day practices.

Often, whether you consume carbohydrate alone or a carbohydrate and protein combination is a matter of convenience. Transporting and packing high-carbohydrate items may be easier than also packing items containing protein. Recovery protein should be high-quality sources such as those found in dairy and soy milk, yogurt, and lean animal proteins. A variety of commercial recovery products are available, which are not necessary for immediate-recovery eating but can be very convenient for replenishing immediately after training.

Of course, rehydration is also a top priority after moderate to hard training because athletes typically replace only three-fourths of their sweat losses by drinking fluids during exercise. Your goal is to fully restore fluid losses from one training session to the next, keeping in mind that thirst is not a reliable indicator of fluid losses. You are already dehydrated when you are thirsty, and the thirst mechanism will shut down before you have sufficiently replaced all your fluid losses. Try to consume up to 20 to 24 ounces (600 to 720 millimeters) of fluid for every pound of weight lost after training. Sixteen ounces (480 millimeters) actually replaces a fluid loss of 2 pounds, but the higher volume of 24 ounces (720 millimeters) will replace both sweat and subsequent urine losses.

Pay attention to what stimulates your desire to drink. You may prefer a sweeter product or perhaps something a bit salty. The temperature of the drink may also affect the volume of fluid you consume. It makes sense that a cool drink would be more palatable, particularly in hot weather, while it may be difficult to drink very large amounts of a very cold beverage.

Some athletes may feel reluctant to weigh themselves before and after every training session. You may also not have a scale available every time you train or would prefer not to get overly focused on a weight number. What you can do is obtain pre- and postexercise weights after specific types of training sessions. For example, you may determine that you replace only 50 percent of your fluid needs during hard training sessions, whereas you meet 80 percent of your fluid requirements during less demanding exercise when it may be easier to reach for and consume fluid. Once you have established the replenishment levels of your best drinking efforts, you can then develop a system for rehydrating after exercise. You may also want to determine what your typical fluid losses are for specific types of environmental conditions. Of course, you can also check the color of your urine to evaluate your hydration efforts. Clear urine (the color of lemonade) can reflect adequate hydration; darker urine (the color of apple juice) indicates inadequate hydration. But on days when you know you are to train or compete in more extreme conditions, you may want to check your weight before and after exercise carefully. During intense training times and in hot-weather training, perform a daily check on your hydration status. After urinating in the morning, check your weight. If your usual weight is down by more than 1 pound (0.5 kilogram), you may not be keeping up with your usual fluid requirements.

Sodium or salt may not only stimulate your drive to drink but can also enhance the rehydration process. Generally, in most athletes, sweating results in large fluid losses and relatively small sodium losses. When you finish exercise, your blood volume and total body water are reduced, while there is a mild increase in blood concentration and its sodium content. When you consume large amounts of plain water after exercise, you will dilute your blood before your full blood volume has been restored. This dilutional effect will shut down the thirst mechanism, and you will urinate to bring the concentration of the blood to a normal level. The end result is that you have produced a large amount of dilute urine before you are fully rehydrated.

You can offset this negative effect by consuming some sodium or salt after exercise. A series of studies determined that rehydrating with drinks higher in sodium produced significantly lower urine losses than low-sodium drinks, indicating that more of the fluid consumed was retained and therefore hydrating. Therefore, it is recommended that when your fluid losses are significant, you replace sodium losses as well. It also appears that some individuals may have greater sodium sweat losses than others, so consuming sodium after exercise may be prudent unless medically contraindicated. Some athletes may actually require up to several grams of sodium over the course of the day, especially when training in hot weather.

If your fluid losses exceed 1 to 2 pounds (0.5 to 1 kilogram) during exercise, you should make a focused effort to drink fluids on schedule and incorporate fluids into your recovery nutrition strategies. Products that contain sodium can also be integrated into your food and fluid choices to facilitate rehydration. If your recovery time is short, and the next training session is to take place in several hours, it makes sense to actively include sodium in your fluid and food choices.

Sports drinks are formulated for tolerable consumption during exercise, not after exercise. Postexercise, a 150-pound athlete requires 75 grams of carbohydrate, which translates to 40 ounces (1,200 millimeters) of a sports drink. Sports drinks are also relatively low in sodium, though higher-sodium formulas are available.

You may consider adding 0.25 to 0.5 teaspoon of salt to your total fluid intake. However, consuming a sports drink rather than a recovery drink may not be your most effective recovery fluid choice, though they are preferable to plain water when rehydration is important.

Recovery products concentrated in carbohydrate, providing anywhere from 50 to 100 grams per 16-ounce (480 millimeter) serving, are also available. Some of these products provide up to 25 grams of protein per serving, too. Sports tubes that supply only protein are also available and can be consumed with a high-carbohydrate food or fluid source. Aim for recovery products that have a higher sodium content.

Other sports nutrition products such as gels and bars can be consumed conveniently after exercise. They should be taken with plenty of fluid, including those that provide carbohydrate.

Experiment with your own low-fat shake and smoothie recipes made from dairy milk, yogurt, soy milk, or juice and fresh or frozen fruit for a hydrating carbohydrate and protein combination.

Limit caffeine-containing beverages after exercise to optimize fluid replacement. Consume alcohol only after fluid balance has been restored, if at all. Incorporate sodium into your recovery meal and snacks and fluids to facilitate rehydration in conjunction with the nutritional recovery process.

The recovery process is a continual effort that takes place after one training session and until the next, but you can get off to a good start by paying close attention to what you consume immediately and within the 2 hours after exercise. Then follow these postexercise nutrition practices with food and fluid choices that match your daily training requirements.

The Big Picture

Daily recovery is essential to replenishing your body fuel, fluid, and electrolyte stores from one training session to the next. The key component to your recovery diet is an adequate calorie intake that allows room for the total grams of carbohydrate needed to replace glycogen losses from that day's specific training. Your total protein requirements should also be met for the day. Fat rounds out your caloric intake. Wholesome and nutrient-dense food choices of carbohydrates, proteins, and fats should be emphasized whenever possible, with sports nutrition products used appropriately and not replacing foods in the diet.

Recovery is also about timing, and nutritional recovery begins when the training session ends (see Table 5.4). Athletes should consume specific amounts of carbohydrates, proteins, fluid, and sodium after intense training sessions. These amounts can also be consumed again in 2 hours to continue the refueling and rehydration process. Meals and snacks should then be timed according to tolerances and the athlete's training schedule and meet the athlete's daily requirements. A more aggressive and structured eating and drinking schedule is required when there is less recovery time, such as when the athlete trains twice daily.

The daily menu for team sport athletes encompasses their overall nutritional needs and food preferences, and the optimal timing of meals and snacks based on their training schedule. Sample menus for training and competition are provided in Part III, specific to each team sport.

PERIODIZING YOUR NUTRITION PLAN

As a team sport athlete, you no doubt realize that your training program very likely changes throughout the year depending on your level of competition and participation in your sport. You have a lot to accomplish in your yearly training program, including enhancing both aerobic and anaerobic conditioning, increasing strength and power, building muscular endurance, and developing quickness, agility, speed, and flexibility. All of these components of your training program complement one another to ultimately improve your performance. At specific times of the year, you may highlight a particular aspect of your program. Certain aspects of your program need to be built before others,

TABLE 5.4 OPTIMAL NUTRIENT TIMING FOR RECOVERY

Training Program	Posttraining Nutritional Strategies within 30–60 minutes	Ongoing Nutritional Strategies
High-intensity training greater than 60 minutes	• Consume 50–75 g carbohydrates. • Choose high-glycemic carbohydrates. • Can have 10 to 15 g high-quality proteins. • Drink 20–24 oz. (600–720 ml) for every pound of weight loss. • Consume sodium-containing fluids in hot weather.	• Consume another 50–75 g carbohydrate in 2–3 hours. • Continue rehydrating to baseline weight. • Include sodium in meals and snacks in hot weather.
Moderate-/high-intensity training greater than 90 minutes	• Consume 50–75 g carbohydrates. • Choose high glycemic carbohydrates. • Consume 10–15 g high-quality proteins. • Drink 20–24 oz. (600–720 ml) fluid for every pound of weight lost. • Consume 250 mg sodium with rehydration.	• Consume another 50–75 g carbohydrate in 2–3 hours. • Continue rehydrating to baseline weight. • Include sodium in meals and snacks in hot weather.
Hot-weather training drills, hard efforts	• Rehydrate with liquid supplement containing carbohydrate and sodium.	• Include sodium in meals and snacks. • Monitor weight and return to baseline.

while others are emphasized when specific training components of your program are de-emphasized. The year-round schedule and cycling of your training program is called *periodization,* and it is designed to optimize performance results and prevent overtraining.

An entire year of conditioning and training is referred to as the *macrocycle,* which is broken down into smaller *mesocycles,* generally off-season, preseason, in season, and postseason. Each mesocycle is broken down further into *microcycles* around which the athlete's weekly schedule is planned.

Generally, the off-season is time to build a base for both aerobic fitness and strength. In the preseason, training shifts to more high-intensity training, speed, and intervals and sport-specific training. During the season, the athlete focuses on preparing for competition, maintaining fitness, and developing any weaker areas. Depending on your sport and whether you are a high school, collegiate, masters, or professional athlete, you may compete several times a week, in weekend tournaments, or only once weekly, all of which affects your training program and recovery time. Postseason is a rest period and varies in length for each sport and athlete.

These cycles in your training program all require adjustments in your diet composition and meal timing. Changes in your diet can occur in a number of ways, depending on the athlete's specific program. For example, you may need to adjust your total caloric intake for lower-intensity training. During the off-season, the overall intensity of your program may decrease, with a focus on aerobic conditioning. Your energy needs for training may lessen without the intensity of preseason training and competition. Volume may also be higher with low-intensity aerobic base building, which in turn can affect carbohydrate and energy requirements.

As you build a strength base, you may require a heavy focus on the nutritional strategies required for muscle building. (These guidelines are reviewed in Chapter 6.) Depending on your program, your energy needs may still be quite high, with a different focus on the timing of your meals and snacks and a modification in the timing of your protein and carbohydrate intake.

Meal timing adjustments can be made depending on your training schedule. After high-intensity, shorter-duration interval training, you should still focus on recovery nutrition and the beginning of glycogen resynthesis. After more moderate training, continue to focus on rehydration, even for workouts that are only mildly dehydrating.

Refer to the guidelines for calories, carbohydrates, and protein, based on the volume and intensity of training to determine how these nutrient requirements can change during the season. Carbohydrate requirements can decrease when volume and intensity drop off and there is less training time. The breakdown of your diet may change, with less emphasis on carbohydrates and a slight shift to increased protein in the strength-building phase and during the preseason.

You should continue to replace fluids during all training sessions and maintain daily fluid requirements. Dehydration can occur during different levels of exercise; it is just the degree of dehydration that distinguishes various types of workouts. Rehydrate during training whenever possible, and rehydrate appropriately after training.

You can replace carbohydrate during sessions lasting longer than 60 minutes with a sports drink that provides 30 to 60 grams of carbohydrate per hour. This may be necessary during longer aerobic conditioning sessions, as well as high-intensity work that depletes muscle glycogen. (Training nutrition guidelines are covered in Chapter 7.)

Your training intensity may continue year-round if you participate in more than one team sport during the year. Energy requirements can decrease during rest periods in your training cycles, just as they may decrease during rest days in your training week.

How nutritional needs cycle throughout the season is unique to each athlete, his or her body composition goals, the individual training program with its training cycles and development of skills, and both aerobic and anaerobic conditioning as you continue to develop the program that best fits your sport and specific training goals. Table 5.5 reviews some nutritional considerations for a training program.

TABLE 5.5 PERIODIZING YOUR NUTRITION PROGRAM	
Training Cycle	**Nutrition Strategies**
Off-season	Moderate carbohydrate, high protein, low fat Nutrition guidelines for strength training Adequate carbohydrate intake for light aerobic conditioning Replacement of fluid losses during training
Preseason	Moderate to high carbohydrate, moderate protein, low fat Nutrition strategies specific to strength-training sessions Replacement of carbohydrate and fluids with a sports drink during interval and high-intensity training Immediate recovery nutrition after high-intensity training lasting longer than 60 to 90 minutes Monitoring weight to assess hydration status
In-season	High carbohydrate, moderate to high protein, adequate fat for energy Fluid and carbohydrate replacement during practice and competition Optimal precompetition meal Recovery nutrition after training and competition Daily hydration
Postseason	Moderate carbohydrate, moderate protein, low fat Basic hydration Replacement of sweat losses Maintaining healthy body weight

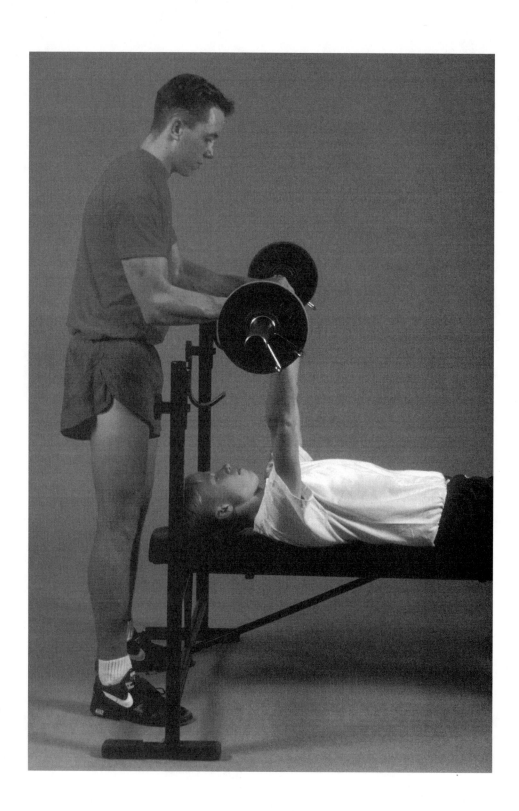

CHAPTER 6

WEIGHT, MUSCLE BUILDING, AND CHANGING BODY COMPOSITION

Team sport athletes come in a variety of shapes and sizes and many athletes participate in their chosen sport from grade school, through high school, into college, and even beyond. As you progress in your sport, you may find that your muscular development increases and your body composition changes. Many team sport athletes may be focused on building muscle and decreasing body fat to improve athletic performance. Some athletes may arrive easily toward the body composition physique that is appropriate for their sport, while other athletes need to work on building muscle and strength and decreasing body fat.

There are smart and sensible ways to attain a lean and strong body. However, many destructive ways can also be used to attempt to attain an overly idealized body composition that may not be realistic for your age, growth and development, level of training, and genetics. It is easy to assume that dropping a few "extra" pounds will improve your performance and that intense training builds muscle strength, but athletic success is not always that simple. Examples abound of athletes at all levels who have restricted their diet or increased their training in an attempt to improve body composition, with the end result ultimately being a decrease in energy levels and performance. It is important that you keep an open mind regarding your "best weight." Don't compromise your recovery and energy to build a few pounds of muscle or to lose a few pounds of fat.

BODY COMPOSITION, WEIGHT, AND PERFORMANCE

Athletic performance in team sports does depend on a number of interrelated factors, including your ability to sustain power and move your body weight at high speeds. Both of these factors can be affected by your body composition. An athlete carrying excess weight or lacking in muscle strength can be at greater risk for injury when performing the skills required for team sports.

When striving to make body composition changes, you should appreciate that you will perform your best at your own optimal body composition, and not at some idealized body composition that would require excessive training efforts and restrictive food strategies. Severe food restriction and excessive training can result in low energy levels, poor-quality training sessions, increased risk of injury, and both short- and long-term health risks.

Some athletes may desire to achieve a certain level of body fat for optimal performance, but strength training or resistance training is a common element of a training program for many team sport athletes. The high level of muscle mass and strength possible with resistance training is an important factor in athletic performance whether on the court, ice, or field. Optimal and effective methods for gaining muscle mass have long intrigued sports nutritionists and the muscle and supplement industries that pay for heavy marketing and promotion of muscle-building products. However, the key ingredients for maximizing muscle building and strength include your genetic potential, an appropriate resistance-training program, and specific muscle-building nutritional strategies supported by solid scientific research.

Let's take a look at some strategies for building muscle and assessing body composition, along with the science, hype, and possible health risks behind some of the supplements marketed to strength-training athletes.

Building Muscle

Hormones in your body, specifically growth hormone, testosterone, insulin, and insulin-like growth factor, largely control muscle growth. Nutrition can very effectively support your efforts to increase lean body mass by affecting these hormone levels and providing your body with the nutritional tools required for optimal muscle building. Much of the nutritional strategies for muscle building center not only on your daily training diet but also on the intake of certain nutrients timed specifically around your weight-training sessions to optimize your muscle-building efforts.

Some of the keys to optimizing muscle-building efforts include the following:

- Consuming enough calories so that your body has the energy required to build muscle
- Taking in enough carbohydrates so that you meet the fuel demand for both resistance training and training for your sport
- Consuming enough protein in your daily diet

- Timing your nutrient intake before and after resistance training, particularly for protein
- Enjoying fluids and carbohydrate during your workout

Nutritional Requirements for Building Muscle

Calories and carbohydrates. When you strength train, you are likely also participating in regular training for your sport and are burning significant amounts of stored body fuel from both types of exercise sessions. During weight training, the stored fuels of creatine phosphate and muscle glycogen serve as important energy sources. When combined with other components of your training program, resistance training can provide a further drain on your body's carbohydrate fuel stores. While you may typically think of increased protein intake in relation to strength training, your first focus should be on consuming adequate energy to build muscle tissue.

The most important nutrition guideline for effectively building muscle is to consume enough calories. Because of the increased energy it takes to build body tissue, falling short on your calorie requirements will impair your rate of muscle building. An additional 350 to 500 calories daily are needed to gain 1 pound of muscle mass per week. Further increases in muscle building require additional calories. Once you gain the muscle and strength that you desire for your sport and performance, it also takes an adequate amount of energy to maintain this increased weight. Keep in mind that these additional calories are the calories required above your energy needs for training and recovery in your sport. The combination of both your team sport training program and weight training can have a significant impact on your energy needs.

Often the perception is that extra calories consumed to build muscle should be protein calories. Although protein is required to build muscle tissue, it is only one of the required tools for the tissue-building process. The amounts of protein that you require as a team sport athlete should be adequate to cover your needs for muscle building, and your protein needs may increase only slightly if at all. In fact, many of the extra calories needed for muscle building should come from carbohydrates in your diet.

Muscle glycogen is an important fuel source during weight training, and an intense session may deplete 30 percent of your muscle glycogen stores. Clearly, when this type of training is combined with your team sport training, muscle glycogen stores can become significantly depleted in a single day or over several days. Regardless of how quickly you deplete these stores, it is important that you replenish glycogen stores adequately after training, whether in the weight room or on the court or field, so that you continue high-quality training sessions.

Protein. Strength training calls for increased carbohydrate intake, but protein is also an important construction material for the repair and growth of your muscle fibers. Strength training causes the breakdown of muscle fibers, which respond by making bigger and stronger muscle fibers to protect against further stress. Protein is one of the major construction materials for this repair process. While this means that athletes who strength train have higher protein requirements than sedentary individuals, the amount of protein that you consume for your regular sport training is likely more than adequate to put you in positive protein balance. *Positive protein balance* means that you consume enough protein to meet all the protein-requiring processes and functions in your body, including synthesizing new muscle tissue.

Your protein needs may increase slightly, if at all, when weight training becomes part of your program. If you do consume protein in excess of what is required for both your strength training and team sport training, this extra protein is burned for energy, which is not a very efficient process, or simply stored as fat. More is not better, and eating twice as much protein as your body requires won't make your muscles twice as big. Strength training also makes your body more efficient at utilizing protein.

Real foods can easily be part of a well-balanced diet that meets your protein requirements for both weight training and team sport training. Stick with the good high-quality sources of protein mentioned in Chapter 2, such as lean red meat, poultry, fish, and skim milk dairy products. You will also obtain protein from some plant foods, all of which contribute to your total protein intake. Fat in your diet should continue to round out your calorie choices just as it would for your regular training diet.

Timing Your Nutritional Intake

After weight training, your body synthesizes new muscle protein and replenishes muscle glycogen. Several research studies indicate that your nutritional intake in the hours before and after weight training can have a significant impact on supporting your muscle-building efforts. Consuming a combination of carbohydrate and protein both before and after weight training may be more effective in improving protein building than just increasing your overall daily protein intake to build muscle.

Consuming some protein prior to your resistance training efforts is probably the most important nutrition strategy to facilitate improved protein synthesis and may be even more effective than what you consume after training. Aim for about 15 to 20 grams of protein, emphasizing high-quality sources such as skim milk dairy products, whey protein, and protein from animal foods, as essential amino acids are the most potent stimulators of muscle protein synthesis. Combine this protein with 35 to 50 grams of carbohydrate, to provide carbohydrate for training.

You can also include both carbohydrate and protein in the next snack or meal that you consume after weight training to continue to facilitate the recovery and muscle-building process. Carbohydrate and protein consumed after resistance training should also work to stimulate both muscle glycogen synthesis and protein synthesis. This form of supplementation increases blood levels of insulin and growth hormone, both of which are tissue-building agents. High-glycemic carbohydrates can be emphasized after resistance training, just as they can after your regular training sessions. Aim for 15 to 20 grams of protein and 50 grams or more of carbohydrates in your recovery snack or meal.

Often your nutritional choices before and after weight training may be related to the practicality of your food and fluid choices and availability. Keep snacks on hand to consume both before and after resistance training. Aim for convenience choices like a low-fat shake or smoothie. Pack protein-containing snacks such as yogurt with fruit, a peanut butter and honey sandwich, or low-fat cheese and crackers. A commercial sports supplement containing a mix of carbohydrate and protein is convenient and meets your nutrition requirements in the hour before weight training.

What you consume during resistance training may also be beneficial to your recovery and the quality of your training sessions. Although ATP and creatine phosphate in the muscle are your primary fuel sources while weight training, muscle glycogen can become somewhat too significantly depleted between training sets, depending on the intensity and duration of your training. Between sets, your muscle will use the glycolysis energy pathway to regenerate ATP stores. Consuming a sports drink for its carbohydrate can help you maintain muscle glycogen stores and provide energy during your workout. These drinks also provide fluid to maintain adequate hydration levels. Of course, consuming plain water during resistance training is also recommended. As with any training session, try to start your workout well hydrated.

Protein Supplements and Weight Training

Protein supplements, currently available in a variety of forms, are a convenient way to consume protein before and after resistance-training workouts. As discussed previously, this nutritional strategy can optimize muscle building because the timing of protein intake is key. This protein can be consumed with moderate amounts of carbohydrate in conjunction with both strength training and after a hard training session or competition for your sport.

Whey protein is an increasing popular protein supplement. Whey is the component of milk that is separated when making cheese and other dairy products. It is a high-quality protein and easy to digest. Whey protein can also be lactose-free in the form of whey protein isolate. Soy protein is also an excellent source of protein, especially soy protein isolate. It is also a high-quality, lactose-free protein choice for vegetarians. Casein is another protein obtained through cheese production. It does not have as strong an amino acid profile as whey protein but is still a good protein source.

Egg protein is obtained from egg whites and considered the reference standard against which to compare other proteins. However, eggs may not be as convenient a protein source as other supplements depending on the timing and location of your training. Other high-quality protein can be obtained from real food sources, such as milk and yogurt, tofu and other soy products, and poultry and lean meats.

Like many other sports nutrition strategies and choices, use of protein supplements before and after resistance training may be a matter of convenience. These products should be taken with a carbohydrate source such as juice. Often, only a small scoop of the protein supplement is needed to provide the required 15 to 20 grams, though higher doses may be encouraged on the label.

Some practical protein and carbohydrate combinations to be consumed before and after weight training include homemade smoothies that use a variety of quality protein ingredients such as soy milk, yogurt, and dairy milk. Fruit juice or fruit can be added for carbohydrate. A generous serving of yogurt with fruit can make a good protein and carbohydrate combination. Low-fat cheese is also a high-quality protein source that can be consumed with fruit or a granola bar.

Your Weight-Training Diet

Your nutritional strategies for optimizing muscle building and increasing strength are complex and interrelated. Consuming adequate calories is key to providing your body with the energy to build muscle. However, your daily protein needs must be met, and the timing of your protein intake is also important, particularly before training and after as well. Weight training is also a fuel-depleting exercise, and consuming carbohydrate before and after training with protein can facilitate energy and recovery, while consuming carbohydrate during training also fuels your efforts.

To gain muscle mass while following a strength-training program, you require an additional 350 to 500 calories daily for a muscle gain of 1 pound per week. These additional calories can come mainly from carbohydrate and some protein. Here are some strategies for obtaining additional calories:

- Adding a bit more protein to sandwiches and dinners
- Topping carbohydrate foods such as bagels with jams and honeys
- Including another snack to your meal plan
- Adding a fruited yogurt, fruit smoothie, low-fat shake, or instant breakfast drink to your meal plan
- Enjoying a pasta or rice salad side with your lunch
- Considering a high-calorie shake or meal replacement
- Making oatmeal and soups with milk
- Mixing wheat germ, sunflower seed, and dried fruit into cereals
- Drinking higher-calorie juices such as apple, cranberry, and nectars, and blends
- Consuming calorie-dense cereals such as muesli, granola, and Grape-Nuts
- Having higher-calorie starchy vegetables such as peas, corn, and winter squash

Stepping on the Scale and Your Body Weight

Just as you may be focused on building muscle for your team sport, you may also monitor your weight and attempt to become leaner in hopes of improving your performance. Often, your efforts at body-composition change result in frequent weight checks on the scale. It is important that you keep the scale in perspective because it provides only a rudimentary measure of your body weight and some of the markers that you may be trying to monitor.

The scale weighs all of you—muscle, fat, bone, water and fluid fluctuations, body organs—and does not differentiate between these body tissues. For this reason, highly muscular athletes may weigh at the high end of their "ideal" weight. Conversely, thin, small-boned people weigh less and are favored by the scale. Obviously your body weight is influenced by much more than what you eat and how much you train. Many of the factors that affect your weight are determined by genetics and thus are basically out of your control.

The best use of a weight scale is to monitor long-term changes over time as they coincide with monitored body composition changes and to measure short-term changes related to your hydration status. As mentioned previously, weight loss after a hard training session provides feedback regarding your level of hydration. It is recommended that

Nutritional Factors in Muscle Building

Daily Diet

Calories: Provide additional 350–500 calories in daily diet to build one pound muscle per week.

Carbohydrates: Fuel source during weight training. Require adequate carbohydrates in diet to replenish glycogen stores for comprehensive training program that includes aerobic and anaerobic conditioning.

Proteins: Increased requirements for muscle building. Protein needs easily met on well-planned diet for comprehensive training program that includes weight training and aerobic and anaerobic training.

Fat: Adequate fat in the diet to maintain hormone levels, including testosterone. Healthy fats should be emphasized for cardiovascular health.

Before Weight Training
One hour before:

- Consume 10–15 g high-quality protein from whey, dairy, or soy sources.
- Consume 25–50 g of carbohydrate.
- Prehydrate with 16–24 oz. (600–720 ml) of fluid.

During Training

During a heavy training cycle:

- Consume 16 oz. (600 ml) of carbohydrate–electrolyte beverage if desired.
- Can consume gel and water for carbohydrate and fluid sources.

After Training

- Consume 10–15 g of high-quality protein from whey, dairy, or soy sources.
- Consume 25–50 g of carbohydrate.
- Rehydrate with 20 oz. (600 ml) of fluid for pound (0.5 kg) of weight loss.

for every pound (0.5 kilogram) of weight lost during exercise, you rehydrate with 24 ounces (720 milliliters) of noncaffeinated fluid.

Long-term weight changes as measured by a scale can provide you with a crude indicator regarding changes in body composition over time or even help you determine if you are keeping up with your energy needs or possibly exceeding your energy needs. Chronic unwanted weight loss can indicate that you are not meeting your caloric requirements and perhaps pushing yourself to an overtrained state. It is also important not to get overly focused on an idealized weight obtained from a height and weight chart, or on the weight and body fat levels of your top competitors. While certain body fat level averages have been measured for specific sports, a number of individual and interconnected factors other than body fat affect an athlete's performance. Averages also indicate that athletes can be successful at varying degrees of reasonable body fat levels, with some competitors at the low end of the body fat range and others at the high end. Top athletes do not always fit the lean and muscular ideal for their sport, and a low body fat level does not guarantee success.

Techniques for Measuring Body Fat Levels

Regardless of the body fat measurement technique that you employ, you should keep in mind that they all measure your body fat indirectly. When choosing a body fat measurement technique, you should consider the following guidelines:

- The technique and formula used to estimate your body fat should be valid for athletes in your sport, gender, and age.
- A reliable technician should perform the technique.
- The same technique should be repeated over time to obtain long-term data and to measure progressive changes.
- The results should be interpreted by a knowledgeable expert who is aware of the limitations of the technique and can advise you appropriately.

Clearly, the measurement of body composition is far from being an exact science. For example, a commonly utilized technique is skinfold testing, which has a standard error of 3 percent. If an athlete were to test at 15 percent body fat, actual body fat levels could range from 12 to 18 percent body fat. Body fat assessments provide a possible range of body fat, rather than an absolute number. When monitoring your body composition over time, it is very important that you do not try to compare various body fat levels measured using different techniques and technicians. Table 6.2 provides the measured body fat levels of athletes from various team sports. Each athlete has his or her own individual body fat level at which that athlete performs best.

The following body fat measurement techniques are the ones most commonly used, but they all contain some inherent error in their technique and provide only an estimate of body composition. No one method is absolutely accurate, and accuracy can vary among techniques. Table 6.1 rates the different percentages of body fat.

Hydrostatic Weighing

Hydrostatic or underwater weighing is a water displacement technique often cited as the "gold standard" of body fat assessment, despite having a standard error of at least 2 percent. Hydrostatic weighing involves being weighed underwater after expelling all

TABLE 6.1 BODY FAT LEVELS FOR HEALTH

Rating	Body Fat Levels
At risk (low levels)	Males: <5% Females: <9%
Below average	Males: 6%–10% Females: 10%–15%
Good	Males: 11%–14% Females: 16%–19%
Average	Males: 15%–18% Females: 20%–25%
Above average	Males: 19%–24% Females: 26%–29%
At risk (high levels)	Males: 25% or more Females: 30% or more

the air from your lungs. Your body density is estimated from the difference between your weight on land and your weight underwater. Your body fat is then extrapolated from this information.

Like all methods, hydrostatic weighing is not error-free. This method assumes a constant fat-free body density and may not be appropriate for all population groups. There is some potential error related to your hydration status and how much air is actually left in your lungs when being weighed underwater.

Underwater weighing can be a bit uncomfortable but is offered at some sports medicine centers and universities. Your health club may have someone perform this technique several times throughout the year. This can be a useful body composition technique as measured over time by a skilled technician.

Air Displacement

Also known as *body plethysmography,* this technique also measures body density, but by air displacement rather than water displacement. Your body fat percentage is calculated based on equations. This technique provides body fat estimations similar to underwater weighing, though more data are needed on competitive athletes. You sit in an enclosed capsule (a Bod Pod) while a computer measures the amount of air displaced.

This is an expensive system but is less inconvenient than underwater weighing. However, this technique may not be widely available but may be at some universities and health clubs.

TABLE 6.2 BODY FAT LEVELS FOR TEAM SPORTS	
Exercise Type	**Protein Requirements per Weight**
Football	Backs: 9%–12% Linebackers: 13%–14% Linemen: 16%–19% Quarterbacks/kickers: 14%
Baseball	12%–15%
Soccer	Males: 10% Females: 12%–22%
Basketball	Males: 7%–11% Females: 20%–27%
Hockey	Males: 8%–15% Females: 15%–20%

Bioelectrical Impedance Analysis (BIA)

Use of bioelectrical impedance has markedly increased over the past 10 years because it is relatively inexpensive, portable, and convenient. BIA is based on the conductive property of different tissues within the body. Because muscles contain a high percentage of water, they conduct current more quickly than fat stores. The BIA machine passes a small and undetectable current through the body and analyzes the resistance to the flow of the current. The slower the signal, the more fat you have.

While BIA is relatively quick and simple, it may overestimate body fat in lean individuals, and results are affected by hydration levels. If you are not well hydrated, you will appear to have a higher level of body fat than you actually have. You should be well hydrated for the test but also not drink fluids 4 hours before the test to empty your bladder. It is best if you do not exercise within 12 hours of the test. Alcohol, diuretics, and caffeine should also be avoided prior to this measurement.

Many individuals are now purchasing a home scale (Tanita scale) that measures body fat with this technique. You should take the readings at the same time of day, be well hydrated, and have an empty bladder. Avoid early-morning readings when you are most likely to be dehydrated.

Skinfold Calipers

The skinfold caliper method is the most widely used technique and the most inexpensive and convenient method for measuring body fat. A skilled technician uses calipers to indirectly measure the double thickness of subcutaneous fat underneath the skin. Several standard skinfold sites have been identified on the body: abdomen, arm, thigh, hip area, and back of shoulder. They must be accurately marked, and the skinfold is then pinched and gently pulled away from the body. The sum of several skinfolds (anywhere from three to seven sites) is plugged into a formula that is then used to estimate total body fat.

This technique has several disadvantages. It requires a skilled technician. It assumes that subcutaneous fat is proportional to total body fat. The formulas for skinfold measurements are also based on body composition measurements from the indirect measurement of underwater weighing. Formulas used for skinfold measurements should be appropriate for athletes and their sport. When formulas for the general population are used, body fat is often underestimated in athletes. Skinfold measurements may also underestimate body fat in very lean athletes.

However, when kept in perspective, this technique can be reliable and accurate. When this technique is utilized, you cannot only calculate the fat but also obtain a number that is the sum of all the skinfolds measured. This absolute number is not formula-dependent and can be monitored over time. For example, a 20-year-old male basketball player may have a three-site skinfold sum of 40 and estimated body fat of 11 percent. A follow-up measurement at several months may show an increase in body weight, while total skinfolds decreased to 36 millimeters. These results would indicate a probable loss in body fat and increase in muscle mass. This trend can be monitored over a month's and year's time, providing useful feedback regarding training and diet.

Tape measure readings can also be combined with skinfold assessment. Measurements are taken at thigh, arm, and abdominal sites. The more skinfold measurement sites required by the formula, the better. You should never compare body fat estimations made over time using different formulas.

Changing Body Composition

Because your body composition is the result of genetics, as well as training and diet, some athletes may fall naturally at an optimal body composition, while others may struggle due to hereditary factors. Extreme efforts to maintain a set body composition may not be worth the energy as intense weight loss approaches may compromise the quality of your diet and training. It is also important to keep a perspective on body fat. Aim for a healthy and appropriate range rather than a specific number. Body fat levels may also change over the course of a season depending on the phase of your training, your age, and the stage of your competitive career.

If you are considering improving your body fat composition, have it assessed by a skilled technician. An optimal goal weight can be determined, but it is important to be realistic regarding how much body fat you want to lose and how quickly you should reach your goal. This goal may require some professional advice.

First, consider your genetics. Experts suggest that 25 to 40 percent of how much fat our body stores is related to our genetics. If you have a history of struggling with body fat loss and maintenance or can say the same of your family members, you should consider a moderate, gentle weight loss goal. Next, look at your lifestyle. Food choices are heavily influenced by your schedule, commitments, environment, and stress levels. It is important for your weight loss and body fat goals to be reasonable, as you have to meet the energy demands of not only training but life and work or school as well.

Dieting Pitfalls

Dieting certainly presents several pitfalls for the team sport athlete. An athlete who is glycogen depleted, electrolyte depleted, low on protein, and dehydrated from dieting will not perform at her best and likely will perform poorly. Rigid dieting and too much calorie restriction can deplete body fuel stores. Intense weight loss efforts can also result in hormonal imbalances, iron deficiency anemia, compromised bone health, and loss of muscular strength and power. Severe dieting can also make you crabby and tired. Dieting just isn't fun.

Food is fuel for your hardworking body, and your body does not respond positively when fuel runs low. A low fuel gauge sends out a slew of appetite-triggering brain chemicals that drive you to eat. What many dieters perceive as a lack of willpower is really the body's drive for self-preservation. Restricting foods can lead to overeating and even binge eating, thwarting weight loss efforts. Besides playing games with the body, dieting wreaks havoc with the mind. Restrictive eating can lead to feelings of deprivation and a preoccupation with food.

Besides triggering overeating, drastic calorie reduction can break down body protein stores for energy. This muscle loss not only hinders your strength and power but also negatively impacts your metabolism. Muscle is what keeps your furnace burning. Your body also responds to calorie restriction by lowering its resting metabolic rate. Eating normally can restore your metabolism, though this may be difficult if you have a history of repeated dieting. Over time your body may become more efficient at utilizing calories and storing body fat.

Healthy Weight Loss Guidelines

A healthy weight for an athlete is about how you feel and perform, not just about how you perceive how you look or the weight reading on the scale. Keeping a healthy perspective on weight can be confusing these days. The ideal in our society has become more muscular and leaner than ever, while as a whole the population has increased in body weight. Often the ideal portrayed in the media is unhealthy and unrealistic and can only be attained through excessive exercise and overly restrictive eating.

Healthy weight loss starts with setting a realistic goal and avoiding quick, unbalanced, and extreme weight loss approaches. Try to accomplish a realistic weight loss in a reasonable amount of time and at an "off-season" time of year. Let's take a look at some sensible weight loss guidelines.

Set a realistic body composition and weight goal. It is very likely that your training program emphasizes both muscle building and maintaining a low level of body fat. Often, real body composition changes do not result in drastic body weight changes, as the scale measures all body tissue, not just body fat. Elicit the advice of a qualified professional who can assess your body composition results and provide recommended changes in body composition that are appropriate for your age, growth and development if appropriate, current training program, and sport.

Set a realistic calorie deficit. Keep in mind that when you attempt to lose body fat, you have to restrict calories; however, when you desire to build muscle, you need to consume adequate calories, so it is important to find a balance between your body composition goals. Females should not exceed a weight loss of 1 pound weekly and males 2 pounds weekly, especially during heavy training periods. Losing 1 pound weekly requires a deficit of 500 calories daily. Greater weight loss requires even more restriction. Losing 2 pounds weekly requires a daily 1,000-calorie deficit, clearly calling for some intense calorie-cutting and calorie-burning efforts, which are not always appropriate during periods of growth and/or heavy training cycles.

Trimming no more than 200 to 300 calories daily may be the safest and most effective long-term weight loss approach. This mild reduction should have no metabolism-lowering effects and will not precipitate feelings of hunger and deprivation. However, if you are stepping up your muscle-building efforts, your best results may be obtained by following the proper training program and the nutrition program that is optimal for building muscle mass.

Keep a food journal to assess your current eating habits. Write down your food intake, times eaten, and portions for 1 week. Record your training sessions, noting the duration and intensity of training in conjunction with your food intake. You can also record your moods, thoughts, and feelings that correlate with your food intake to determine some of your eating triggers such as stress or fatigue. It may also be helpful to make a note of your energy levels and recovery during and after various types of training sessions.

Assess your intake. Make sure that you are following the principles of postexercise recovery nutrition. Monitor your hunger and fullness patterns. Do you often wait until you are ravenous before eating? Do you get overfull at meals? Do you eat for comfort or in reaction to stress fairly often? Do you have significant drops in your energy levels during the day?

You may be surprised at how much you actually consume during the day. Writing your food down can also be very helpful in keeping you on track while you are trying to lose weight and, more important, improve the quality of your diet and nutritional strategies, because it makes you accountable and conscious of your food choices.

Have a healthy strategy or plan for reducing your caloric intake and improving your diet. A number of effective ways to reduce your caloric intake and improve your diet are possible. It is important that you do eat well postexercise and practice the recovery nutrition guidelines reviewed, as well as time your meals and snacks appropriately before training. If you eat out frequently or eat too much fast food, you may be consuming a large amount of hidden fat in your diet.

Other techniques for reducing fat intake include choosing leaner meats, switching to low-fat dairy products, minimizing added fats and those used in cooking, and decreasing the frequency of sweets. You can also cut back on high-calorie fluids such as alcohol, sodas, and perhaps juices.

Pay attention to portions when you eat out or grab items on the run. A bagel or muffin can easily provide more than 300 calories.

Plan ahead. Preparing meals ahead of time can help you avoid fatty restaurant foods. Learning how to shop for quick, low-fat, and nutritious foods is extremely helpful in improving your diet and changing your body composition. You can also pack healthy snacks such as fresh fruits and vegetables. Programming your food environment for success or learning how to manage the environment in which you make your food choices will go a long way to supporting you in reaching your weight loss goals.

Eat balanced meals at the right times. Having real meals will leave you feeling satisfied. Make sure that you consume meals throughout the day, and don't set yourself up for periods of intense hunger. Have a full breakfast and lunch, and don't consume all your calories in the evening. Your body works best on a steady supply of fuel throughout the day. As you can see from the nutrition guidelines outlined for pretraining eating, recovery nutrition, and nutrition strategies designed to optimize muscle building, eating small, frequent meals is ideal and effective.

Have some protein and fat with your meals and snacks. These foods will keep you feeling full longer and help prevent the hunger that leads to an unplanned trip to the vending machine. Choose lean proteins and small amounts of healthy fats. Look at your food journal to determine what times of day you get too hungry. Add a bit more protein or fat to the preceding meal or snack if hunger sets in quickly at specific times.

Pay attention to hunger and fullness. Your body's inner, physiological signals are one of the best ways to gauge when it is best to start eating and when your body has had enough food at that particular meal. Of course, you must also plan when you eat around your training and schedule, but paying attention to your hunger and fullness can also provide some valuable direction regarding your food intake and portions. You can also use the 20-minute rule to wait and see if your meal has been filling and satisfying.

Enjoy the meal, and have some treats. Food is not only fuel but also a source of enjoyment. This means sitting down and enjoying your meals whenever possible, eating slowly and savoring the food, and making sure that favorites are included in your diet on a regular basis.

The Spectrum of Disordered Eating

When you train and compete, being able to quickly move your body over a given distance for a set amount of time offers a performance advantage. So having a lower level of body fat is considered to be a mechanical advantage. However, athletes can become overly focused on their weight and body fat levels. Because athletes may be driven, goal oriented, perfectionistic, and highly competitive, some of the qualities that promote athletic success may manifest in unrealistic weight and body fat goals, and a high degree of importance on losing a few pounds. Pressure to lose this weight may come from a number of outside sources including trainers, coaches, athletic peers, and ideals promoted in the media. Female athletes seem especially at risk of being dissatisfied with their body image, though males are also susceptible.

The estimated prevalence of eating disorders in athletes ranges greatly depending on the screening technique used, the athletes studied, and how an eating disorder was defined. Estimates in female athletes range from a low of 1 percent to a high of 62 percent, and from 0 percent to 57 percent in male athletes. Despite these wide-scale ranges, most experts agree that eating disorders pose a significant health risk to too many athletes. It is also important to appreciate that there is a full spectrum of disordered eating that differs from the full-blown eating disorders of anorexia nervosa, bulimia nervosa, and eating disorders not otherwise specified (EDNOS). *Disordered eating* is a broader term that describes misguided and unhealthy strategies for weight loss or even occasional bingeing and purging.

There are many gray areas in the area of disordered eating, and it can often be difficult to differentiate when a true eating disorder begins. Often behavior that begins as an attempt to lose weight takes on a life of its own and develops into unhealthy groups of behaviors known as disordered eating. Disordered eating represents a full spectrum of eating behaviors, with poor eating habits at one end and full-blown anorexia nervosa and bulimia nervosa at the other end.

While full-blown eating disorders are not exceptionally high in most sports, studies indicate a high prevalence of disordered eating behavior and distorted concerns regarding body weight, body fat, and body shape among athletes. Some common disordered eating behaviors may include skipping meals, weighing constantly, eating very little fat, and fearing that specific foods may promote unwanted weight gain. Binge eating, as characterized by consuming large amounts of food while feeling out of control, can be part of disordered eating.

Another term, *anorexia athletica,* describes a syndrome characterized by disordered eating and compulsive exercising. It is associated with an intense fear of gaining weight, despite being at normal or below normal weight, and is characterized by food restriction, often less than 1,200 calories per day, and excessive exercise. Bingeing, self-induced vomiting, and use of laxatives and diuretics may also occur. Some athletes are able to stop these behaviors when participation in a sport stops. But for other athletes, this behavior continues to develop into a full clinical eating disorder.

Eating disorders are complicated and multifactorial. Psychological and emotional issues such as anxiety and depression, an inability to cope with family and personal problems, life stresses, biochemical imbalances, and the pressure to be thin or lean from both sport and society may be involved. Some triggers associated with eating disorders in athletes include traumatic life events such as relationship problems, recommendations to lose weight, prolonged periods of dieting, and a large discrepancy between actual weight and a self-defined ideal weight. It is possible that individuals at high risk for eating disorders may gravitate toward certain sports, but being involved in a sport may also trigger the eating disorder in a susceptible athlete. Some risk factors that are more specific to athletes than the general population include prolonged periods of dieting or weight cycling, an increase in training volume, stress related to their sport and training such as the loss of a coach, weight loss pressures from coaches and trainers, lack of guidance on appropriate weight and body composition goals, and healthy weight management strategies.

While eating disorders in men and male athletes is not as high as in females, it is still a concern, and the figures available may underestimate the true prevalence of eating

Eating Disorders

Anorexia Nervosa

- Resistance to maintaining body weight at or above a minimally normal weight
- Intense fear of gaining weight or becoming fat even though underweight
- Distortion in the way in which one's body weight or shape is experienced, denial of the seriousness of current low body weight
- Infrequent or absent menstrual periods in females who have reached puberty

Physical characteristics of anorexia nervosa

- Hair loss and growth of fine body hair
- Low pulse rate
- Sensitivity to cold
- Stress fractures, osteopenia, or osteoporosis
- Overuse injuries
- Abnormal fatigue
- Gastrointestinal problems

Bulimia Nervosa

- Recurrent episodes of binge eating, characterized by a sense of lack of control, and an excessive amount of food within a short period of time
- Purging behavior such as self-induced vomiting, misuse of laxatives, diuretics, enemas, or other medications
- Binge eating and purging behavior occur on average at least twice weekly for 3 months
- Self-esteem is inappropriately influenced by body shape and weight

Physical characteristics of bulimia nervosa

- Frequent weight fluctuations
- Difficulty swallowing and throat damage
- Swollen glands
- Damaged tooth enamel from gastric acid
- Electrolyte imbalances and dehydration
- Menstrual irregularities
- Diarrhea or constipation

Eating Disorder Not Otherwise Specified (EDNOS)

This category includes disorders of eating that do not meet the criteria for a specific eating disorder.

- Binge eating disorder and episodes of binge eating without the use of compensatory behavior as seen in bulimia nervosa
- Repeatedly chewing and spitting out, but not swallowing large amounts of food

- The criteria for anorexia nervosa are met except that the individual has regular menstrual periods
- All the criteria for bulimia nervosa are met except that the frequency of binge eating and purging behavior occur less than twice weekly and for less than three months
- Regular purging behaviors occur after consuming small amounts of foods

Muscle Dysmorphia

This term describes a form of body image disturbance described in male body-builders and weight lifters.

- Preoccupation with not being sufficiently lean and muscular
- Preoccupation with muscularity causes significant social impairment
- Characterized by excessive exercise, preoccupation with food, abuse of steroids, and abuse of dietary supplements aimed at increasing body size or decreasing body fat

Anorexia Athletica

This term has been used to describe a condition that is not a full-blown eating disorder.

- Characterized by disordered eating and compulsive exercise

- Intense fear of weight gain despite weighing below the expected weight for age and height
- Weight loss is achieved by food restriction and extensive compulsive exercise
- May involve self-induced vomiting and use of laxatives and diuretics

Binge Eating Disorder

This disorder is currently a subset of EDNOS, but is expected to be classified as a separate diagnostic entity. It is the recurrent episodes of compulsive eating during a discrete period of time, and characterized by a large amount of food and a sense of lack of control. Binges episodes are characterized by:

- Eating more rapidly than normal
- Eating until uncomfortably full
- Eating large amounts when not physically hungry
- Eating alone because of embarrassment of the volume of food
- Feeling disgusted, depressed, or guilty after eating
- Marked distress regarding binge eating
- Bingeing occurs two days weekly for six months

disorders in men. Males who develop disordered eating are more likely to previously have been overweight or even obese, and the fear of gaining weight may relate to this past experience. Male athletes may also diet in order to improve performance or in response to an injury that limits training.

In addition, male athletes may have a recently identified body image disorder called *muscle dysmorphia*. Muscle dysmorphia is characterized by an intense preoccupation with body size and degree of muscularity. Individuals with this disorder attempt to increase body size and may abuse performance-enhancing drugs or dietary supplements that promise to increase muscle mass or decrease body fat. This disorder is more common in male weightlifters and bodybuilders.

Several common warning signs may signal the start of an eating disorder. They include repeated concerns about body weight, refusal to maintain even a minimal weight, periods of severe calorie restriction, and excessive physical activity that is not part of a balanced training program. Other warning signs may include food rituals, self-induced vomiting, and abuse of laxatives and diet pills. Many of these behaviors by themselves do not prove the presence of an eating disorder, but they justify further attention to the possible presence of a problem. The sidebar, Eating Disorders (page 122), describes some of the characteristics of full-blown eating disorders.

Disordered eating and eating disorders can result in poor performance related to glycogen depletion, dehydration and electrolyte depletion, and loss of lean body mass. Nutrient deficiencies can result, as can increased risk of infection, illness, and injuries. Other health-related effects are decreased metabolism, gastrointestinal complication, menstrual dysfunction in females, and decreased bone mineral density. To avoid these harmful effects, an athlete with an eating disorder requires the help of a team of skilled professionals trained in treating this condition, including a physician, dietitian, and psychologist or therapist.

EVALUATING NUTRITIONAL SUPPLEMENTS
Sales and Marketing of Ergogenic Aids

The term *ergogenic* means "to produce work." Nutritional ergogenic aids are promoted as increasing muscle size, increasing strength, promoting fat burning, and improving speed. For example, it is claimed that several ergogenic aids such as carnitine "enhance fat burning." Creatine is reported to enhance muscle building when taken during a strength-training program.

Apparently many consumers have believed the promise that nutritional ergogenic aids promote, as nutritional ergogenic aid sales have become a serious and lucrative business. U.S. sales from one such product, creatine, increased from $30 million in 1995, to $180 million in 1998, to a high of $400 million in 2001. In fact, sales for the entire dietary supplement industry sales, which include these ergogenic aid products, grew to nearly $18 billion in 2002, of which sports nutrition sales exceeded $6 billion for that same year.

With all sports nutrition product sales, not just ergogenic aids, in the United States expected to have surpassed $7.2 billion in 2004, athletes have clearly embraced a wide selection of these products as an important component of their training programs.

One study of female collegiate varsity athletes determined that more that 60 percent of them used some type of nutritional supplement at least once a month. Good health was the reason most frequently cited for supplement use. Over one-third of the female athletes took a multivitamin and mineral supplement with iron, plus some use of amino acids and protein supplements and herbal products.

Chapters 5 and 7 outline practical uses for products such as sports drinks, gels, and bars, and high-carbohydrate and meal replacement supplements that are backed by both research and the practical experience of athletes. Using these products knowledgeably and appropriately carries minimal risk and some clear performance benefits that support your training and competition goals. However, some sports drinks and recovery drinks may also contain ingredients that are not necessary or even safe for some athletes to consume, especially young and developing athletes.

Ergogenic aid sales are a serious business for both male and female athletes. It is important that when you ingest a product in the quest for top performance, you have verified that it is legal, effective, and safe. Unfortunately, many of these products are backed solely by strong and enticing claims, anecdotal hearsay, high-profile athlete and coach testimonials, and referenced "research" that has not been published in full in a reputable scientific journal. In reality, the majority of these supplements have *not* been thoroughly and appropriately tested. Moreover, many of the supplements that are tested independently of the manufacturers who supply them don't live up to their performance claims. But despite this lack of plausibility, it can be tempting to top off all your hard work with an easily ingested supplement that promises a quick and effective performance boost.

With new products coming out monthly, athletes need to be discerning when evaluating nutritional ergogenic aids or performance enhancers. It is important that you can make knowledgeable choices about these products. Keep these tips in mind before you use them:

- Understand how the ergogenic aid purportedly functions.
- Know the summary of the current research support on the supplement.
- Be aware of any safety concerns surrounding the product.
- Know whether the product is a legal supplement for athletes.

Chances are you may try a supplement because it is widely talked about on your team or is surrounded by enticing marketing claims for building muscle, burning fat, and increasing energy output. But these supplements are never going to be an effective substitution for a solid training program and an optimal training diet.

Another important consideration when evaluating the safety of these supplements is the age of an athlete. The American Academy of Pediatrics does not recommend high-performance supplements in the diet of child athletes. These supplements are also routinely tested on adults (if at all) and not on young and growing bodies or athletes of high school age. Studies of collegiate athletes are limited, as are long-term safety data. What safety information is available would not address safety issues in high school athletes. Some supplements are also banned by the National Collegiate Athletic Association (NCAA).

Regulation of Dietary Supplements and Nutritional Ergogenic Aids

Athletes are bombarded with claims of the magical effects of nutritional ergogenic aids on performance. Advertising and claims surrounding these products have increased exponentially since the Dietary Supplement Health and Education Act (DSHEA) was passed in 1994. DSHEA significantly changed how all dietary supplements such as vitamins, minerals, herbs, amino acids, metabolites, and even hormones were tested, marketed, labeled, and manufactured.

Unlike regulation of makers of a drug or food additive, supplement manufacturers are not required to prove that a dietary supplement works. Under DSHEA, manufacturers are responsible for making sure that products are safe. The government does not review these products before they are put on the market, but the Food and Drug Administration (FDA) can take action against any unsafe dietary supplement products. However, the FDA cannot evaluate the thousands of products on the market and makes selective use of time and resources. It is more likely that it will respond only to products that have resulted in significant adverse health effects that occur on a large scale.

You may also notice on the label a somewhat loosely defined "nutrition support claim." These claims may relate to the "structure and function" of the body and "general well-being." Although a certain set of conditions must be met to make these claims, they do not require prior FDA approval. Manufacturers must be able to substantiate that the claim is "truthful and not misleading," but they cannot promise to prevent or cure a disease. Some nutrition support claims may include "maintains a healthy circulatory system" or "helps maintain a healthy intestinal flora." Note that supplements providing these types of claims must also state, "This product is not intended to diagnose, treat, cure, or prevent any disease."

The FDA also recommends that the discerning consumer realize that it is up to each company to decide how its manufacturing practices will prepare and package supplements, thereby affecting their purity, safety, potency, and therefore overall quality. According to the FDA, a consumer can contact the manufacturer and request product safety information and research support, which would preferably not be in-house published data. They can also question whether the firm has a quality control system in place and whether any adverse event reports have resulted from the use of their product.

Starting in 2003, the FDA is in the process of developing Good Manufacturing Processes (GMPs) in coordination with the supplement industry. Two Web sites, www.consumerlab.com and www.nsf.org, currently list products that have been evaluated for appropriate quality control. Both of these sites also test products for banned supplements and can certify for athletes that products do not contain them. Some supplement companies have their own GMPs in place and may be regulated under the National Nutrition Foods Association at www.nnfa.org.

You should also review the "Supplement Facts" labels on the package of dietary supplements. Unlike conventional foods, the dosage on labels is not standardized. So remember that higher amounts than needed or are safe may be recommended. The label will provide the following:

- Statement of identity
- Net quantity of ingredients
- A structure function claim statement
- Directions for use
- Other ingredients listed in descending order of predominance by common name or proprietary blend
- Name and address of packer, manufacturer, or distributor

Unfortunately, even if companies are accused and fined regarding false claims on dietary supplements, they may not be deterred from promoting new products. Often fines may be rendered insignificant by a large volume of sales generated while claims are investigated.

Is It Effective?

Valid scientific testing of a nutritional ergogenic aid costs time, money, and resources. Tests of a supplement's effect on performance should be conducted with well-trained athletes and can be specific to the type of sport. For these and other reasons, much of the supplement industry forgoes testing and relies heavily on testimonials, anecdotes, and untested scientific theories, rather than research studies to promote their product. But a theory is not proof. A theory is a hypothesis or intriguing idea that requires testing. "Scientific breakthroughs" may be new and interesting ideas with little or no basis in fact.

A scientific trial remains the best way in which to examine the effectiveness of ergogenic aids on performance. Here, athletes' experiences can be helpful to researchers, who desire to focus on potentially effective substances. Scientists can use them to determine what products are worth testing and what dosages are appropriate for test protocols. Testing should closely mimic real athletic performance conditions as much as possible. Researchers should control for age, level of training, and nutritional status. Various dosages, supplementation periods, types of exercise, and performance testing may need to be incorporated.

Studies should control for the placebo effect as much as possible by incorporating a double-blind design. In this approach, subjects receive both the substance being tested and a placebo. To minimize bias, subjects and researchers don't know which product is being administered when. In addition to a placebo trial, there may be a control (no treatment) group. These are only some of the needed features of well-designed testing that satisfy the scientist but not always the athlete. A large change in performance is required for outcomes to be considered statistically significant. In many cases, however, changes produced by nutritional supplementation are likely to be smaller. Although a 1 to 3 percent change may not be statistically adequate, it may be useful in elite competition. Researchers also report the overall performance effect within a group. Positive results of individuals within a group may be diluted by the negative or neutral responses of other subjects. Not all subjects respond in the same way to a particular substance.

Unfortunately, even well-designed studies can be quoted out of context. Research findings are extrapolated to inappropriate conclusions. Companies often state that they are in the process of conducting research. Other times they say that research is "in-house" or has simply never been published in reputable peer-reviewed journals. And even well-designed preliminary studies require verification through additional sound research. Unfortunately, even studies published in reputable journals can provoke criticism when placed under close scrutiny. Additionally, patented nutritional ergogenic aids may also look impressive. Yet patents are not granted based on the effectiveness of the product, but rather on its distinguishable differences. Patents can be obtained with a theoretical model rather than objective double-blind research.

Is It Safe?

False claims aside, the next step in determining if you should use an ergogenic aid is safety concerns. As previously mentioned, supplement manufacturers are not required to prove a product's safety. Negative effects from products may be acute, mild, or temporary, but they can also be serious and chronic. Some dietary supplements may be toxic or decrease the absorption of other nutrients, especially in high doses, where the "more is better" belief prevails. Ironically, independent testing has also found that many supplements do not contain the ingredients marked on the label. Often products are watered down or contain other unlisted ingredients that may be harmful or illegal. Hopefully this concern will be resolved when all companies comply with adopted GMPs.

Is It Legal?

As a competitive athlete, particularly if you may be drug tested, you do not want to inadvertently take a dietary supplement that contains a banned substance. The past several years has seen a significant increase in the number of positive tests at the elite and professional level, claimed to be the result of a contaminated or mislabeled dietary supplement. All athletic governing bodies have some regulation regarding the use of ergogenic aids. Products banned by the NCAA are listed at www.ncaa.org. Even if you avoid illegal products such as ephedra or androstenedione, reading labels is not a 100 percent guarantee of avoiding banned products. Cross-contamination can occur in the manufacturing process, and the purity of these supplements is often questioned.

Specific nutritional ergogenic aids can benefit athletes under certain conditions. However, the supplement industry is an extremely profitable business that relies on theories and testimonials to market products. Ergogenic aid theories may even be extrapolated from clinical research on disease states or nutrient deficiencies. To say that this product will then produce a performance improvement is not a scientific breakthrough but a leap in logic. Even with proven ergogenic aids, it is important to keep their role in perspective. While they may produce small performance improvements, ergogenic aids are no substitute for proper training, nutrition, and psychological preparation.

SUPPLEMENT RESEARCH SUPPORT, SAFETY, AND PRACTICAL ISSUES

This section reviews several popular nutritional ergogenic aids for scientific validity as determined by quality research. Any safety concerns and any practical issues regarding use of these supplements will also be reviewed in this section. Not surprisingly, many sports physiologists and sports nutritionists do not provide overwhelming support for the majority of these supplements. They would rather that you trained and ate properly, as this approach very effectively improves performance! Many professionals also have concerns about younger and developing athletes taking supplements that have not been proven safe, as supplement testing is usually done in adults.

Types of Ergogenic Aids

Many ergogenic aids marketed to team sport athletes are designed to increase muscle mass and strength and decrease body fat. Some ergogenic aids are also reported to improve performance by increasing power output during exercise.

Ergogenic Aids that Affect Body Composition

Creatine. With sales at $400 million dollars in 2001, creatine is clearly a supplement that came out of the starting blocks and shifted into high gear. Fortunately, creatine is one of the best-researched ergogenic aids, making it possible for sports nutritionists to provide clear and confident recommendations regarding this sports nutrition supplement.

Creatine is often advertised as a steroid alternative, but it is really more comparable to glycogen loading. Just as carbohydrate ingestion maximizes glycogen content of the muscle, "creatine loading" can increase muscle creatine stores. Your normal intake of creatine is about 2 grams daily (perhaps less for vegetarians), and it is also synthesized in the liver and kidney. Creatine is an essential fuel of the ATP creatine phosphate system. Loading the muscle with creatine is designed to increase ATP resynthesis. This power system typically stores enough fuel to last 6 to 10 seconds. Creatine can also buffer lactic acid and transport ATP to be utilized for muscle contraction.

Muscle biopsies have confirmed that rapid loading can be achieved with 25 to 30 grams of creatine daily divided into five to six doses. A more gentle loading protocol is 3 grams daily over 28 days. Unlike carbohydrate, creatine appears to remain trapped in the muscle without supplementation for 4 to 5 weeks. About 30 percent of individuals who creatine load appear to be "nonresponders." Ingesting about 75 to 100 grams of carbohydrate has been demonstrated to enhance creatine accumulation in the muscle. You should also be aware that a 2- to 5-pound weight gain is associated with creatine loading. Scientists believe this to be water gain, as urine output decreases during the loading phase.

Though not documented in the scientific literature, anecdotal reports abound that creatine loading is associated with muscle cramping and GI upset. When loading with creatine, make sure that you consume plenty of water to help prevent any side effects. Taking more than 30 grams of creatine daily over 5 days offers no additional benefits for loading. As is often the case with many nutritional supplements, more is not better. In fact, there are some concerns that chronic and high doses of creatine can lead to liver and kidney damage. People with existing kidney disease should not take creatine.

We know that creatine ingestion can load the muscle, but how does it affect performance? Creatine loading appears to increase the rate of creatine resynthesis during recovery (20 seconds to 5 minutes) from bouts of high-intensity exercise (6 to 30 seconds). Creatine loading delays fatigue during activity that includes repeated, all-out surges of energy interspersed with rest periods.

One creatine-loading study in female soccer players found that despite the increased body weight seen with loading, they improved performance of some repeated sprint tasks and agility tasks that mimic soccer play.

Creatine could potentially assist other team sport players. Creatine loading appears to benefit resistance training, allowing more repetitions to be performed and consequently increases in strength. Of course, resistance training is commonly part of a team sport athlete's training program.

It is not recommended that you supplement for more than 60 days, and it should be at a low dose of 3 grams during this time period. Creatine loading may also only be necessary once or twice yearly due to the cyclical nature of your training and the muscle's ability to hold creatine for several weeks.

Creatine is currently legal. However, there have been some concerns of cross contamination of creatine products in recent years, as athletes ingesting this supplement have tested positive for banned prohormone products. No creatine studies have been done with high school athletes or athletes who are still growing and developing. Many high schools and colleges likely have their own policy regarding creatine supplementation in their athletes. The NCAA does not allow use of creatine.

Beta-Hydroxy-Beta-Methylbutyrate (HMB). HMB is primarily marketed to strength and power athletes and is one of the fastest-selling supplements on the market. Team

TABLE 6.3 SUMMARY OF ERGOGENIC AIDS			
Supplement	**Claims**	**Scientific Data**	**Safety**
Creatine	Supports training for increased muscle mass	Well supported by scientific data	Can be used safely by adults when following scientific protocols
HMB	Builds muscle strength and inhibits breakdown of muscle and protein	Limited human data supporting claims; several studies found no benefits	Doses at 3 g taken for 6–8 weeks appear safe
Protein supplements	Facilitates muscle building	Can consume 10–15 g high-quality protein in conjunction with carbohydrate before and after weight training	Can consume protein from real foods, supplements not required; exceeding recommended dose provides no additional benefits
Amino acids	Facilitate muscle building and exercise recovery	Not supported by well-designed research	Can upset balance of amino acid metabolism when taken in large doses
Ribose	Improved muscle recovery, energy and endurance enhancer; rebuilds ATP	Published research is limited; current data far from conclusive	Not enough safety data
Glutamine	Supports the immune system; promotes protein synthesis	May benefit athletes with a true glutamine deficiency; more data required	Often incorporated in many sports nutrition supplements; too much could upset amino acid balance

sport athletes who weight train and want to facilitate muscle recovery may be interested in this supplement.

HMB is not actually a nutrient but a metabolic by-product produced in small amounts when the amino acid leucine is metabolized. You produce only about 0.2 to 0.4 gram of HMB daily. HMB was first developed by scientists and then patented by the company that produces HMB, which has sponsored much of the research on HMB.

Much of the initial HMB research was done on animals, but there are also human data. Although some data have indicated greater increases in muscle mass and fewer markers of muscle damage, these studies did not always control for diet, which can have a significant impact on muscle gain in conjunction with weight training. Several

TABLE 6.3 SUMMARY OF ERGOGENIC ACIDS, *CONTINUED*			
Supplement	**Claims**	**Scientific Data**	**Safety**
Carnitine	Metabolic fat burner	Not supported by well-designed research	L-carnitine form only; can be consumed at 1–2 g daily for six months
Chromium	Builds muscle and burns fat	Not supported by well-designed research	Not to exceed 200 µg daily
Pyruvate	Improves endurance; promotes muscle building and fat loss	Not tested on athletes; not supported by research	Not much safety data
Prohormones	Promotes muscle building	Illegal products	Banned by the USADA and IOC; long-term safety concerns and possible adverse health effects
Weight loss supplements	Promotes body fat loss and weight loss	Many ingredients not supported by well-designed research; risks may outweigh benefits	Risks of supplements may be serious; some ingredients may be banned
Caffeine	Promotes endurance; may improve power output for shorter distances	Good data on endurance exercise; limited data on power sports indicate need for more research	Can be used safely in moderate doses; high doses are not required for ergogenic effect
MCT oil	Provides fuel during training and spares muscle glycogen; enhances fat burning.	Tested mainly for endurance exercise; not supported by well-designed research	May cause mild gastrointestinal symptoms

studies found no ergogenic benefit from HMB supplementation. One study on collegiate football players showed no improvements in muscle strength and body composition with HMB supplementation. Another study in elite male rugby players found that both aerobic and anaerobic capacity was unaffected by HMB supplementation, as well as a combination of HMB and creatine supplementation.

Further published data on this supplement are needed. A daily dose of 3 grams appears to be safe when taken for a 6- to 8-week period.

Amino acids. Marketing of amino acid supplements is heavily targeted to strength athletes and team sport athletes who benefit from building muscle mass. Supporters of amino acid supplementation claim that these products are more readily digested and absorbed than the protein found in foods. This statement is simply false, as your body is well equipped to handle protein from whole foods by secreting a number of enzymes that renders amino acid absorption at a high level of effectiveness. It is true that the timing of your protein intake before and after weight training can facilitate muscle building and recovery. However, full muscle recovery entails following specific nutrition guidelines to obtain enough calories and protein in your daily training diet. Purchasing expensive amino acid supplements simply isn't necessary.

It is also important for you to appreciate that amino acid or protein metabolism is very complex. This process is affected by a variety of factors, including amino acid concentration in the blood, competition with other available amino acids, and the presence of other nutrients. Amino acid mixtures could potentially lead to nutritional imbalances, as an excess of one amino acid may negatively affect the absorption of another.

Amino acid supplement dosing may also be misleading. A bottle listing up to 500 milligrams in a capsule actually contains less than 1 gram of amino acids, whereas only 1 ounce of chicken contains 7,000 milligrams, or 7 grams, of amino acids in the form of whole protein. Clearly, amino acid supplements cannot meet the dosing found in a compact source of natural protein.

The amino acids arginine, lysine, and ornithine are often sold individually or in combination as "legal anabolic compounds" and "recovery agents." Claims surrounding these products include promoting release of growth hormone and a subsequent increase in lean body mass and decrease in body fat. These claims surfaced after two studies found that infusing these amino acids directly into the bloodstream stimulated the release of human growth hormone, which is involved in building muscle tissue.

The effects of oral supplementation on human growth hormone are very questionable. Several well-controlled studies have verified that oral supplementation is not comparable to intravenous infusion. Other studies utilizing oral supplementation have been criticized for their design. One study that provided a large oral dose of arginine and ornithine found a slight increase in growth hormone release. However, this was most likely stimulated by the resistance training rather than the amino acid intake. High oral dosages of these amino acids are also associated with gastrointestinal problems.

Arginine, lysine, and ornithine are available individually or in mixtures in powder or tablet form. Dosages used in several research studies were 2 to 3 grams, and 6 grams may cause gastrointestinal distress. High doses of amino acids may also inhibit absorption of other amino acids. Doses used in several studies are also easily obtained by consuming high protein foods. Use of these supplements or any other amino acid supplement combination is unlikely to be beneficial and they are not recommended.

Ribose. Ribose is hyped as a supplement that can improve muscle recovery, boost energy, enhance endurance, support cardiovascular fitness, and rebuild ATP. A sugar formed from the conversion of glucose, it is considered the starting substance for ATP production and is part of the metabolic pathway that results in ATP resynthesis.

However, published research on the effect of ribose in athletic performance is relatively limited. Ribose did benefit one group of men who suffered from cardiac ischemia, which is not applicable to athletes. Three published studies measured sprint or repeated high-intensity exercise in trained male athletes. Ribose supplementation did not affect power output. Another study that combined the ribose supplements with creatine and glutamine found no improvement in muscular strength and endurance or in body composition.

Ribose is for sale, so safety must be considered. Ribose has not been used for long periods of time, though doses of up to 20 grams appear to be tolerated. Higher doses may result in gastrointestinal side effects. Manufacturer recommendations are often 3 grams prior to and 3 grams after exercise. The patent holder recommends that it be consumed with carbohydrate on an empty stomach. Current data are far too limited to safely recommend a cycling or maintenance dose. In fact, much more data and solid proof are required before this supplement can be recommended.

Glutamine. Glutamine is an amino acid synthesized in the muscle tissue. It is the most abundant amino acid in the body and used as a fuel source by the cells of the immune system. Impaired glutamine status has been associated with the overtrained state in athletes. Overtrained athletes are thought to be more susceptible to upper respiratory tract infections and other infections.

Blood glutamine levels fall during endurance exercise and remain lowered during the recovery phase several hours after exercise. Glutamine depletion is thought to become cumulative if recovery between sessions is inadequate, as overtrained athletes have lower blood glutamine levels. However, adequate daily carbohydrate consumption is thought to possibly be the most effective means for preventing glutamine depletion.

The theory maintains that glutamine supplementation could help prevent the immune problems suffered by overtrained athletes. Research data, however, are not consistent in proving this true. Only one study has reported that supplementation reduced the incidence of infection the week following a heavy exercise session. What is likely is that glutamine supplementation benefits those athletes with a true deficiency and that it is not a general cure for immune system problems.

Another theory regarding glutamine supplementation is that it promotes protein synthesis and helps maintain positive protein balance in the muscle by preventing protein breakdown. Glutamine may also stimulate the synthesis of muscle glycogen.

Obviously glutamine performs some very important functions in the body. However, more research on glutamine supplementation in athletes is needed.

Carnitine. Often promoted as a "metabolic fat burner," carnitine is a nonessential nutrient formed in the liver from two amino acids. Your skeletal muscles contain at least 90 percent of the carnitine in your body. Carnitine is of interest to athletes because it carries fat into the cells to be burned for energy during exercise. If carnitine supplementation did increase fat burning and decrease your body's reliance on glycogen and blood glucose, it could enhance performance.

Carnitine is unlikely to be an effective ergogenic aid, as carnitine supplementation does not appear to increase muscle carnitine levels (as measured by muscle biopsies). Glycogen sparing with carnitine supplementation was also not found in the studies conducted on its use. Only one study found a slight increase in muscle carnitine content after supplementation with 2 grams daily. Other studies found no improvements in exercise performance with carnitine supplementation. Two studies that did find a positive performance effect have been criticized for their methodology and design.

Carnitine supplementation appears to be safe if you consume the L-carnitine form of the nutrient only. DL-carnitine can be toxic as it depletes L-carnitine and may lead to a deficiency. A 2- to 4-gram daily dose can be consumed for one month, though 1- to 2-gram doses have been taken for 6 months.

Chromium. Chromium is a trace mineral, often marketed as a legal alternative to anabolic steroids and human growth hormone. Scientists have long known that chromium enhances the effects of the hormone insulin, which regulates glucose metabolism. Adults with impaired glucose regulation have been measured to have positive responses with chromium supplementation. Insulin also promotes the uptake of amino acids into muscle cells and regulates protein metabolism. This protein-building function has linked chromium to an increase in muscle mass.

Proponents of chromium supplementation for athletes maintain that many are chromium-deficient and that a supplement would improve protein building. Other proponents believe that high chromium doses could stimulate greater than normal muscle building. It has not been firmly established that athletes are chromium-deficient; however, the North American diet is high in refined grains, which may trigger a higher release of insulin and require more chromium in the diet than is normally consumed.

Studies on chromium supplementation have produced mixed but mostly negative results. The more recent and better-designed studies monitored and controlled for exercise training and carefully measured body composition. These studies found no significant gains in muscle mass with chromium supplementation. Earlier studies, which showed some positive results, were not as carefully controlled. Higher doses of chromium in several studies have also not shown significant gains in muscle mass.

With high sales of chromium picolinate and large doses recommended by manufacturers, safety concerns regarding chromium supplementation have been raised. There is not much long-term data on chromium doses beyond 200 micrograms. Because chromium is a mineral, concern has been raised about large chronic doses. Minerals often compete with one another for absorption, and one study did find that iron status was compromised with chromium supplementation.

Clearly adequate chromium intake is important. Especially good sources are whole-grain breads and cereals, mushrooms, asparagus, apples, raisins, cocoa, peanuts, peanut butter, and prunes. Various sports nutrition supplements such as recovery drinks and bars are often supplemented with chromium, and many regular multivitamin–mineral supplements also contain it. Try not to exceed 200 micrograms daily from supplemental sources. Most diets likely do not exceed 50 micrograms of chromium daily.

Overall, chromium's ability to build muscle mass in athletes appears highly doubtful. Supplementation in safe doses is only appropriate to correct a deficiency and compensate for an inadequate diet.

Pyruvate. Pyruvate is commonly sold as DHAP, which is a combination of dihydroxyacetone and pyruvate. This supplement is promoted to improve endurance exercise, promote fat loss, and increase muscle mass.

Studies that have tested pyruvate on endurance performance need to be put in perspective. These studies used a small number of untrained subjects exercising at moderate intensity and may not have much relevance to team sport athletes. In addition, several of the study protocols used 25 grams of pyruvate combined with 75 grams of dihydroxyacetone. Many commercial preparations contain much smaller doses. However, these studies did measure an increase in endurance with the supplement.

Pyruvate does not appear to have much validity as a fat burner, either. One often-quoted study restricted participants to a 1,000-calorie diet daily and no activity. It would be impractical and incorrect to apply these data to an athlete participating in team sports.

Prohormones. Prohormones are widely sold as dietary supplements and currently banned by the International Olympic Committee (IOC) and U.S. Antidoping and other sport governing bodies. These products include the "andro" and the "nor" prohormones. Andro products, namely androstenedione, are testosterone precursors, and they transform to this hormone in the body. Other androgenic products include androstenediol and dehydroepiandrosterone (DHEA). Nor products are precursors to the steroid nortestosterone (nandrolone), which is similar in structure to testosterone. Available nor prohormones are 19-norandrostenediol and 19-norandrostenedione. These nor products break down to the same metabolites used to detect nandrolone usage. Andro prohormones may lead to an elevated testosterone/epitestosterone ratio. All of these substances carry the risk of a positive drug test and potential negative side effects.

Prohormones are easily purchased in the United States and over the Internet because they are classified as dietary supplements. Often these supplements are geared toward building muscle, recovering, and "maintaining hormone levels."

Since the late 1990s, a rash of elite athletes have tested positive for the steroid nandrolone. Many of these athletes have claimed that it occurred through inadvertent ingestion of the dietary supplements that contained nor hormones. Athletes can read labels carefully to avoid these banned products, but it is becoming clear that this may not be enough. A study conducted at the UCLA Olympic Laboratory checked urine tests after supplementation with androstenedione and 19-norandrostenedione. As expected, the 19-nor produced nandrolone metabolites exceeding IOC limits. But the results of the andro supplementation were especially concerning. This test actually produced nandrolone metabolites in the urine! At least 20 of 24 positive urine samples exceeded IOC limits. Based on these findings, researchers tested several andro supplements and seven of eight tested capsules contained varying amounts of 19-nor. Researchers speculated that the supplements had been contaminated with 19-nor in the manufacturing process. Many supplement companies use the same equipment to blend, encapsulate, and bottle both prohormone and nonprohormone products. Quality control is entrusted to supplement companies.

Other than inadvertently testing positive, some of these prohormones may carry unwanted side effects. One study that supplemented with andro did not find higher testosterone levels or increased muscle strength but actually an increase in blood estrogen and reduction in the good HDL cholesterol in male subjects. These side effects could result in potentially serious health effects. A second study tested andro combined with an herbal product designed to decrease estrogen production. The estrogenic profile was not reduced from the herbal supplements despite claims from the manufacturer.

Of course, you should not take prohormones because they are illegal. But read labels carefully to ensure that they are not inadvertently consumed in any products that you purchase, and beware that cross-contamination is a real concern. It may be prudent to purchase supplements from companies that do not.

Weight Loss Supplements

Weight loss supplements are surrounded by strong claims such as promises to speed up metabolism, burn fat, and decrease appetite. While several ingredients found in weight loss supplements are legal (and ineffective), some weight supplements are banned substances and may be dangerous to use.

Until 2004, the most widely purchased weight loss supplement was ephedra. Because it was the supplement with the highest incidence of reported side effects, the FDA has also banned this substance. Ephedra, also known as ephedrine or ma huang, stimulates the central nervous system and improves appetite control. However, because of its stimulant nature, reported side effects include nervousness, headache, heart palpitations, dizziness, insomnia, and anxiety. Prior to the FDA ban, ephedra was also a banned substance in sport, and its use will result in a positive test.

Another banned weight loss supplement with serious safety concerns is phenylpropanolamine (PPA), also known as norephedrine. This product claims to suppress appetite and stimulate metabolism. However, it can also increase the risk of bleeding and stroke, and its safety risks far outweigh its effectiveness. The FDA has warned consumers to stop use of a product that contained PPA. In addition to PPA, this dietary weight loss supplement also contained caffeine, another herb called yohimbine, and diiodothyronine, a form of thyroid hormone. The FDA received multiple reports of liver injury or liver failure with use of this product over a 2-week to 3-month period.

Many weight loss supplements are currently marketed as being ephedra-free. However, these supplements may also contain banned products such as citrus aurantium or bitter orange, which is banned by both the NCAA and the IOC, and pseudoephedrine, which is also banned by the IOC. Many other ingredients in weight loss supplements lack a solid research backing. Some weight loss supplement ingredients that you should avoid include caffeine, cola nut, ginseng, and willow bark. Many of these supplements may contain high amounts of caffeine and be strong stimulants, just like ephedra, and can produce potentially dangerous side effects.

Ergogenic Aids for Training
Caffeine

One of the oldest known drugs, caffeine belongs to a group of compounds known as methyl-xanthines. Caffeine is found naturally in coffee beans, tea leaves, cocoa beans, and cola nuts. Caffeine-containing foods are a natural part of many athletes' diets from coffee, tea, chocolate, and soft drinks. Many of these products provide 30 to 100 milligrams per serving.

Although it appears that caffeine does provide some muscle glycogen-sparing effects, this impact appears to be limited to the first 15 to 20 minutes of exercise. Researchers are not certain exactly how caffeine produces this effect. The classic theory is that caffeine elevates free fatty acids in the blood, which exercising muscles use for energy, while conserving muscle glycogen. Caffeine may also impact the enzyme that breaks down glycogen. Besides sparing glycogen, caffeine also stimulates the central nervous system (increasing alertness), blood circulation, and heart function and releases epinephrine, all which could enhance a variety of performance-related functions. Caffeine also stimulates calcium release from the muscle, which triggers muscular contraction.

Recent, well-designed studies using elite athletes have found that caffeine can effectively enhance performance when consumed in relatively low amounts. Doses as low as 1.5 to 2.0 milligrams per pound (3.3 to 4.4 milligram/kilogram) of weight are effective. The optimal dose appears to be at 2.25 to 2.7 milligrams per pound (5 to 6 milligrams/kilogram). Consuming higher caffeine amounts provides no additional performance benefits and may result in adverse side effects such as rapid heart rate, nervousness, and gastrointestinal discomfort. Most studies have had subjects ingest caffeine 1 hour prior to exercise.

It is important to appreciate that not all athletes react to caffeine in a similar manner. Some individuals may not have a performance response to caffeine, whereas others may not respond to caffeine with improved performance. Caffeine's diuretic effect has long been debated, but it appears that it is essentially insignificant. Studies indicate that caffeine does not increase urine output during exercise. Athletes who wish to use caffeine as an ergogenic aid during competition should experiment during training. The positive effects of caffeine during intermittent high-intensity exercise and power exercise are less defined due to limited data.

MCT Oil

Available for clinical use for several years, MCTs have been promoted to athletes for some time. Because of their smaller size (compared to long-chain triglycerides), MCTs empty from the stomach more quickly and are more easily absorbed. In fact, they are absorbed as quickly as glucose and transported to the liver where they are metabolized. Their ergogenic benefit would result in providing quick fuel during exercise and sparing muscle glycogen during extended training.

Of the several studies conducted with MCT oil, one found a performance improvement, while the others did not. One study did determine that the amount of MCT oil that can be tolerated within the gastrointestinal (GI) tract might be limited. GI symptoms ranging from mild to severe can result. Consuming carbohydrate prior to exercise (as is recommended in this book) could also negate the effects of MCT supplementation. MCT oil is also promoted as a metabolism enhancer and fat burner. However, these claims are not supported by research. Overall, this supplement is not recommended to team sport athletes.

The NCAA and Nutritional Supplements

The NCAA currently has a policy regarding sports nutrition supplements that it is not permissible for an institution to provide any nutritional supplements/ingredients to student athletes unless it is a non-muscle-building product and is included in one of the four classes of permissible supplements. Permissible supplements include vitamins and minerals, energy bars, calorie replacements drinks, and electrolyte replacements drinks. A listing of nonpermissible supplements include amino acids, chrysin, condroitin, creatine and creatine-containing compounds, ginseng, glucosamine, glycerol, HMB, L-carnitine, melatonin, Pos-2, protein powders, and tribulus. However, a supplement that contains protein is permissible if it does not contain more than 30 percent of its calories from protein and falls under one of the four permissible categories.

The NCAA is concerned with the lack of quality control in the production and manufacture of nutritional supplements. Supplements geared toward muscle building have been found to be contaminated with substances currently on the NCAA banned drug list. In one study funded by the International Olympic Committee, approximately 15 percent of 600 over-the-counter supplements were found to contain nonlabeled ingredients that could result in a positive doping test. The NCAA promotes the superiority of a well-balanced diet over nutritional supplements and is concerned about the long-term safety of some of these products.

Currently, student athletes wishing to take muscle-building supplements must obtain them on their own. Athletes still require sound nutrition advice from qualified sports nutritionists and information on the scientific data behind these products, rather than advertising claims and professional athlete endorsement. It is not worth risking eligibility to take products that may offer no real benefit beyond nutritional strategies of adequate calorie and protein intake and optimal nutrient timing.

The NCAA encourages students to refer to the Resource Exchange Center (REC), which is sponsored by the National Center for Drug Free Sport, at www.drugfreesport.com/rec.

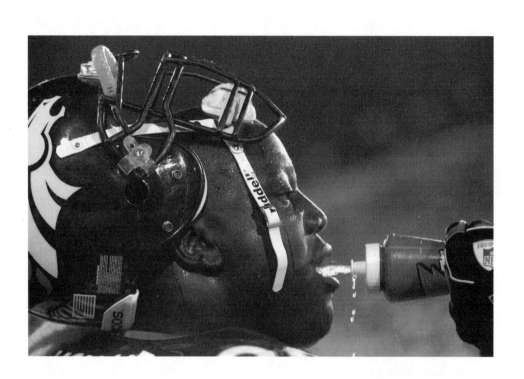

CHAPTER 7

EATING FOR PERFORMANCE AND COMPETITION

What you eat and when you eat are of the utmost importance for the team sport athlete. Recent sports nutrition research has focused on the importance of optimal nutrient timing for improving the quality of training and preparing for competition. In this chapter, we'll consider nutritional concerns before, during, and after competition as well as for the most effective training sessions.

NUTRITION BEFORE TRAINING AND COMPETITION

Ideally, you will consume a training and recovery diet designed to take you in top nutritional form from one team practice or weight-training session to the next. However, real life can sometimes (or perhaps often) get in the way of recharging your fuel stores to the optimal levels required for quality training. A hectic training schedule, especially when combined with work or school, often leaves little time for eating, let alone preparing meals. For some team sport athletes, multiple daily training sessions and other life commitments often result in brief windows of time during which the recommended amount of fuels must be quickly consumed. Even with the most optimal training diet, paying attention to the foods and fluids you consume in the 4-hour period before training can improve your performance. Focusing on the fuel consumed in the several days or 24 hours before competition can also significantly impact the quality of your game.

Team sport athletes also have various options regarding the performance-enhancing fluids and sports nutrition supplements that can be consumed during practice and competition. During training and competition, team sport players want to maximize power, speed, agility, and the skills necessary to perform their sport. These skills require ample body stores of carbohydrate and fluid. Mental sharpness during and especially at the end of a game is also an important consideration for team sport athletes.

When training for your sport, the longer and harder your training session, the greater the risk of developing glycogen depletion and dehydration. Remember that your full supply of glycogen stores provide anywhere from 1,400 to 1,800 calories worth of fuel. At moderate to high intensities, you burn through this fuel in less than 90 minutes. During intermittent training at high intensities, you can burn through this fuel even more quickly and have significant glycogen depletion in under 1 hour. Once you experience muscle glycogen depletion, fatigue sets in as you cannot respond to the demands of your training. Even with plenty of fat stores still remaining, you may need to decrease your exercise intensity, or you may not even be able to complete the training session. Your fat stores cannot supply fuel quickly enough to sustain the high intensities seen in team sport training, and consequently your muscle fibers don't receive the fuel needed to contract during exercise.

Blood glucose, maintained by your liver glycogen stores, is also your brain's only fuel source. When you run low on blood glucose, you cannot focus on the exercise task at hand. You may experience light-headedness, poor concentration, and irritability and not perform the skills for your sports as easily or precisely. Exercise will seem much harder, and coordination will suffer. Your judgment may also become impaired and affect your technique, an all-important consideration for all team sports. You may also have to slow down considerably or stop exercise altogether as the blood glucose supplied by your liver is also an important fuel source for your muscles when they become depleted of glycogen.

While glycogen depletion can become a significant factor in limiting performance at moderate to high intensities, other body nutrient stores may also become depleted. Fluid depletion or dehydration is also an important concern and can impede your training efforts. Dehydration can slow down high-intensity exercise efforts, impair your mental concentration, decrease muscular endurance, and result in overheating, possibly to dangerous levels. Depending on environmental conditions, the event, and the individual athlete, significant electrolyte depletion can also occur and stop your training in its tracks. Of particular concern is hot-weather training or two-a-day practices before an athlete has become acclimated to warmer weather. Significant depletion of electrolytes, particularly sodium, can occur during these practices, so you need specific nutritional strategies to prevent performance-limiting or even life-threatening symptoms.

Team sport athletes who want to complete their training program or compete at their best benefit from several preexercise nutrition strategies designed to minimize the fuel, fluid, and electrolyte depletion that can occur during high-intensity intermittent exercise. Making the most of specific food and fluid choices before training or competition offers several important performance advantages:

- Starting training or competition with optimal fluid levels to help delay or minimize dehydration
- Refilling liver glycogen stores and decreasing risk of developing hypoglycemia during exercise
- Topping off muscle glycogen stores and delaying glycogen depletion while training and competing
- Providing fuel and fluid during the early part of exercise
- Settling your stomach and preventing hunger pains during training and competition
- Providing a psychological edge and comfort level particularly during competition

Fueling Up before Exercise

Clearly, stocking up on your liver and muscle glycogen stores before exercise is essential prior to demanding training sessions. Nutritional strategies recommended before exercise vary depending on how close to training or competition you need or have to eat. You may carefully time your meals prior to competition, yet your school, work, or practice schedule may dictate when you need to eat before practice. For the sports of baseball and football, preexercise eating may simply be a matter of the foods and fluids that work best from a tolerance and psychological perspective, as well as providing high-quality fuel.

Preexercise eating starting on a rest day before a soccer match, basketball game, or hockey game can significantly fuel up the athlete for the energy drain ahead. Training, of course, is also your dress rehearsal for competition. Knowing what you tolerate and like right before a hard practice means that you will have ironed out these important details for the day of competition. Proper planning and eating ensures you have no unexpected surprises that result in your spending the day coping with unpleasant gastrointestinal symptoms, rather than performing your best on game day.

Nutritional strategies leading up to the competition are especially important. The guidelines reviewed here for competition nutrition can also be applied to pretraining eating. Of course, prior to competition, you want to be especially careful of your tolerances, choices, and portions.

The Day before the Event

Team sport athletes usually do not have the luxury of tapering training several days before competition as you may play several games weekly or practice leading up to competition. However, you may have a rest day or light training day before an important game or match. This time period can recharge not only the athlete mentally but also her body's fuel stores. Keeping up with your energy needs during hard training cycles and during the competition season can be challenging in most team sports, and recharging the batteries the day before competition may be necessary for your best game performance.

Training sessions and competitions can take place in the early morning after liver glycogen stores become 80 percent depleted from the overnight fast. Because liver glycogen is an important source of blood glucose during exercise, exercising in this fasted state can cause an unwanted drop in blood glucose. Having a high-carbohydrate dinner and perhaps even a light snack high in carbohydrate will fill your liver with glycogen the night before, somewhat diminishing the effect of low liver glycogen in the morning. Just make sure that any late-night noshes are easy to digest. Research also indicates that muscle glycogen stores return to normal with 24 hours of rest and a high-carbohydrate diet, if there is no significant muscle damage from training earlier in the week.

The day before and especially the night before competition, you do not want to try any new and unusual foods that could result in gastrointestinal upset. Go to bed comfortably full, not stuffed. Avoid consuming large amounts of protein and fat, which take longer to digest and could push out carbohydrates. Be especially careful to limit fiber-containing foods and gassy foods such as broccoli and beans, and avoid alcohol. Practice having various meals the night before an important morning training session. Make simple meals that can be ordered in most restaurants for when traveling. Pasta dishes low in fat are a common favorite among athletes, but other choices also work well. Try rice-based dishes, stir-fried noodles, baked potatoes, and white breads. You probably want to avoid salads and other raw vegetables and raw fruits the night before an important training session or race.

For your 24-hour rest and glycogen-loading day before important games, here are a few guidelines to consider:

- Consume 3 to 5 grams of carbohydrate per pound of body weight (6 to 8 grams/kilogram) in the 24 hours before competition, with levels generally topping off at about 400 to 500 grams daily for female athletes and 600 to 700 grams daily for male athletes.
- Your calorie needs may decrease in this 24-hour period due to light or no training, but the proportion of carbohydrate from your diet should increase.
- If training is not tapered, be especially diligent with consuming the optimal amount of carbohydrate and calories the day before an important competition.

- Be aware that for every gram of glycogen that you store in your body, you also store up to 3 grams of water. This can result in a weight gain and helps to delay dehydration during the event.
- Light exercise the day before competition keeps your muscle light and can reduce the stiffness that comes with the fluid stored in your muscles from storing high level of glycogen.
- If needed according to your tolerances, emphasize low-fiber and compact carbohydrate sources to minimize gastrointestinal upset and to ensure that you consume the prescribed amounts.

The sidebar below emphasizes some good high-carbohydrate food choices that are also low in fiber. Portions of these foods providing 30-gram carbohydrate portions are also provided. Starches, cereals, and breads are fairly concentrated carbohydrate sources, and fruits and fruit juices are also good sources of carbohydrates. Sports nutrition supplements such as sports bars, gels, concentrated carbohydrate drinks, and liquid meal replacements can also fit nicely into your meal plan.

Preexercise High-Carbohydrate, Low-Fiber Foods

30 Grams of Carbohydrate per Serving

Bagel, 2 oz. (60 g)

Bread, white, 2 slices

Pita pocket, 1.5 rounds

Dinner rolls, 2

English muffin, 1

Muffin, low-fat, low-fiber, 3 oz. (90 g)

Tortillas, 2

Cooked cereal, 1 c. (240 ml)

Apple, 1.5 medium

Applesauce, sweetened, 1/2 c. (120 ml)

Grapefruit, peeled, 1 large

Canned fruit, 1 c. (240 ml)

Cold cereal, low-fiber, 1.5 oz. (45 g)

Graham crackers, 6

Saltines, 8

Rice, cooked, white, 2/3 c. (200 ml)

Pasta, cooked, 1 c. (240 ml)

Pretzels, white flour, 1.5 oz. (45 g)

Potato, baked, no skin, 1 medium

Sweet potato, no skin, 4 oz. (120 g)

Apple juice, 8 oz. (240 ml)

Carrot juice, 10 oz. (300 ml)

Grape juice, 6 oz. (200 ml)

Cranberry juice cocktail, 8 oz. (240 ml)

Milk, skim, 20 oz. (500 ml)

Yogurt with fruit, 1 c. (240 ml)

Having a sound menu plan in mind can lessen any stress associated with making food choices the day before an important competition. You may want to consider having moderate portions of proteins and fats when replenishing carbohydrates on a rest day or light training day. This prevents unneeded calories from being consumed and leaves room for the important carbohydrates. Consuming between-meal snacks can help in reaching the required carbohydrate amounts. The Precompetition High-Carbohydrate Menu sidebar provides a sample menu ranging from 400 to 600 grams of carbohydrate daily. For the lower carbohydrate level, trim or eliminate the snacks on the menu.

Eating before Training or a Game

You will have to experiment in training to determine your favorite foods and fluids to consume before practice, and to especially determine your best choices before compe-

Precompetition High-Carbohydrate Menu

Breakfast
1 c. (240 ml) orange juice
1 c. (240 ml) corn flakes
1 large banana
1 c. (240 ml) skim milk
2 slices toast
1 tsp. (8 ml) margarine
2 tbsp. (40 ml) Jelly
147 g carbohydrate, 750 calories

Snack
6 oz. (200 ml) yogurt with fruit
20 g carbohydrate, 150 calories

Lunch
3 oz. (100 g) of lean turkey
2 slices of white bread
3/4 oz. (20 g) of pretzels
1 large pear
8 oz. (240 ml) apple juice
105 g carbohydrate, 585 calories

Snack
Energy bar
40 g carbohydrate, 200 calories

Dinner
2 c. (480 ml) cooked rice
3 oz. (100 g) ground turkey
1 c. (240 ml) cooked peas
2 slices bread
160 g carbohydrate, 961 calories

Snack
12 oz. (360 ml) frozen yogurt
2 Fig Newtons
102 g carbohydrate, 460 calories

Total: 574 g carbohydrate, 3100 calories

tition. Often your eating schedule for training is dictated by practice times and your work or school schedule. You may thus need to plan meals and snack around various practice sessions, such as in early morning or late afternoon, or a midday game start. Your preexercise eating plan may need to be very specific regarding the timing of meals and snacks in regards to game time, and consuming the proper portions. Based on your chosen timing, you can focus on the proper balance of portions. Table 7.1 offers some timing suggestions.

Three to Four Hours before Exercise

Depending on your race time, personal tolerances, and experience, you should consume a light to large meal in the 3 to 4 hours before practice or competition. Many seasoned athletes have identified this time interval as optimal for prepractice or precompetition eating, as you can achieve a good balance between adequate food consumption and plenty of digestion time. The main focus of this preexercise meal should be to replenish your liver glycogen stores. This valuable fuel falls to low levels overnight, especially if you spent your sleep tossing and turning from precompetition nerves. With the right timing and portions, eating 3 to 4 hours before exercise will provide the following benefits:

- Restore liver glycogen to normal levels.
- Store carbohydrate in the muscle as needed if portions are large enough.
- Have some carbohydrate stored in the gut for absorption and release during exercise.
- Avoid feeling hungry during practice or competition.

The morning of competition, it is especially important to choose foods that you enjoy and tolerate and that also provide both a physiological and psychological edge. For every hour you allow yourself to digest, consume just under half a gram of carbohydrate for every pound that you weigh (approximately 1 gram/kilogram weight). You can consume 2 grams per pound (4 grams/kilogram) of carbohydrates 4 hours before exercise and 1.5 grams per pound (3 grams/kilogram) 3 hours before exercise.

For example, if you decide to eat a larger meal 4 hours before a basketball game or soccer match, you can consume 2 grams of carbohydrate per pound weight (2 grams/kilogram). For a 150-pound athlete, this translates to 300 grams of carbohydrates (and 1,200 calories). It would probably be easiest on your stomach if a good portion of this fairly substantial meal consisted of dense low-fiber foods and some liquid carbohydrate

TABLE 7.1 MEAL TIMING PRIOR TO TRAINING AND COMPETITION

Timing	Carbohydrate/Food Recommendations	Sample Foods	Start Times
Night before	High-carbohydrate meal 300 grams carbohydrate Low in fiber Plenty of fluid	Pasta dishes Rice dishes Lean protein Easy on fat Cooked vegetables	• Essential for early starts • Helpful for any start time
3–4 hours prior	Carbohydrates: 1.5–2 g/lb. wt. (3–4 g/kg) Low-fat proteins Low fat Low fiber Plenty of fluids	150-pound athlete: 225–300 g of carbohydrate Cereals, bread, crackers, milk, yogurt, fruit, juices, jelly, muffins, bagels	For mid-morning starts: • Eat at 7:00 a.m. for 10:00 a.m. start Mid-afternoon starts: • Eat at 10:00 a.m. for 2:00 p.m. start For evening starts: • Eat at 4:00 p.m. for a 7:00 p.m. start after adequate carbohydrate meals
2 hours prior	Carbohydrates: Up to 1.0 g/lb. wt. (2 g/kg) Minimal low-fat protein Low fat and fiber Plenty of fluids	150-pound athlete: 130–150 g carbohydrate Cereals, bread, milk, yogurt, fruit, juices, jelly, crackers meals throughout	For mid-morning starts: • Eat at 8:00 a.m. for 10:00 a.m. start For mid-afternoon start: • Eat at 12:00 noon for 2:00 p.m. start after a large morning breakfast For late starts: • Eat at 6:00 p.m. for 8:00 p.m. start after adequate carbohydrate the day
1 hour prior	Carbohydrates: 0.5 g/lb. wt. (1.0 g/kg) Emphasize liquids Easy-to-digest carbohydrates Avoid protein, fat, and fiber	Sports drinks, concentrated carbohydrate drinks and gels, sports bars, tolerated fruits	For early starts: • Eat at 6:00 a.m. for 8:00 a.m. start For mid-morning starts: • For 10:00 a.m. start, have snack/liquid at 9:00 a.m. in addition to 6:30–7:00 a.m. meal
Immediately prior	Carbohydrates	Sports drinks Energy bars if exercise starts at moderate intensity for at least 30 minutes	For any start time

sources. You can obtain 300 grams of carbohydrate by consuming one large bagel topped with 2 tablespoons (40 ml) of jelly, a fruited yogurt, and 32 ounces of a concentrated sports drink. The small amounts of protein in the yogurt may help keep you full a bit longer. You can also add a bit of peanut butter or cream cheese to your bagel if a small amount of fat is well tolerated. Of course, smaller meals may be only what some athletes tolerate close to exercise, particularly competition. Every athlete needs to iron out their individual tolerances in terms of foods, portions, and timing.

Eating 3 to 4 hours beforehand can be appropriate for several exercise start times. An early morning breakfast can be consumed at 6:00 to 7:00 a.m. for a 9:00 to 10:00 a.m. start time. For a later start time, such as 2:00 p.m., you may want to consume a large breakfast of easily digested foods at 10:00 a.m. Often your pregame meal strategy must include a planned sleeping and wake-up time, both a preexercise meal or snack, and even some food and fluid choices in the hour leading up to a game. Some sample preexercise meals are provided in Table 7.2.

TABLE 7.2 PREEXERCISE HIGH-CARBOHYDRATE, LOW-FAT MEALS

2 slices toast or small bagel
1 large banana
2 tbsp. (40 ml) jelly
8 oz. (240 ml) juice
	1.5 c. (360 ml) concentrated
	   carbohydrate beverage
	
	1 slice of toast
		1 carbohydrate gel
		24 oz. (750 ml) of
		   sports drink

120 g carbohydrate **520 calorie:**	**90 g carbohydrate** **380 calories**	**95 g carbohydrate** **380 calories**

Chicken, 2 oz. (60 g)
Bread, 2 slices
Fruit juice, 16 oz. (480 ml)
Pretzels, 2 oz. (60 g)
Carbohydrate supplement,
   16 oz. (480 ml)
	Pasta, 2 c. (480 ml) cooked
	Marinara sauce, 1 c. (240 ml)
	Bread, 2 slices
	Frozen yogurt, 12 oz. (360 ml)
	Fruit juice, 8 oz. (240 ml)
	Margarine, 2 tsp. (13 ml)
		Pancakes, 4 medium
		Fruit topping, 1/2 c.
		   (120 ml)
		Syrup, 1/2 c. (120 ml)
		Fruit juice, 8 oz.
		   (240 ml)

220 g carbohydrate **1,030 calories**	**235 g carbohydrate** **986 calories**	**270 g carbohydrate** **1,200 calories**

Cooked cereal, 2 c. (480 ml)
Instant breakfast drink,
   1 serving
Banana, 1 large
Orange juice, 8 oz. (240 ml)
Carbohydrate beverage, 24 oz.
   (720 ml)
	Rice, 3 c. cooked (720 ml)
	Cooked vegetables, 1 c. (120 g)
	Shrimp, 4 oz. (120 g)
	Sorbet, 1 c. (240 ml)
	Soft drink, 12 oz. (360 ml)
	Oil, 2 tsp. (14 ml)
	Carbohydrate beverage, 16 oz.
	   (480 ml)
		Fruit smoothie:
		8 oz. yogurt (240 ml)
		8 oz. milk (240 ml)
		8 oz. juice (240 ml)
		1 c. fruit (240 ml)
		
		Bagel, 1 large
		Jam, 2 tbsp. (40 ml)
		Energy bar, 1 whole

300 g carbohydrate **1,410 calories**	**300 g carbohydrate** **1,600 calories**	**225 g carbohydrate** **1,185 calories**

Two Hours before Exercise

Consuming food 3 to 4 hours before exercise may not always be possible due to scheduling and very early start times (rising at 5:00 a.m. for an 8:00 a.m. practice to eat does not sound very appealing). Because of timing constraints, eating 2 hours before training and competition may be your preferred or best timing choice. One good food rule for preexercise eating is the closer to exercise you plan to eat, the smaller the meal consumed. Try to keep your intake of carbohydrate to 1 gram per pound of body weight in this time interval (2 grams/kilogram). A 150-pound athlete could consume 150 grams of carbohydrates or less. With this close meal timing, it is likely even more important that liquid carbohydrate choices are part of your meal. Breakfast shakes, liquid meal replacements, and sports supplements often provide over 50 grams of carbohydrate per serving. A juice smoothie may work well, as do easily digested energy bars.

Eating 2 hours prior to exercise could be good timing for an early or midmorning start. It can also work well for tricky early afternoon start times. Following a large breakfast that is well digested with a small to moderate snack 2 hours before exercise to provide fuel and prevent hunger during competition and training works well for many athletes who plan ahead for afternoon or evening start times.

Eating an Hour before Exercise

A variety of scenarios could necessitate the need for food 30 to 60 minutes prior to exercise. Rising in the extremely early hours of the morning simply to eat food and fuel up for an early start time may not be feasible or desirable. Scheduling may also result in a long time gap between the last meal and the start of a training session, and hunger and limited fuel during training and competition may become a significant issue. It may also be helpful to eat closer to longer training sessions in which the added fuel provides a performance benefit.

From an athlete's perspective, whether or not you consume carbohydrate 30 to 60 minutes prior to exercise needs to be individualized to your tolerances and practice or competition schedule. Deriving a performance benefit from ingesting fuel 30 to 60 minutes prior to exercise is most likely to occur when the carbohydrate you consume replenishes compromised fuel stores. So consider consuming carbohydrate within an hour before exercise if you have not eaten for 4 hours or more or prior to early-morning training when liver glycogen is low. Eating an hour before intense training sessions can also prevent hunger and provide extra calories for team sport athletes who have very high energy requirements.

Some controversy over the years has surfaced in athletic circles regarding carbohydrate consumption in the hour before exercise. The concern was that carbohydrate consumption in the hour before exercise can result in hypoglycemia or a decrease in blood glucose levels during exercise. Many scientific studies have confirmed that consuming carbohydrate in the hour before exercise does not impair performance and can actually *help* performance. These studies, however, used exercise test protocols that mimicked steady-state endurance exercise, not the intermittent exercise of many team sport training programs. What was also interesting about these studies was the individual blood glucose responses seen in subjects. A small number did experience hypoglycemia.

If you are concerned that you are a carbohydrate-sensitive athlete during the 1 hour prior to exercise, you may find a few sensible strategies useful. Consuming a high enough amount of carbohydrates may simply offset any lowered blood glucose levels and hypoglycemic symptoms. Amounts of 70 grams or more seem to maintain blood glucose levels in individuals susceptible to exercise hypoglycemia. Individuals not susceptible to hypoglycemia can consume anywhere from 50 to 100 grams of carbohydrate prior to exercise, depending on what they prefer and what feels comfortable. You can also consider a carbohydrate source with a lower glycemic index, though this often requires the consumption of real foods very close to exercise rather than easily digested sports nutrition products. Common sense would indicate that consuming a carbohydrate beverage or gel might be more practical than chowing down on a big bowl of lentils the hour before exercise. Many of these products, such as gels, bars, and sports drinks, provide anywhere from 30 to 50 grams of carbohydrate per serving. You may choose one of the items or any combination of them in portions that you tolerate.

Regardless of your start time, a precompetition (or pretraining) meal or snack can provide some performance benefit. While the main part of your intake will be carbohydrate, small amounts of protein, and perhaps fat, may be tolerated if appropriately timed. Determine your optimal preexercise meal through experimentation during training, not on race day.

The Glycemic Index

Some athletes may choose to include low- to moderate-glycemic index foods in their prepractice or precompetition meal regardless of the timing. Some athletes believe that incorporating these carbohydrate choices will keep their blood glucose levels steady over the next few hours and through practice and competition. While research regarding pre-exercise eating and low-glycemic foods has not fully supported this belief, choosing low-glycemic foods in the several hours before exercise certainly does not hurt performance.

Athletes who feel that they perform better when consuming low- to moderate-glycemic intake carbohydrates can incorporate these foods into their preexercise meal. As was also discussed in Chapter 1, adding protein and a small amount of fat to a meal can also blunt the glycemic effect of the meal. Small amounts of lean protein and fat can help maintain steady blood glucose levels and prevent hunger during exercise. Athletes should also consider that consuming a carbohydrate source during practice and competition when breaks allow can offset any drops in blood glucose, making the types of carbohydrates that you consume before exercise less important.

Timing and Portions

The bottom line is that you should focus on pregame or prepractice nutrition that is appropriate for your game time start and training schedule. Rest or light training the day before a game provides the opportune strategy for replenishing muscle glycogen stores to full levels that provide fuel during exercise. On game day, you can decide on the prerace meal timing that best suits your preferences and tolerances. Specific amounts of carbohydrate consumed at set times prior to exercise have been shown to enhance performance by increasing liver glycogen stores and providing fuel during the early part of exercise.

Athletes who feel that they are sensitive to consuming carbohydrates in the hour before exercise can make sure that they ingest over 70 grams of carbohydrates to offset any hypoglycemia. Your best strategy is to plan ahead and know what size meals to consume at what times leading up to training or competition.

Hydration before Exercise

Dehydration is one of the most significant problems that occurs during practice and competition, and it can put a halt to your team training long before you feel the effects of fuel depletion. Despite your best attempts to drink adequately during practice and competition, you are unlikely to match 100 percent of your fluid losses. Depending on your sport, you may have limited opportunities to drink fluids. Significant dehydration can especially occur in team sport athletes who have very high sweat rates, when there is little opportunity to drink during practice or games, or when environmental conditions are extreme.

Just as strategies to maximize muscle glycogen stores offer a performance advantage, so are techniques for maximizing fluid stores before exercise. But hyperhydrating is not considered to be as optimal as drinking during exercise to replace fluid losses. However, if you anticipate that it will be difficult to drink during training and especially during competition due to limited fluid availability and lack of opportunities to drink, prehydrating could be a very practical move on your part. Even when training practices allow time to replenish fluids and the athlete is consciously making the effort to hydrate during exercise, fluid intake typically replaces only about 80 percent of sweat losses.

At all costs, avoid starting practice or a game in the dehydrated state. Your goal during practice and competition is to keep up as much as possible with fluid losses, so starting out dehydrated already puts you behind on your fluid intake efforts. One of the best gauges of your hydration efforts during exercise is to weigh yourself before and after training. Every pound (0.45 kilogram) of weight lost represents 16 ounces (480 milliliters) of fluid loss. However, to compensate for urine losses when rehydrating, you should consume 20 to 24 ounces (600 to 720 milliliters) of fluid for every pound (0.45 kilogram) decrease in weight. Techniques for drinking more during exercise will be discussed later in this chapter.

It is important to plan ahead and begin your next training session as well hydrated as possible. To prepare for the next day's training, consume 16 ounces (480 milliliters) of fluid before bedtime. Your early-morning intake should then consist of 16 to 24 ounces (480 to 720 milliliters) of caffeine-free fluid. Prior to training, you should attempt to consume 8 to 10 ounces (240 to 300 milliliters) of fluid every hour during the day. About one hour before exercise, you can hyperhydrate by consuming 16 to 32 ounces (480 to 960 milliliters) of fluid. At this time, fluids providing carbohydrates and small amounts of sodium, such as sports drinks, are likely to be the best choice and may have some hydration advantages over water. You can fill your fluid stores further by drinking another 8 to 16 ounces (240 to 480 milliliters) 20 minutes prior to training.

Similar guidelines can be followed prior to competition, although you may decide to stop drinking 30 minutes prior to the game. This strategy should allow you to empty your bladder if needed and not compromise your hydration status if you have consumed adequate fluid in the hours leading up to competition.

In summary, you will be adequately hydrated if you focus on these simple guidelines:

- Consume 16 ounces (480 milliliters) of fluid before bedtime.
- Consume 8 to 10 ounces (240 to 300 milliliters) of fluid every 1 to 2 hours during the day.
- Prehydrate 1 hour before exercise by consuming 16 to 32 ounces (480 to 960 milliliters) of fluid.

- Consume another 8 to 16 ounces (240 to 480 milliliters) 20 minutes prior to exercise if possible.

NUTRITION DURING TRAINING AND COMPETITION

Athletes in team sports can significantly drain fluid stores, electrolytes, and carbohydrate stores during moderate- to high-intensity training. That's why consuming adequate fluid, carbohydrate, and electrolytes during training and competition is beneficial. This practice can bring you these benefits:

- Delays and minimizes dehydration
- Maintains blood glucose levels
- Offsets muscle and liver glycogen depletion
- Fuels your brain
- Offsets electrolyte losses, particularly sodium

Fluid Requirements

As an athlete participating in team sports, your performance during both training and competition is greatly affected by your hydration levels. Dehydration can easily develop during practice, both indoors and outdoors, and negatively affect your performance long before fuel depletion drains your efforts. For example, football players that begin practices in the hot months of summer need to acclimate and replace fluid losses carefully to prevent such side effects as a rise in body temperature, increased heart rate, and the extreme case of heat stroke. Even losing as little as 1 to 2 percent of body weight, or 2 to 3.5 pounds (1 to 1.5 kilograms) during practice from fluid loss can slow down your training efforts both indoors and outdoors; of course, it can be a performance-limiting factor during competition, too.

It is also important for a team sport athlete to appreciate that dehydration can affect their mental concentration and ability to perform the skills required for their sport. Clearly dehydration does not support your top performance if it affects movement control, decision making, and concentration.

Moderate to severe dehydration in which 3 to 4 percent of body weight is lost can also result in gastrointestinal upset. Consequently, when you make the effort to drink more after you have become dehydrated, your rehydration efforts can result in stomach discomfort.

The longer and harder the practice, the greater the risk that sweat losses can impair your performance. Your sweat losses are also affected by your genetic makeup, fitness level, and degree of acclimatization to heat; the environmental temperature in which you are training; and the amount and type of clothing that you are wearing. You will also have greater sweat losses in hot and humid weather, particularly before you are fully acclimated. There are many good reasons for preventing dehydration, including avoiding the following detrimental physiological effects of dehydration:

- Increased heart rate
- Lowered body temperature
- Decreased blood volume
- Increased perception of effort
- Compromised mental concentration
- Compromised fine-motor skills
- Delayed stomach emptying of fluids
- Increased risk of GI upset

Because sweat losses can vary greatly from athlete to athlete, sweat loss averages can range from 1 to 1.5 quarts (approximately 1 to 1.5 liters) per hour and even reach 2 to 3 quarts (approximately 2 to 3 liters) per hour during hot weather and demanding training sessions and competition. A high level of fitness also promotes a more efficient sweat response, and the better trained you are, the more you will sweat. Athletes cannot train themselves to adapt to, or to tolerate dehydration; it is best prevented or minimized as much as possible.

Just as there is much individual variability in sweat rates among athletes, there is also much variability in efforts to replace fluids during exercise. While your ideal goal is to match your fluid intake to your fluid losses, most athletes fall short and replace only 50 to 80 percent of their fluid losses during practice sessions. Even with strong efforts to match your fluid losses, your GI system may only be able to absorb a certain volume of fluid per hour. Often, whether or not you can maintain adequate hydration status during exercise is a matter of practicality rather than scientific theory. Consuming the recommended amounts can be challenging due to your practice schedule, logistics in obtaining fluids when training and competing, limited opportunities to drink, availability of fluids, taste preferences, and GI tolerances. Fluid replacement efforts in team sports are also greatly affected by the position played and scheduled breaks during training. Of course, during competition, players must make the most of any opportunities to drink, such as during breaks in play, time off the field or court, quarter or halftime breaks, or breaks between periods.

Clearly you need to assess the drinking opportunities and fluid availability for your own sport and practice sessions. You may choose to pack some of your own fluids for training and competition, or request that the coaching staff and trainer have specific products on hand. Once the proper products are available, behaviors and practices that promote adequate fluid consumption are up to the athlete. Regardless of how they reach you, you are more likely to consume fluids that taste good and are the right temperature. Commercial sports drinks often appeal to hot and sweaty athletes. In addition to their flavor, which may stimulate you to drink more, sports drinks are a source of fuel and electrolytes in the form of carbohydrate and sodium chloride. Here are some hydration strategies designed to maximize your fluid intake during practice:

Consume 4 to 8 ounces (120–240 ml) of fluid during every 15 to 20 minutes of exercise. Practice, practice, practice. Try to drink at regular intervals, and take big gulps as larger volumes empty from your stomach more quickly. Cooler fluids are more appealing and should assist you in drinking a greater volume.

Start drinking early. This strategy is particularly important if breaks in practice occur at greater time intervals. Even if you start exercise adequately hydrated, it does not pay to practice "catch-up" drinking. Once you are dehydrated, fluids will empty from your stomach more slowly. In extreme situations, dehydration may lead to GI upset, including a bloated stomach. Because fluids are emptying slowly, you will feel dehydrated (you are dehydrated) and may compensate by attempting to drink more, further aggravating any stomach upset.

Monitor your sweat rates during training. It is important that you note the rate at which you lose fluid during different types of training sessions and environmental conditions. Practice drinking during training sessions that simulate competition conditions. Monitor your weight before and after exercise to assess how effectively you replace fluids. The sidebar, Estimating Fluid Lost, outlines some strategies for determining your own specific fluid losses.

Develop a taste for various sports drinks. While you may discover that you have a favorite sports drink brand and flavor that you can consume during training, practice with the products and flavors that are also available to you during competition and get accustomed to their taste and feel during training. This allows for greater flexibility and improved drinking on competition day. Bring your own products if that works with the team plan.

Coaches and trainers should provide the necessary support for athletes to maintain good hydration levels. Fluid should be nearby and easily accessible. Players should have their own individual squeeze bottle to drink from during practice. Fluids can be frozen the night before and thawed during practice to keep fluid temperature cool for hot outdoor practices. Athletes should be encouraged to drink on a schedule and given opportunities to drink during practice.

Monitor your hydration status by checking urine volume and color. Athletes should empty several full bladders of urine daily. The lighter the color of your urine, the better your hydration levels. Dark urine suggests that you may be dehydrated.

Prehydrate before practice and rehydrate after practice. Despite all your good intentions, behavior strategies, and support from the coaching and training staff, it is best if you start every practice session well hydrated. This ensures that you can minimize your fluid losses during practice. Rehydrating also allows you to start the next training session with optimal fluid levels.

Estimating Fluid Losses

This technique for estimating fluid losses is fairly accurate, especially in warmer-weather training. Check your sweat losses for various types of training sessions, whether indoor or outdoor training with your teammates or weight-training sessions, to better estimate and meet your sweat losses.

1. Check your weight before and after training and calculate your weight loss.

160–158 lb. (73–72 kg)

2-lb. weight loss during training (0.9 kg)

2. Know the amount of fluid that you consumed during the training session. Fifteen oz. of fluid weighs about 1 pound (an easier estimate is 1,000-ml fluid equals 1.0 kg body weight). You can also weigh the bottle before and after your training session to determine the actual weight of the fluid you consumed during training.

Let's say you consume 60 oz. (1,800 ml) of fluid during a 2-hour practice. This fluid weighs 4 lb. (1.8 kg).

3. Add the weight you lost with the weight of the fluid you consumed.

2-lb. weight loss during training, plus you consumed 4 lb. of fluid during training.

This equals 6 lb. of fluid lost.

(0.9 + 1.8 kg = 2.7 kg)

4. 6 lb. equals 90 oz. fluid divided by 2 hours = 45 oz. per hour for sweat losses.

(2.7 kg equals 2,700 ml fluid divided by 2 hours = 1,350 ml/hr)

In this example the athlete sweats about 45 oz. or 5.5 c. of fluid per hour (1,350 ml). Sweat rates can vary from 24 oz. or 3 c. of fluid per hour (720 ml) to 80 oz. or 10 c. (2,500 ml or more) per hour.

Fuel Requirements

Due to the high-intensity, intermittent nature of longer training sessions seen in team sports, especially basketball, hockey, and soccer, fuel replacement as well as fluid replacement during practice and competition are also important considerations. Carbohydrate consumed during exercise can maintain blood glucose levels and provide fuel to glycogen-depleted muscles. Carbohydrate consumption may also provide the opportunity for glucose to be stored in less active muscle fibers during rest periods. For example, when you exercise at a low intensity, muscle fibers that fuel higher-intensity efforts may be replenished.

Your brain may also benefit from carbohydrate intake during longer practice sessions and hard competition as consuming only water during high-intensity exercise decreases blood glucose levels. Because your brain counts on glucose for fuel, this will result in some negative central nervous system effects. Having adequate blood glucose to fuel your brain helps you to maintain the high level of skill that you require for training and competing in your sport. Carbohydrate intake can prevent or reverse symptoms of glucose deprivation such as fatigue, perception of increased effort, and poor coordination. Carbohydrate is also thought to prevent an increase in brain serotonin levels that can occur during prolonged exercise. Serotonin produces feelings of drowsiness and fatigue in the brain.

Much of the research on carbohydrate intake during exercise has centered on endurance sports and continuous activity. But studies also demonstrate that besides providing performance benefits for exercise lasting about 90 minutes and fueling your brain, carbohydrate may also improve performance during high-intensity exercise lasting about 60 minutes. Several studies over the past decade measured the performance effects of consuming a sports drink during exercise performed at 80 to 90 percent VO_2max and lasting about 1 hour. Results indicated that the sports drink provided a performance benefit.

In addition to these studies looking at endurance exercise of 60-minute duration or greater, several additional studies measured the performance effects on intermittent high-intensity exercise lasting about 1 hour, more closely matching the type of training conducted for team sports. Consuming a sports drink at rest intervals allowed the activity to continue longer. Researchers speculated that the carbohydrate drinks provided the fast-twitch muscle fibers, which operate at higher intensities, some fuel to work with at rest intervals between high-intensity efforts. More research of this type is needed, but for now many players in team sports have clearly enhanced performance by consuming both fluid and carbohydrate during practice since the energy demands of training reduce muscle glycogen and fluid reserves.

Sports Drinks

Both fluid and carbohydrate are required during moderate- and high-intensity practices that last over 1 hour. In order for your body to receive both carbohydrate and fluid in a timely and well-tolerated manner, several steps in the digestion and absorption of sports drinks must be considered. First, when you consume these nutrients, they must empty as quickly as possible from your stomach. Next, they enter your small intestine, where they must be absorbed as quickly as possible and then enter the bloodstream. Carbohydrate is then available as fuel for your exercising muscles, and the fluid maintains your blood volume and offsets sweat losses.

In an effort to provide the most scientifically sound formulation, sports drink research has looked at each one of these steps to see where the flow may actually slow down or speed up. If your sports drink gets bogged down in any one of the steps, it takes the fluid and carbohydrate that much longer to reach you. Consequently, the sports drink is not as performance enhancing. It has been determined that the two factors that determine how quickly a sports drink leaves your stomach are the volume of fluid in your stomach and the concentration of the carbohydrate in the drink.

Concentration

The greater the carbohydrate concentration of the fluid, the longer it takes to empty from your stomach. Research has determined that carbohydrate solutions of about 4 to 8 percent concentration empty from your stomach very efficiently and deliver an optimal balance of both carbohydrate and fluid. Conveniently, most sports drinks fall into this range, at about 6 to 8 percent carbohydrate. This drink concentration allows fluid to reach your bloodstream pretty much as quickly as water, but it still delivers performance-boosting carbohydrates at a rate that is tolerated when you exercise. Drinks of these concentrations seem to be well tolerated by most athletes, and tolerance to these products can also improve with practice. In contrast, drinks of 10 to 12 percent concentration, such as soft drinks and fruit juice, are emptied more slowly from the stomach, though they do provide carbohydrates and energy. However, these drinks are not as hydrating and should be diluted if they are consumed during exercise.

Volume

Volume affects the degree of stomach distention and consequently gastric emptying. Increased stomach distention will result in liquids emptying from your stomach more quickly, with about 50 percent of stomach contents being emptied every 10 minutes. To maximize emptying, try to start exercise with a comfortably full stomach and drink at regular intervals of about 10 to 15 minutes if possible. How much fluid an athlete can empty from his stomach is highly variable. However, emptying rates of 24 to 40 ounces, or 3 to 5 cups (720 to 1,200 milliliters), per hour are common. The most important strategy is to consume fluid whenever the opportunity presents itself. Aim to consume one 20-ounce (600-milliliter) squeeze bottle for every hour of practice. Refill your bottle as needed depending on the duration of the practice session.

Intestinal Absorption

Studies measuring intestinal absorption rates have determined that sports drink solutions are as readily absorbed as water. Different forms of carbohydrates are absorbed across the intestinal wall, utilizing various transport mechanisms. Again, avoid higher-concentration drinks, as they draw water into the intestinal tract before being absorbed.

The wide variety of sports drinks products available provides a wide variety of carbohydrate sources. These include glucose polymers (maltodexterin), glucose, sucrose, and fructose. Many drinks have a mix, allowing various carbohydrate types to be transported simultaneously. These carbohydrate mixes all appear to have a moderate to high glycemic index, handy for quickly raising blood glucose levels and giving you a quick burst of both brain power and energy when consumed.

Glucose polymers do not seem to offer any absorption advantages over glucose, but they are popular because they have a milder rather than overly sweet taste. Fructose is the only beverage not used in high amounts or solely in a sports beverage. Large amounts of fructose are not well absorbed and can lead to GI upset. But drinks that contain some fructose should provide easily tolerated concentrations and additional flavor.

More recently, some sports drinks have been surrounded by claims concerning the drink's effect on blood glucose levels, and insulin, in relation to the type of carbohydrate in the drink and the glycemic index of the product. While there is virtually no research comparing the performance effects of sports drinks with various glycemic index levels, the high glycemic effect of most sports drinks would quickly raise blood glucose levels and provide quick fuel for the athlete during training and competition. The number of sports drinks with a lower glycemic index is limited, the glycemic index of many sports drinks is not available, and research is lacking in just how the glycemic index of a drink affects training and performance. Just as has been measured with various food choices, the glycemic index of a carbohydrate source or drink is not necessarily related to whether or not the carbohydrate source is a "simple" or "complex" carbohydrate. Maltodrextin, which is often promoted as a complex carbohydrate source, has a high glycemic index, while the simple sugar fructose has a very low glycemic index. Often, the choice of a sports drink comes down to personal tolerances and preferences, and what drink is available to the athlete and team. Appendix C provides a listing of the glycemic index of various sports drinks and various carbohydrate sources that are currently available.

Recently, some sports drinks containing protein have entered the market. Research regarding protein-containing sports drinks and performance in team sports is limited. More well-designed research studies and data are needed regarding these products.

Amount and Timing of Carbohydrate

Basically the amounts of sports drinks you consume should mimic the water intake guidelines described previously, or about 4 to 8 ounces (120 to 240 milliliters) every 15 to 20 minutes. Drinking at regular intervals can usually take place during practice, but competition does not always present as many opportunities to drink. Performance benefits begin when about 30 grams of carbohydrate per hour is delivered. However, 50 to 60 grams may be optimal to meet fuel needs during higher-intensity exercise and after some muscle glycogen depletion has occurred. Every athlete has his or her own personal tolerances and carbohydrate requirements that maintain optimal energy levels during practice.

Check labels and instructions of your favorite sports drinks. Then determine what volume you would need to consume in an hour to obtain 30 to 60 grams of carbohydrate. Experiment to determine what fluid consumption volume best enhances your performance and maintains adequate hydration levels. As far as timing is concerned, large single feedings and smaller, regular intakes of a sports drink are both beneficial. Basically, drink whenever possible as the nature of your practice permits or during specific breaks during competition. Quarter and halftimes, or breaks between periods, present the best times to consume sports drinks. Players can also refuel and rehydrate on the bench by consuming the fluid volumes tolerated. Consuming carbohydrate after depletion has set in can help, but consuming the carbohydrates early on in order to prevent fatigue is smart and prudent. Don't wait until the signs and symptoms of a low fuel tank register before consuming your carbohydrate sports drink.

Form of Carbohydrate

In addition to liquid carbohydrate, semiliquid and solid carbohydrate sports supplements are also consumed by athletes before, during, and after exercise, though tolerances to these products can vary depending on the intensity of exercise and timing of the carbohydrate supplement. Obviously, carbohydrate drinks offer the advantage of hydration and fuel. Although sports drinks are practical, team sport athletes may appreciate the more concentrated carbohydrate gels, for situations when energy needs outweigh the desire for fluid. These products, however, should be consumed with some fluid. More solid items such as energy bars may take the edge off hunger during practice, though most athletes prefer to avoid solid items during high-intensity competitions.

Fluid and carbohydrate choices can be somewhat individualized. Often it is possible that fluid needs are of greater significance than energy needs out on the football field or baseball diamond on a hot, humid day. If carbohydrate needs are a greater priority during the end of an intense practice, then a gel taken with water or a more concentrated sports drink may provide the shot of energy you need.

The Electrolyte Edge

Though your sweat is mainly water, it does contain a number of electrolytes, including sodium, potassium, and calcium. However, the main electrolyte lost in sweat is sodium. Electrolyte losses in sweat can also vary greatly among athletes, mostly in regard to salt or sodium content. But, because electrolytes are the major solid component of sweat, research has focused on replacement needs of these nutrients during exercise. Sodium and potassium have been most frequently studied, though chloride is also a consideration. Sodium has recently become an important consideration for athletes who train in the heat and humidity and who may be susceptible to muscle cramping. Football players who have several practices daily in the heat and soccer players who compete in hot and humid conditions are just two examples of team sport athletes who may be experiencing muscle cramping related to high sodium losses. Data suggest that cramp-prone athletes are "salty sweaters" and experience significantly higher sodium losses during training than their noncramping counterparts.

A recent study that examined the sodium sweat losses of cramp-prone football players found that they had two to three times the sweat losses of players who did not experience muscle cramping. The cramp-prone athletes increased their salt intake around practice and subsequently did not experience muscle cramping.

What these data demonstrate is that some athletes may have high sodium losses despite being acclimatized to hot and humid weather. Players wearing heavy equipment can aggravate these sweat and sodium losses further. It is possible that heat cramps in some athletes may be connected to sodium balance. Well-conditioned athletes may also have a high amount of sodium in their sweat due to genetic influences. Sodium losses are so individual that they can range from 150 to 1,800 milligrams in 1 quart (960 milliliters) of sweat.

While restricting sodium may be a useful health strategy in sodium-sensitive and sedentary individuals susceptible to high blood pressure, it may not be the best strategy for the team sport athlete susceptible to muscle cramping and one training in hot and humid weather. Several hours of sweating daily during training can add up to significant sodium losses in some athletes. These sodium losses need to be replaced with a diet moderate in salt. Salt intake can be increased by light use of a salt shaker and consumption of salty foods such as pretzels, soups, low-fat chips, and pickles. Sports drinks also have varying levels of sodium, and athletes prone to cramping can choose those higher in sodium. After practice, it is also important to replenish your body with both fluid and sodium. For every pound (0.5 kilogram) of weight lost during practice, consume 20 to 24 ounces (600 to 720 milliliters) of fluid.

Obtaining adequate fuel and fluid during training sessions and competition takes practice, experience, and experimentation. Here are some practical tips for making the most of your fluid and fuel intake during exercise:

Have a plan and drink on a schedule. Have a squeeze bottle of fluid ready and available at practice so that you can consume it during breaks in training. Check your intake every hour to determine if you are keeping up with the required fluid amounts.

Know your sweat losses by monitoring your weight before and after practice. It is not necessary to consume more fluid than your body requires, but do try to consume adequate fluid during practice to minimize sweat losses. If you lose more than 2 pounds during an hour or longer practice, you need to drink more. Gaining weight during practice indicates that you are consuming too much fluid.

Start exercise well hydrated. Drink 16 to 20 ounces (480 to 600 milliliters) of fluid in the hour before exercise. Start practice with a comfortably full stomach. This will speed up gastric emptying, as will drinking fluid every 15 to 20 minutes.

Use a sports drink during moderate- to high-intensity practice sessions lasting longer than 60 minutes. Research indicates that this combination of fluid and carbohydrate improves performance by replacing sweat losses and providing carbohydrate fuel for your muscles.

Consume 30 to 60 grams of carbohydrate per hour from a sports drink during moderate- to high-intensity training. This amount will ensure that you do not become dehydrated and provide fuel as glycogen stores become depleted. Most sports drinks provide 14 to 20 grams of carbohydrate per 8-ounce (240-milliliter) serving. One full squeeze bottle would provide 35 to 50 grams and should be consumed over 1 hour of practice.

Start drinking early on during practice and competition. Minimizing a fluid deficit makes more sense than reversing dehydration during exercise. Your brain also derives benefits from the carbohydrate consumed, and the carbohydrate spares liver glycogen stores that can be broken down for use later in exercise.

Experiment carefully with other sources of carbohydrate. During intense practice sessions and at quarter and halftime breaks, a more solid form of carbohydrate such as a gel may be appealing and provide needed carbohydrate fuel to prevent depletion. Gel servings usually provide up to 50 grams of carbohydrate per gulp. Just remember to consume gels with plenty of water; otherwise they empty from your stomach slowly, as they are a concentrated carbohydrate source.

Know your sweat losses in different environmental conditions and at different times during the season. Monitor your weight before and after practice in various temperatures and at different times of the year. Train yourself to drink the proper volumes to replace sweat losses in various situations.

Have a squeeze bottle at each practice session, and consume fluids from it regularly. The coaching and training staff should have policies in place that make fluids readily available to team sport athletes.

Drink during the warm-up, and have a regular fluid intake when on the bench. Drink a small amount of fluid at each break in play.

Coaches and trainers should remind players to drink regularly, especially those with high fluid losses and low intakes during practice.

Experiment with various sports drinks to determine your favorite flavor and best tolerance. Consuming a variety of flavors may minimize the occurrence of taste fatigue during long exercise sessions and competitions. You may find that different products appeal to you in various athletic conditions. In hot and humid weather, you may favor a product with little or no flavor. Know what works for you under various exercise, temperature, and race conditions.

Pay attention to signs of dehydration. Frequent gastrointestinal problems may indicate that you are not drinking enough. Gastric emptying is delayed when you are dehydrated. It may appear that you do not tolerate a particular product, when what is actually occurring is that the product is unable to empty from your stomach and subsequent drinking causes distention.

Learn to recognize the signs and symptoms of hypoglycemia. Feeling lightheaded or experiencing an inability to focus or dizziness can all indicate that blood glucose levels are running low. Be proactive and try to increase your intake of carbohydrate with sports drinks or gels.

Refine your drinking technique. Practice drinking in all types of training situations. Know your limits regarding exercise intensity and the ability to tolerate certain volumes of fluid ingestion. Push your limits and maximize your fluid intake to maintain fluid balance.

Pay attention to your sodium intake if you are susceptible to muscle cramping. Emphasize salty foods and salt foods to taste. Choose higher-sodium sports drinks. When you consume a wide variety of sports nutrition supplements over the course of a day or even a week, it is important to consider the other nutrients they provide, such as vitamins and minerals. Note your intake in the context of your entire day's food intake, and be careful not to oversupplement on vitamins and minerals through use of these products and individual supplements.

TIMING MATTERS

Nutritional recovery does take 24 hours and is impacted by what foods and fluids you consume in the hours after exercise and in your daily diet. But, clearly there are specific sports nutrition strategies that occur in the hours leading to the training session and during training and competition that benefit team sport athletes. Consuming properly timed meal(s) or snack(s) at various intervals in the 4-hour time period before practice or competition boosts fuel stores for exercise and supports optimal performance. Replacing fuel and fluid that become depleted during practice and competition is also crucial for top performance. Effective strategies are specific to each sport; moreover, fluid and fuel choices vary from athlete to athlete. Experiment until you find just the right combination for your unique needs.

Practical Uses for Sports Nutrition Products

Sports Drinks

- Consume 16 to 24 oz. (480–720 ml) in the hour before exercise.
- Consume 4–8 oz. (120–240 ml) every 15–20 minutes if practice schedule allows.
- Consume 8 oz. (240 ml) during practice breaks whenever possible.
- Consume after exercise with high carbohydrate food or supplement.
- Consume at halftime or play breaks whenever possible.

Sports Gel

- Consume one packet in the 30–60 minutes prior to training or competition.
- Consume at breaks during practice and competition.
- Consume as part of recovery nutrition snack.

Sports Bar

- Include in prepractice, precompetition snack.
- Consume as part of daily training diet for concentrated carbohydrate source.
- Consume as part of your immediate postexercise nutritional recovery plan.
- Consume during long game days for easy-to-digest source of carbohydrate.

High-Energy Carbohydrate Drink

- Consume as part of a pretraining, precompetition meal or snack.
- Consume as part of immediate post-exercise recovery nutrition.
- Consume as part of a high-energy meal plan.

High-Carbohydrate Protein Drink

- Consume before and after resistance training for quality protein combined with carbohydrate.
- Consume as part of a pretraining, pre-competition meal.
- Consume as part of a high-energy training plan.

Sports Shake

- Use as preexercise meal or snack for a carbohydrate and protein source.
- Include in a precompetition menu for easily digested nutrients.
- Eat as recovery snack after practice or weight training.
- Include as part of a high-energy training plan.
- Use for quick meal for convenience due to the athlete's schedule.

CHAPTER 8

CREATING THE OPTIMAL TRAINING DIET

As a dedicated team sport athlete who strives for optimal energy for training and full recovery, you must translate sound scientific recommendations into everyday food choices. The proper food choices can replenish your body fuel stores, build and repair muscle tissue, promote good health, and leave you feeling satisfied with your diet.

YOUR DAILY MEAL PLAN

Much of the success of your daily eating plan will hinge on consuming adequate calories, carbohydrates, and proteins that match your training program for that day (and the next day) and rounding out your meals and snacks with the correct balance of fats. As described in Chapters 5 and 6, how you time your meal and snacks around your team training and weight-training sessions is also crucial.

Meal planning is not as complicated as it may sound. In fact, you will be amazed at how quickly you can adopt some new food strategies and incorporate them into your daily life of training and eating once you have a program and some structure in place. You will find that planning and organization make this part of your life easier and more effective. Just as you plan ahead to ensure that all the necessary equipment and clothing are available for practice, you must also plan to ensure that the optimal foods and required sports nutrition supplements are available to support your training program that day. Table 8.1 summarizes the range of nutritional requirements for calories, carbohydrate, protein, and fat for team sport athletes. This table also outlines the total calorie, carbohydrate, protein, and fat requirements of a 160-pound (73-kilogram) athlete who has completed some hard training that day.

Of course, your energy needs can vary depending on the intensity of your training, whether you are in a serious muscle-building phase, and whether you are going to practice more than once daily. Your daily energy requirements can also vary not only day to day but during different times of the season. A qualified sports dietitian can assist you in determining your nutritional requirements during different phases of your training program. (You can also refer to Table 5.1, to estimate your energy requirements.)

TABLE 8.1 NUTRITIONAL REQUIREMENTS FOR TEAM SPORT ATHLETES			
Calories **(cal/lb. weight)**	**Carbohydrate** **(g/lb. weight)**	**Protein** **(g/lb. weight)**	**Fat** **(g/lb. weight)**
Mild: 12–14 (26–31) **Moderate:** 15–17 (33–37) **High:** 18–24 (40–53) **Very high:** 24–29 (53–64)	**Mild/Moderate:** 2.25–3.0 (5–6.5) **Moderate/High:** 3.0–4.5 (6.5–10) **High/Very High:** 4.5–5.5 (10–12)	**Moderate:** 0.45 (1) **High:** 0.5–0.75 (1.2–1.6) **Very High:** 0.8–0.9 (1.8–2.0)	> 0.5 g/lb. (> 1g/kg) depending on energy needs
160-lb. (73-kg) **athlete with high** **activity level:** 2,800–3,800 calories	560 g carbohydrate (60% calories)	128 g protein (13% calories)	115 g fat (27% calories)

Note: Parenthetical notations convert grams to kilograms.

After you determine your nutritional needs for training, how these recommended nutrients' amounts are translated into specific food choices and serving sizes can initially be one of the most difficult aspects of adopting your optimal high-performance diet. In real life, an individualized plan can differ from athlete to athlete depending on medical history, age, gender, food preferences, training and life schedule, and culinary skills. But food charts can be very helpful in making carbohydrate servings more accessible and carbohydrate is often an important theme of your diet for several reasons:

- Running low on liver and muscle glycogen can impair your training efforts long before depletion of other body fuels slow you down.
- Your carbohydrate intake is directly linked to the amount of glycogen you store in your liver and muscles, and these stores are relatively limited depending on your training that day.
- On certain training days you require significant amounts of carbohydrates to replenish your muscle glycogen stores, and if you don't consume these amounts, your muscle glycogen stores may not be adequate to properly fuel your subsequent training efforts.
- Consuming these carbohydrates takes planning as the amounts you require often exceed what is found in an everyday diet, and if you leave your diet to chance, your intake may be inadequate.

- You need to consciously choose wholesome carbohydrates in the North American food environment.
- Timing of your carbohydrate intake is also essential to your training and recovery.
- During various cycles of your training program, you still need a diet that provides at least 50 percent carbohydrate calories, and needs may increase to 60 percent during various training cycles. This means that the total grams of carbohydrate that you need to consume can fluctuate.
- Many team sport athletes participate in more than one sport and may participate in their sport year-round through various clubs and leagues, requiring a well-planned sports nutrition diet for much of the year.

Food tables providing 10- to 30-gram carbohydrate portions can make meal planning for your training diet smoother and more effective. You receive carbohydrates from several food groups: the bread, cereal, and grain group; the fruit and fruit juice group; the vegetable group; the milk and yogurt group; and of course miscellaneous carbohydrate foods provided by snack items, desserts, and other carbohydrate toppings. You can match up the number of servings you require from these carbohydrate-containing groups to meet your requirements for training and recovery. On days when your carbohydrate needs are especially high, grains and starches are likely to comprise a good portion of your diet. They are concentrated food sources and provide 30 grams of carbohydrate per serving. As discussed in Chapter 1, try to choose lightly processed or whole-grain sources as much as possible. Many items from the grain group, such as pretzels and crackers, also make good snack choices.

Fruits, dried fruit, and fruit juices, which also supply 30 grams per serving, are your next great source of carbohydrate and are excellent food choices for maintaining good health due to the abundant nutrients they supply. Vegetables are also sources of carbohydrate, though not as high per portion as grains and fruits, at 10 grams per serving. However, few foods can match vegetables for their high nutrient content.

Dairy milk and yogurt, and other milks such as soy milk and rice milk, are also good sources of carbohydrate ranging anywhere from 12 to 40 grams per serving. Yogurts can be especially high in carbohydrate when they come mixed with fruit and sugars.

One last source of concentrated carbohydrates are sweets and desserts, which also supply 30 grams per serving. Sweets should not routinely replace more wholesome carbohydrate choices in your diet, but they are a great source of additional carbohydrate. They offer the advantage of being dense and less filling than some higher-fiber, more wholesome choices, and when your carbohydrate requirements are especially high, these foods are handy choices when your requirements exceed 500 grams daily. For very heavy training days, you can also consider adding some sports nutrition products high in carbohydrate to your food plan.

But, of course, team sport and weight-training athletes cannot live and should not live on carbohydrate alone. Choosing quality proteins and healthy fats will provide you with essential nutrients and balance out your meals and snacks. Proteins and fats also keep you full longer and even out blood glucose levels during the day. Protein foods are ranked according to their fat content so that you do not exceed healthy limits of total fat and saturated fat in your diet. Plant proteins and milk and dairy sources are emphasized for vegetarian athletes. Fats are organized according to the types of fat they provide, so that you can choose healthy essential fatty acids and foods high in monoun-saturated fat.

Table 8.2 outlines some of the serving recommendations for various calorie levels. This table is intended to be a framework from which you can base your own individual food choices. You may find that you prefer to do a bit of shuffling around with the suggested food groups and number of servings to suit your own health goals and personal tastes. For example, some of the suggested daily plans may be too high in dairy foods for your own tastes. These plans can be modified and the carbohydrate intake maintained by adding the equivalent grams of carbohydrate servings from fruits and juices or perhaps by substituting soy milk for dairy milk. You may also wish to have fewer grain servings and increase the number of servings from fruits and fruit juices to match your carbohydrate requirements on certain training days. On some training days, your carbohydrate needs may be less than the proportion outlined in the sample menus. However, regardless of your personalized food plan and preferences, you need to reach the recommended carbohydrate amounts for optimal recovery and can add up the carbohydrate in the manner that best suits you. Of course, the nutrition guidelines presented in Chapters 1 and 2 should also direct you in making quality food choices as often as possible.

FOOD JOURNALS: TRACKING YOUR INTAKE

One useful tool for helping you to determine whether you are meeting your energy and nutrient requirements is a food journal. You may already be familiar with keeping records regarding your training program and have learned what a good feedback tool a journal provides for fine-tuning your training program. To reap similar benefits from

TABLE 8.2 SERVING SUGGESTIONS FOR CALORIE LEVELS				
	Calorie Levels			
Food Groups	**2,000 calories**	**2,400 calories**	**2,900 calories**	**3,400 calories**	**4,000 calories**
Grains	6	7	8	10	12
Fruits	3	3	4	5	6
Vegetables	2	3	3	3	3
Milk/yogurt/ soy milk	2	2	2 (milk) 1 (yogurt)	2 (milk) 1 (yogurt)	3 (milk) 1 (yogurt)
Protein	6	6	6	7	8
Fats	3	4	5	6	8
Menu breakdown	315 g carb 84 g protein 45 g fat	350 g carb 112 g protein 60 g fat	450 g carb 114 g protein 70 g fat	550 g carb 120 g protein 80 g fat	650 g carb 150 g protein 89 g fat

keeping a food journal, it is best if you write down your food choices and portions while eating or immediately after eating. Don't forget to note snacks, supplements, and any fluids consumed. With help from the food lists provided, you can assess a number of items regarding your food intake.

For starters, add up the amount of carbohydrate grams you consume in a day and determine whether your intake matches your training efforts. Note carbohydrate amounts from food labels, and use the food lists provided to estimate carbohydrate amounts per serving. You can also tally your total serving intake from the carbohydrate-containing food lists and see how your choices match up with the meal plans provided. You can see not only whether your daily totals are adequate but also whether the amount of carbohydrate you consume before and after exercise is appropriate to support your training and recovery.

Record the amount of fluids and carbohydrate that you consume before, during, and after practice. Determine whether you meet the recommended fluid amounts and whether you take ample opportunity to consume fluids and carbohydrates during breaks in training. Note how your energy levels during training may fluctuate depending on your carbohydrate and fluid intake.

Look through the day's intake to ensure that you are consuming adequate sources of concentrated and high-quality lean proteins. If you are vegetarian, check that your portions of plant proteins are full portions so that your body receives all the required amino acids. Check that protein is included in your recovery foods and fluids and that you also consume high-quality protein before and after training.

Determine whether the fats you consume are derived from healthy monounsaturated, liquid unhydrogenated polyunsaturated, and omega-3 fatty-acid food choices. Check that you consume good sources of essential fatty acids in your diet.

Measure your intake of hydrating fluids for the day and before and after training. Make sure that you are well hydrated before exercise and that you consume enough fluid to replace sweat losses after exercise.

Check for hidden fats, such as those found in muffins, pastries, and high-fat crackers. Try to minimize your intake of these foods whenever possible.

Pay attention to your eating patterns. Note if you become too hungry at some times during the day, and adjust your mealtimes accordingly. Pay attention to any eating that may occur due to boredom, stress, and other issues not related to hunger.

Make sure that you are timing your foods appropriately before and after training. Check that you are consuming quality protein with carbohydrate before and after weight training. It is also important that you practice recovery nutrition strategies after intense training with your team.

Tables 8.3, 8.4, and 8.5 will help in sports nutrition meal planning. Table 8.3 provides serving and carbohydrate amounts for the major foods that can comprise a well-balanced sports nutrition diet. Table 8.4 ranks the protein foods according to fat content so that you may choose the leanest choices available and limit your intake of saturated fat. In Table 8.5, the fats are also grouped according to types of fat, to help you make the healthiest choices possible.

PLANNING YOUR DAILY MEALS

Meal planning does not need to be a frustrating experience. The necessary tools depend on who is responsible for preparing your meals and what types of food choices are presented to the athlete. Of course, younger athletes require the support of their parents in providing healthy food choices for their growth and training program. High school athletes can take responsibility for their food choices away from home, including lunches and snacks at school, as well as when eating out with friends. Collegiate athletes often have a wide range of choices available at the dorm food service, and many schools now support their athletes with a training table. Athletes living on their own can shop for and prepare their own healthy meals, and it isn't necessary to employ your own personal chef for quick, gourmet meals, though professional athletes may do just that. Regardless of your living situation and resources, like your training program,

TABLE 8.3 CARBOHYDRATE-CONTAINING FOODS

30-g Carbohydrate Servings for Cereals, Starches, Grains

Breads

Bagel	1/2 large or 2 oz. (60 g)
Bread crumbs	1/2 c. (120 ml)
Bread sticks	2 oz. (60 g)
Bread	2 slices or 2 oz. (60 g)
Corn bread	1 square or 2 oz. (60 g)
Dinner rolls	2 oz. (60 g)
English muffin	1 whole or 2 oz. (60 g)
Hamburger bun	1 whole or 2 oz. (60 g)
Pita pocket	1 round or 2 oz. (60 g)

Cereals

Bran cereal	2/3 c. (160 ml)
Cereal, cold, unsweetened	1.5 oz. (45 g)
Cream of wheat, cooked	1 c. (240 ml)
Grits, cooked	1 c. (240 ml)
Granola, low-fat	1/2 c. (120 ml)
Grape-Nuts	1/3 c. or 5 Tbsp. (100 ml)
Oatmeal, cooked	1 c. (240 ml)
Puffed cereal, 3 c.	Shredded Wheat, 1/4 c. or 1.5 oz. (45 g)

Grains

Barley, raw	1/4 c. (60 ml)
Bulgur, cooked	3/4 c. (180 ml)
Buckwheat, raw	1/4 c. (60 ml)
Muffin, low-fat	3 oz. (90 g)
Pasta, cooked	1 c. (240 ml)
Pancakes, 4-in. diameter	3
Pancake mix, dry	1/3 c. (80 ml)
Pretzels	1.5 oz. (45 g)
Rice, cooked	2/3 c. (160 ml)
Rice milk	1 c. (240 ml)
Tortilla, corn or flour	2
Saltines	8 crackers, 1.5 oz. (45 g)
Crackers	1.5 oz. (45 g)

Starchy vegetables

Baked beans, cooked	3/4 c. (180 ml)
Corn, cooked	3/4 c. (180 ml)
Kidney beans, cooked	3/4 c. (180 ml)
Peas, cooked	1 c. (240 ml)
Potato, baked	1 medium or 5 oz. (150 g)
Sweet potato, baked	4 oz. (120 ml)

30-g Carbohydrate Servings for Fruit

Apple	1.5 medium
Applesauce, unsweetened	1 c. (240 ml)
Applesauce, sweetened	1/2 c. (120 ml)
Apples, dried	7 rings
Apricots, fresh	8 medium

TABLE 8.3 CARBOHYDRATE-CONTAINING FOODS, *CONTINUED*

Banana	1 large
Blueberries	1-1/2 c. (360 ml)
Cantaloupe, raw pieces	2 c. (480 ml)
Dates, dried	1 fruit
Figs, dried	3 whole
Fruit salad	1 c. (240 ml)
Grapefruit	1 large
Grapes	30 or 1 c. (240 ml)
Kiwifruit	3 medium
Mango	1 medium
Nectarine	2 small
Orange	2 medium
Papaya	1 whole
Peach	2 medium
Pear	1 large
Pineapple, fresh, pieces	1-1/2 c. (360 ml)
Plum	3 medium
Raisins	1/3 c. or 3 tbsp. (60 ml)
Raspberries	2 c. (480 ml)
Strawberries	2-1/2 c. (600 ml)
Watermelon	3 slices or 3 c. (720 ml)

30-g Carbohydrate Servings for Fruit and Vegetable Juices

Apple juice	8 oz. (240 ml)
Carrot juice	10 oz. (300 ml)
Cranberry juice cocktail	8 oz. (240 ml)
Grape juice	8 oz. (240 ml)
Grapefruit juice	8 oz. (240 ml)
Orange juice	8 oz. (240 ml)
Pineapple juice	8 oz. (240 ml)
Vegetable juice cocktail	24 oz. (720 ml)

10-g Carbohydrate Servings for Vegetables

Artichoke	1 medium
Asparagus, boiled	1 c.
Beans, green, boiled	1 c.
Beet greens, cooked	1-1/4 c.
Broccoli, boiled	1 c.
Broccoli, raw	2 c.
Brussels sprouts, boiled	3/4 c.
Cabbage, cooked	3/4 c.
Carrots, raw	2 medium
Carrots, cooked	2/3 c.
Cauliflower, cooked	3/4 c.
Kale, boiled	1-1/4 c.
Mushrooms, cooked	1 c.
Mustard greens, cooked	1-1/2 c.
Peppers, sweet, raw	2 c.
Summer squash, cooked	1 c.
Spinach, boiled	1-1/2 c.
Tomato, raw	2 medium

TABLE 8.3 CARBOHYDRATE-CONTAINING FOODS, *CONTINUED*

12- to 50-g Carbohydrate Servings for Milk and Yogurt

Milk, buttermilk, 1%	8 oz. (12 g) (240 ml)
Milk, nonfat	8 oz. (12 g) (240 ml)
Milk, 1%	8 oz. (12 g) (240 ml)
Milk, 2%	8 oz. (12 g) (240 ml)
Yogurt, nonfat	8 oz. (15 g) (240 ml)
Yogurt, low-fat	8 oz. (15–20 g) (240 ml)
Yogurt, with fruit	8 oz. (30–45 g) (240 ml)

30-g Carbohydrate Servings for Sweet and Baked Goods

Angel food cake	1/12 whole
Chocolate milk	8 oz. (240 ml)
Cake	1/12 whole
Cookie, fat-free	4 small
Fruit spreads, 100% fruit	2 tbsp. (40 ml)
Gingersnaps	6 cookies
Graham crackers	6 squares
Granola bar, low-fat	1 bar
Honey	2 tbsp. (40 ml)
Ice cream	1 c. (240 ml)
Jam or jelly	2 tbsp. (40 ml)
Pie	1/8 whole
Pudding, regular	1/2 c. (120 ml)
Sherbet	1/2 c. (120 ml)
Sorbet	1/2 c. (120 ml)
Syrup, regular	2 Tbsp. (40 ml)
Vanilla wafers	10 wafers
Yogurt, frozen, low-fat	2/3 c. (160 ml)
Yogurt, frozen, fat-free	1 c. (240 ml)

meal planning does require forethought, organization, and flexibility. With practice, your meal-planning skills will become second nature. Some of the fundamentals of meal planning when preparing your own meals are as follows:

Have a well-organized and well-equipped kitchen. Make sure that you have all the convenience items that you need, including a microwave, streamer, toaster oven, microwave-proof cookware, and a slow cooker. Other handy items include a large stove-top skillet or wok, a rice cooker, a lasagna dish, and sharp knives. Knowing where all your items are located and feeling comfortable in your kitchen will make putting together quick and easy meals that much easier.

Have a stock of some foods and snacks and use what limited cooking resources are available. For collegiate athletes, keeping some dry snack items and sports

TABLE 8.4 PROTEIN FOOD CHOICES

Very Low-Fat (<2 g Fat/oz.*)	Low-Fat (3–4 g Fat/oz.)	Medium-Fat (4–5 g Fat/oz.)	High-Fat (6–8 g Fat/oz.)	Very High-Fat (>8 g Fat/oz.)
Fish				
White Fish	Dark Fish	Tuna and salmon		Any fried fish
Grouper	Salmon	packed in oil		product
Tuna	Mackerel			
Haddock	Sardines			
Sole				
Halibut				
Bass				
Shellfish				
Crab				
Shrimp				
Lobster				
Clams				
Cheese				
Fat-free cheese	Low-fat	Feta cheese	Mozzarella	American,
Cottage cheese,	Cheeses	Mozzarella,	Neufchâtel	processed
1%		part-skim		Cream cheese
Cottage cheese,		Grated Parmesan		Brie
2%				Cheddar
				Edam
				Monterey
				Muenster
				Limburger
				Swiss
Beef				
Round, choice,	Round, choice,	Round, choice,	Roast beef	Short ribs
90% lean	85% lean	73% lean	Meatloaf	Corned beef
	Rib-eye, choice	Round, choice,		Prime cuts
	Flank steak, choice	80% lean		
	Porterhouse, choice			
Pork				
Ham, lean,	Sirloin roast	Pork butt	Italian sausage	Pâté
95% fat-free	Center loin chop			Pastrami
Pork tenderloin	Boneless rib roast			Bacon
Boneless sirloin	Center rib chop			Pork sausage
chop	Blade steak			
Top loin chop	Canadian bacon			
Lamb				
Leg, top round	Loin chop	Roast lamb		Ground lamb
Leg, shank, half	Loin roast			
	Rib chop			

TABLE 8.4 PROTEIN FOOD CHOICES, *CONTINUED*

Very Low-Fat (<2 g Fat/oz.)	Low-Fat (3–4 g Fat/oz.)	Medium-Fat (4–5 g Fat/oz.)	High-Fat (6–8 g Fat/oz.)	Very High-Fat (>8 g Fat/oz.)
Legumes (per c.)				
Black beans	Chickpeas	Tofu	Soybeans	
Kidney beans				
Lentils				
Lima beans				
Pinto beans				
Poultry				
Turkey breast	Chicken, dark,	Ground turkey,	Duck, roasted,	
Chicken, white,	no skin	mixed meat/skin	w/skin	
no skin	Chicken, dark,			
Turkey, dark,	w/skin			
no skin	Turkey, dark,			
	w/skin			
	Duck, roasted,			
	no skin			
Other				
95% fat-free	86% fat-free	Eggs	Luncheon meat	Knockwurst
luncheon meat	luncheon meat		Bologna	Bratwurst
Egg whites	Egg substitute		Turkey/chicken	Beef/pork
Egg substitute			Hot dogs	hot dogs
			Salami	Peanut butter

*Note: 1 ounce equals 30 grams, making a low-fat protein <2 g fat per 30 grams.

TABLE 8.5 SOURCES OF FAT

Polyunsaturated Fat, 5-g Serving	Monounsaturated Fat, 5-g Serving	Saturated Fat, 5-g Serving
Margarine, stick, tub, or squeeze, 1 tsp. (7 ml) lower-fat, 1 tbsp. (20 ml)	Avocado, medium, 1/8	Bacon, cooked, 1 slice
	Oil, canola, olive, peanut, 1 tsp.	Butter, stick, 1 tsp. (7 ml)
	Olives, black, 8 large (7 ml)	whipped, 1 tsp. (7 ml)
Mayonnaise, regular, 1 tsp (7 ml)	Nuts	reduced fat, 1 tbsp. (20 ml)
reduced-fat, 1 tbsp. (20 ml)	almonds, cashews, 6 nuts	Cream, half-and-half, 2 tbsp. (40 ml)
	peanuts, 10 nuts	
Nuts, walnuts, 4 halves	pecans, 4 halves	Sour cream, regular, 2 tbsp. (40 ml)
Oil, corn, safflower, soybean, flaxseed, walnut, 1 tsp. (7 ml)	Peanut butter, 2 tsp. (14 ml)	reduced fat, 3 tbsp. (60 ml)
	Sesame seeds, 1 tbsp. (20 ml) (60 ml)	
Salad dressing, regular, 1 tbsp.	Tahini paste, 2 tsp. (14 ml)	
Sunflower seeds, 1 tbsp. (20 ml)		
Pumpkin seeds, 1 tbsp. (20 ml)		

nutrition products on hand can be useful and supplement on-campus food appropriately. You should be able to keep some perishable items refrigerated in your room, and some dorms have limited cooking facilities on the floor.

Plan out your week's meal ideas beforehand. Think ahead to what meals you will need to cook, pack, or eat out based on that week's schedule. Determine how many dinners you will cook that week, and leave room for healthy takeout, eating out, and leftovers. Think about where you will be for lunch. Do you need to pack a full lunch or some extras like pretzels and fruit? Determine whether your training schedule requires you to have energy bars or carbohydrate drinks on hand. Perhaps you need quick recovery nutrition items to tide you over until your next full meal. You may want to be very specific and have certain days of the week designated for specific types of meals. For example, Monday night could be chicken, Thursday is fish, and Friday is stir-fry. Try to vary the types of vegetables and sides you consume. Sometimes it is easier to obtain variety when dinner is prepared for an entire family. When cooking for just one to two persons, try to obtain variety on a weekly basis, switching the grains, fruits, and vegetables you consume.

Understand the choices available to you in your food environment. Just as people purchasing food and preparing their own meals can plan ahead, you can also be aware of the foods offered at your school and various locations on campus. Have a strategy for choosing lower-fat items and making healthy choices. Look ahead to menus that may be posted regarding main entrees. Have a list of backup healthy meals that are offered on a regular basis. Pack snacks to consume between classes and before practice as needed.

Keep nonperishable stock food items amply supplied. Having a well-stocked cupboard of items such as rice, pasta, whole grains, instant couscous, and other dry items can save you in a pinch when fresh food supplies run low or during busy training weeks. Some quick meals made from these ingredients include black bean burritos (freeze the tortillas), pasta and tomato sauce, stir-fry made from frozen chicken, instant rice, frozen vegetable mixes, and canned chili with bread or crackers. A suggested stock list is provided in Table 8.6. College athletes can keep a stock of healthy snacks in their room.

Go grocery shopping every week for fresh items. Have a designated grocery shopping day and time, and make it part of your weekly schedule. Based on your food plan for the week, put together a shopping list. Don't wait to shop when it is convenient, as it may never be convenient! You also don't want to set yourself up for several quick trips to the store to grab a few needed items. In the long run, this habit will cost you more time. Try to find a supermarket that can supply all the items you need. You will know where all your regular items are located and save time. Go during off-peak times to avoid crowds, and don't mull over items that are not on your shopping list. If you can't make it to the supermarket some weeks, try an increasingly popular alternative and find a grocery store or online grocery system that accepts phone, fax, or Internet orders and delivers.

Keep a running list of items that need to be replenished. Have a pad and pen handy. When you notice that items are running low or are used up, add them to your list. Trying to remember everything you need while shopping at the grocery store may not be the best strategy for a busy athlete.

Batch-cook meals, make extra portions, and freeze single servings. This strategy can be a great time-saver. You can set aside a lighter training day to cook items such as soups, chilies, and lasagnas. When cooking regular meals, making an extra one to two portions for the next day can save dinner preparation time or provide you with a nice midday meal. Freeze single-item portions in plastic containers for future heavy training days.

Pack meals, snacks, and food supplements for the next training day the night before. If your next day's schedule is full, consider packing your foods and snacks the night before. Having some portioned items and fresh food in the fridge will make this task as simple as possible. Plan snacks that can be eaten on the run.

Acquire a repertoire of quick and easy to prepare meals. Anyone can become a proficient cook, and it does not have to be a time-consuming project. Be on the lookout for quick and simple recipes. Ask friends for some of their quick meal ideas. Focus on recipes like stir-fry, risotto, burritos, and pasta ideas.

Take advantage of food shortcuts. You can purchase chicken tender strips, beef stir-fry strips, frozen precooked shrimp, and rotisserie chickens. Try frozen vegetable stir-fry mixes, precut fruits, preseasoned and cut tofu, ready-to-heat soups, instant couscous mixes, fresh pastas (you can freeze them), and canned beans, chickpeas, and other legumes.

Although you may not always have full kitchen facilities available to you when training and competing in college, some options are possible for storage in your dorm room. Often a small refrigerator or hot plate is available. Some items that you can keep on hand are peanut butter, whole-grain bread, jam, instant soup and grain cups, fresh fruit, and granola bars. Stocking up your dorm room with healthy foods can mean making good choices when snacking in the evening and packing healthy snacks for between meals.

TABLE 8.6 SIMPLE SUGGESTIONS FOR STOCKING YOUR PANTRY

For the Freezer	For the Refrigerator	For the Cupboard
Chicken tenders	Fresh fruit	Pasta
Cooked shrimp	Fresh vegetables	Rice
Lean ground beef	Juices	Couscous
Lean pork fillets	Milk	Quinoa
Cubed meat for stir-fry	Yogurt	Pilaf
Soy and garden burgers	Eggs	Tabouleh
Textured vegetable proteins	Reduced-fat cheese	Canned beans and chickpeas
Variety of breads	Prewashed salad greens	Canned tuna
Waffles	Minicarrots	Peanut butter
English muffins	Oranges, apples, bananas	Instant stuffing mixes
Muffins	Lean deli meats	Low-fat crackers
Tortillas	Fresh pasta	Cold cereal assortment
Frozen vegetables	Soy and rice milk	Oatmeal and farina
Stir-fry mixes	Sauces and condiments	Dried fruit
Sorbet	Salsa	Granola bars
Frozen fruit	Lean deli meats	Canned soup
Precooked pasta and rice	Tub margarine	Nuts and sunflower seeds
Egg substitute		Pretzels
		Instant soup and grains
		Fig Newtons
		Seasoning mixes

Breakfast, Lunch, and Snacks

Breakfast is one of the most important meals of the day. It revs up your body's metabolism and fills up liver glycogen stores that have become depleted overnight. It may even be an important recovery meal after a solid early-morning practice session. By skipping breakfast, eating a medium-size lunch, and feasting at dinner, you may not only be compromising your recovery but also be cheating your body of important nutrients. Skipping breakfast is also a terrible weight management strategy that can set you up for increased hunger and overeating later in the day.

Breakfast will keep your digestive juices flowing, but it may keep you feeling satisfied for only 3 hours or so until you are hungry again. If this occurs, place a midmorning snack into your eating plan. If your energy needs are high, try to have a substantial breakfast. Eat up on calorically dense cereals such as granola and muesli. A large glass of juice will also add a substantial amount of calories and carbohydrates. Adding some protein to your breakfast can do a nice job of keeping you comfortably full until the next meal. Depending on your schedule, you may consume breakfast on the fly. Quick choices can include a fruit smoothie made with yogurt and granola. Quick packs include yogurt, bananas, dried fruit, bagels, and muffins.

Breakfast Ideas

- Cooked oatmeal with raisins, cinnamon, and low-fat milk
- Open-face English muffin halves with broiled cheese and fruit
- Egg substitute omelet with vegetables, toast, juice, and milk
- Yogurt with fresh fruit and a low-fat muffin

- Whole-grain cereal with milk and fruit
- Fruit smoothie made with yogurt, fresh or frozen fruit, and granola
- Whole-grain bread with peanut butter, banana, and honey
- Any leftovers that sound appealing

For many athletes, lunch will be brought from home, purchased at a restaurant or fast-food establishment, or chosen from a cafeteria-style menu. Like all your meals and snacks, lunch should provide some quality carbohydrates and be balanced out with protein and fat. Eat lunch when hunger first sets in, as this is a sign that your body needs fuel.

Packing a lunch takes a little extra time and planning but is well worth the effort. You can ensure that you have lean proteins and the right type and amount of fats. Sandwiches are always a good place to start when last night's leftovers seem too repetitive. Some good protein options are lean beef, hummus, turkey or chicken, tuna, and low-fat cottage cheese. Liven up that same old turkey sandwich with add-ons such as avocado, lettuce leaves, cucumber, tomato, sprouts, and low-fat cheese. High-carbohydrate items that you can include with your lunch are fruits, pretzels, raw vegetables, yogurt, low-fat chips, low-fat crackers, and vegetable and bean soups.

Snacks are also a very important part of an athlete's diet. When your energy needs are high, snacks give you a nice calorie boost. They also provide some fuel before training sessions and keep hunger at bay until you can sit down for a full meal. Many athletes swear by snacking. Plan some serious snacking into your diet. If there is a particular time of day when you experience an energy low or hunger, snacking may make all the difference.

LABEL-READING TIPS

Nutritional information on labels can help you determine the nutritional breakdown of foods. First check the ingredient list. You may want to include more whole-wheat flours

Smart Snacks to Keep Your Tank Topped Off

- Cereal, with or without milk
- Peanut butter and jelly sandwich
- Hard and soft pretzels
- Baked potato with low-fat cheese
- Crackers with peanut butter
- Muffins and bagels with jam and low-fat cream cheese
- Sports bars, breakfast bars, low-fat granola bars
- Yogurt with fruit

- Bowl of soup with crackers
- Pasta or bean salad
- Fresh fruit, low-fat cheese, and nuts
- Cottage cheese and fruit
- Instant breakfast mix and fruit
- Tuna salad and crackers
- Hummus and crackers or pita bread
- Fruit smoothie
- Milk chug and fruit

and other whole grains into your diet. Ingredients are listed in the labels by weight from the most to least.

Pay attention to the serving size on the label and compare it to the amount that you actually eat. Portions you consume may be double those on the package, and you should adjust the nutrition information accordingly. You can also use the label to evaluate if a food will significantly impact your carbohydrate intake by checking the total grams of carbohydrate listed. You can then determine what portion of that particular food would provide 30 grams or more of carbohydrate to help you meet your training requirements.

Total fat grams, as well as calories from fat, are also listed. To determine the percentage of calories from fat, divide the fat calories per serving by the total calories per serving and multiply by 100. Keep higher-fat foods in perspective. Your fat intake needs to be considered in the context of an entire day. Your total day's intake should provide 20 to 25 percent fat calories, which allows for some healthy foods that may be a bit higher in fat. Some foods such as dried pasta will be very low in fat, while others such as margarine provide a high amount of fat.

The Daily Values for various vitamins and minerals provided on the nutrition label are based on a 2,000-calorie intake. The percentage of the Daily Value can tell you if a food is high or low in a nutrient such as calcium, fiber, iron, or vitamin C. A food is considered to be a good source of a nutrient if it provides 20 percent of the Daily Value.

Besides increasing your intake of foods high in specific nutrients, you can also use the Daily Values to avoid excess fat, saturated fat, and cholesterol.

EATING OUT

If you're like many North Americans, you probably eat out several times weekly. Lunch is the meal most frequently eaten away from home, followed by dinner, and then breakfast. Currently, more than 45 percent of money spent on food in the United States goes to restaurant meals and other foods purchased away from home. You may eat out at restaurants, in a cafeteria, on campus, at work, and even in the car.

Regardless of where you eat your meal out, the basic strategies are the same. Watch out for hidden and added fat, and keep a close eye on the portions. Despite your high energy requirements for endurance training, not all restaurant meals fit nicely into your nutrition plan. They may be too high in fat to become a frequent indulgence, and they may not provide the healthy ingredients that you require. It is important to learn what healthy food choices are available at your favorite restaurants. Ask questions about how foods are prepared, and don't hesitate to request modifications or changes. Often you can creatively outsmart the menu and enjoy your meal as well.

Fast Food

Fast food can provide excessive amounts of protein and fat through supersize burgers and grease-laden French fries. But it is possible to make choices that fit into a sports diet at some fast-food establishments. Have the small hamburgers that provide only 2 to 3 ounces of meat. Order baked potatoes over French fries whenever possible. Broiled chicken sandwiches are decent choices, while chicken pieces are generally fried. The same goes for fish sandwiches, as they come dripping with plenty of unwanted oil. Order skim milk or juice instead of soda. Salads and vegetables may be on the menu, but watch out for dressings. Limit sauces and toppings whenever possible.

Many fast-food establishments now provide good sandwich choices. You can choose lean roast beef, ham, turkey, or chicken and limit oils, mayonnaise, and cheese. Go for baked chips and pretzels when offered. Chicken fajitas or tacos make some good lower-fat choices. You can also choose frozen yogurt and low-fat milk shakes.

Other fast-food choices that can fit into your sports nutrition plan include vegetarian thin-crust pizza. Some establishments also have a soup and baked potato bar. Bean burritos and soft tacos are also available, as are chili, bagels, English muffins, waffles, pancakes, and cereals.

Navigating the Fast-Food Lane

Most fast-food choices tend to be high in calories, fat, and sodium, while being low in fiber and vitamins A and C. Menus tend to be high in protein choices and lacking in fruits and vegetables. Here are some fast food-tips for athletes who want to make the best choices possible.

- Always avoid the largest sizes of sandwiches, burgers, fries, and drinks. These portions are too large to be regularly be part of a healthy sports diet. Order smaller versions of these items.
- Chicken and fish are only good choices if grilled, broiled, or baked. Often these proteins are breaded and deep-fried and can contain more fat than a burger.
- Fast-food establishments that offer lower-fat sandwiches are likely to be your best choice.
- Portion distortion has become a big part of our fast-food culture. Choose the smaller items on the menu. Often they provide all the protein and calories that you need for your training diet.

Dairy Products. Choose low-fat milk, frozen yogurt, and low-fat milk shakes. Avoid whole milk products and hard ice cream.

Starches and Grains. Choose the small order of fries, low-fat muffins, bagels, cereals, baked potatoes, and pancakes and waffles. Avoid large fries, croissants, hash browns, and pastries.

Meats and Main Dishes. Choose grilled chicken, plain small hamburgers, chicken fajitas, bean burritos, bean chili, vegetable pizza, and chicken, turkey, vegetarian, and ham sandwiches. Avoid fried chicken and fish sandwiches, large hamburgers and cheeseburgers, fish or chicken nuggets, and pizza with meat toppings.

Salad Bar. Choose lettuce, pasta with marinara, raw vegetables, low-fat dressing, vegetable soups, fresh fruit, and baked potatoes with vegetable toppings. Avoid cream soups, high-fat dressings, potato salad, and tuna salad.

Sauces. Choose ketchup, mustard, and barbecue sauce. Avoid mayonnaise and cream sauces.

Ethnic Cuisine

Chances are that if you eat out frequently, you enjoy many types of ethnic cuisine that are increasingly popular and available. These cultural edibles can fit into a healthy training diet if you know what choices to make and avoid consuming hidden fat.

Italian Cuisine

Italian food is a popular favorite and can be consumed at a variety of settings—upscale, family-style, pizza, or fast food. With an emphasis on grains and vegetables, Italian eating can be healthy. Some lighter, lower-fat choices would be starches such as spaghetti (not cheese filled), risotto, and polenta (both prepared low-fat); vegetable choices such as tomato-based sauces, zucchini, and other vegetables prepared without fat; and lean meats such as skinless chicken, veal, shrimp, and grilled fish. You can also try condiments such as herbs, cooking wines, vinegar, garlic, and crushed red peppers. Fill up on minestrone soup, and top pasta with marinara or red clam sauce. Order your dressing on the side, and have Italian ice for dessert. You can also make some special requests, including removing the olive oil from the table and having the skin taken off chicken.

Plenty of heavier choices are offered at Italian restaurants, too. Starches such as garlic bread and focaccia contain fat, as do fried vegetables and meats such as salami, proscuitto, and sausage. Watch out for high-fat cheeses and dishes prepared with cream, butter, and even olive oil, which still contains plenty of fat calories. Go easy on the antipasto plate and the olive oil served with bread. Alfredo sauce, Italian sausage, lasagna, and parmigiana dishes are all high in fat because of the ingredients and methods of preparation.

Mexican Cuisine

Mexican cuisine may also be on your list of ethnic favorites. Like Italian food, this cuisine contains both light and heavy choices. Many staples of Mexican cuisine can be considered low-fat items such as whole beans, refried beans prepared without oil, tortillas, rice cooked without oil, grilled vegetables, and salsa. Grilled proteins such as shrimp, fish, or chicken are good choices, as are whole black beans. You can also fill up on gazpacho, marinated vegetables, and burritos (easy on the cheese).

Some heavier choices at Mexican restaurants would be tortilla chips, chimichangas, and taco shells. Avocados (including prepared as guacamole) and olives are also high in fat. You should also watch out for chorizo, cheese, sour cream, and oil used in cooking as they may contribute a significant amount of fat and saturated fat to your diet.

Chinese Cuisine

Chinese cuisine, providing a variety of regional cooking styles, is a frequent favorite at mall eateries and small neighborhood restaurants. Although there are light choices in Chinese cooking, there are also many high-fat pitfalls. To keep your meal on the light side, look for stir-fried vegetables. You have a variety to choose from: peapods, bamboo shoots, water chestnuts, cabbage, baby corn, and broccoli.

Lean proteins that are found in Chinese dishes include vegetable dishes with shrimp, chicken, tofu, and lean cuts of beef and pork. Dishes may also contain low-fat fruits such as pineapple and orange sections. Condiments such as mustard, soy sauce, ginger, sweet sauce, and garlic will not increase the fat content of your meals.

Chinese cuisine also contains plenty of high-fat choices. Everyone is familiar with the fatty breaded and fried sweet-and-sour dishes. Fried rice has twice the calories as steamed rice, with all the additional calories coming from oil. Fried noodles and egg rolls can also up your fat intake. Try to stay away from fried seafood, pork, spare ribs, and duck with skin. Stir-fry dishes that contain nuts and peanuts will also be much higher in fat, as will any choices in which oil is used heavily. Request that your dish be prepared with as little oil as possible, and try to split entrées as portions are often large.

Thai Cuisine

Thai food is quickly becoming one of the most popular and frequented types of Asian restaurants. Besides offering hot and spicy dishes, Thai restaurants feature some healthful low-fat choices. Again, make special menu requests that keep down the fat content of the dishes.

Thai tends to be a healthier food choice than Chinese cooking and does employ similar cooking techniques such as stir-frying. Ingredients are also similar, with an emphasis on rice and noodles and certain vegetables and proteins. It is very important to gravitate toward leaner proteins that are cooked stir-fry–style, such as chicken, shrimp, and even thin strips of pork or beef. Sometimes proteins are prepared by deep-frying, so ask questions and make sure that you understand what is on the menu. However, dishes are usually stir-fired, steamed, or braised. You can also request that dishes be prepared light on the oil. Vegetable oil is usually used, but coconut oil is more traditional. Large portions can also be shared family-style. Nuts and peanuts can be added to dishes in small amounts. Soups at Thai restaurants can be vegetable based and filling. Some menu items may load up on vegetables and use light sauce for cooking. Tofu or bean curd dishes are also widely available.

At Thai restaurants, try to avoid fried or deep-fried items, crispy noodles, coconut milk soup, and duck meat. Dressing can be requested on the side, so inquire about the type and amount of oil, and choose leaner proteins.

Middle Eastern Cuisine

Middle Eastern food fare is distinguished by such tasty dishes as hummus, tabouli, baba ganoush, and shish kebabs. Some central ingredients include chickpeas, olives, wheat and pita bread, grains such as rice and couscous, legumes, tomato, and onion. Stuffed dishes, either meat-based or vegetarian, are common, and olive oil is the predominant oil used. Common protein-containing foods include yogurt, lamb, beef, and eggs. Foods can be grilled, fried, or stewed.

Middle Eastern food can be a good match with a healthy sports diet. There are plenty of carbohydrates to choose from, protein portions can be kept to reasonable levels, and vegetables fill the menu. As with many other cuisines, you need to watch out for hidden fats. Watch out for excess olives, olive oil (though it is a healthy type of fat), salad dressings, marinades, and sauces. Try to avoid fried foods such as falafel, and, of

Protein and the Vegetarian Athlete

Team sport athletes do have increased protein requirements, and vegetarian athletes should appreciate that a portion of a quality plant is not as concentrated a source of protein as an animal protein. The key to obtaining enough protein in your diet is to first consume enough calories, so that the protein you do consume is not processed for energy. Second, an emphasis must be placed on high-quality and concentrated plant protein sources. Certain grains, dried peas and beans, lentils, nuts, and seeds are some of the best sources. Soy products such as tempeh and tofu are one plant protein essentially equivalent to animal protein.

Although it is not necessary to combine or complement various plant proteins at the same meal as was once thought, you should make a concerted effort to obtain adequate plant proteins in your diet throughout the day. The body will make its own complete proteins over the course of the day, if you consume enough calories. If your calorie intake falls short, some of the protein you do consume may be processed for energy, rather than be utilized for important protein functions. Table 8.7 lists some good plant protein sources.

TABLE 8.7 PROTEIN SOURCES OF PLANT FOODS		
Food	Portion	Protein (g)
Tempeh	1 c. (240 ml)	39
Soybeans, cooked	1 c. (240 ml)	29
Seitan	4 oz. (120 g)	21
Tofu, firm	4 oz. (120 g)	20
Lentils, cooked	1 c. (240 ml)	18
Kidney beans, cooked	1 c. (240 ml)	15
Lima beans, cooked	1 c. (240 ml)	15
Chickpeas, cooked	1 c. (240 ml)	15
Black beans, cooked	1 c. (240 ml)	15
Pinto beans, cooked	1 c. (240 ml)	14
Quinoa, cooked	1 c. (240 ml)	11
Soy yogurt	1 c. (240 ml)	10
Soy milk	1 c. (240 ml)	10
Tofu, regular	4 oz. (120 g)	10
Peanut butter	2 tbsp. (40 ml)	8
Sunflower seeds	1/4 c. (60 ml)	8
Peas, cooked	1 c. (240 ml)	8
Bulgur, cooked	1 c. (240 ml)	6
Bagel	1 medium	6
Pasta or grain	1 c. cooked (240 ml)	6
Almonds	1/4 c. (60 ml)	5.5
Brown rice, cooked	1 c. (240 ml)	5
Bread, whole wheat	2 slices	5
Potato	1 medium	4.5

course, desserts such as baklava are high in fat. Tahini, which is ground sesame paste, is all fat.

Typically, you have many health salads to choose from; just ask for dressings on the side. You may find healthy lentil soup on the menu. You can also order a series of appetizers and even split some larger entrées. Look for lower-fat items such as chickpeas, tomatoes, onions, and green peppers; grilled meat or kebabs; and charbroiled or stewed items. Go easy on cheeses, oils, and fried items.

Pizza

Pizza is a popular and inexpensive meal out or easily ordered in for lunch, dinner, or a late-night snack. Cold leftover pizza is also good the next day. Pizza starts with dough, then tomato sauce, and then usually high-fat cheese. Vegetables offer a variety of toppings, as do fatty meats such as pepperoni and sausage. It is unlikely that you will find low-fat cheese at most pizzerias, though some gourmet varieties may use a variety of cheese and even leaner proteins such as chicken. Overeating is one of the biggest problems with pizza. It is easy to have more than two slices, and some varieties offer a thick-crust version or an extra-cheesy deep-dish variety.

Besides portion control, you can also make special requests when ordering your pizza. Ask for half the cheese or even cheeseless pizza. You can also ask for extra vegetable toppings and tomato sauce. A sprinkle of cheese such as grated Parmesan can go a long way to adding flavor and not many calories on a cheeseless pizza. Try to avoid fatty proteins such as sausage whenever possible. When ordering salad at pizzerias, ask for dressing on the side.

Seafood

Seafood restaurants are everywhere, and fish is served in a wide variety of restaurants, from some of the most pricey to greasy fast-food fare. A range of choices is possible, from the low-fat, such as mesquite grilled, to the ultra-fat-laden Lobster Newberg. Of course, the fast-food varieties that are breaded and deep-fried are filled with fat as well. All fish prior to preparation is relatively low-fat, even the "fattier" varieties that are full of the healthy omega-3 fatty acids.

Common good appetizer selections, if they are not breaded and deep-fried, include oysters, sushi, shrimp cocktail, clams, and mussels. When choosing fish on the menu, keep in mind the dish's preparation. Blackened fish tends to be low-fat. Inquire about the sauces used to prepare the fish, and avoid cream sauces. Request that the chef go easy on clear sauces that contain oils. Marinated and stir-fried varieties are usually good menu choices, as are teriyaki and any steamed variety. Fish can come with rice or potatoes, prepared low-fat or high-fat. Again, make menu inquiries and substitutions as needed.

Lunch Spots

Lunch is the meal consumed out most frequently, mainly due to timing and convenience. Aim for low-fat items, such as clear, noodle, or vegetable-based soups. Request salads easy on the cheese, with dressing on the side. Look for roasted or grilled chicken items, and request sandwiches to order whenever possible. Watch out for fatty sides such as French fries, onion rings, and potato and macaroni salads. Pretzels are lower-fat, as are fruit sides and low-fat yogurts.

Salad Bars

Visits to the salad bar are often well intended but can result in surprisingly high-fat meals. Besides those healthy raw vegetables such as spinach, tomatoes, broccoli, and green peppers, there are plenty of items mixed with fat or sitting in oil. Some of the less

Protein Tips for Vegetarians

- Include a protein-rich food at all meals and snacks.
- Add milk or fortified soy milk or the yogurt equivalent to every meal or snack.
- Use nuts butters, hummus, and low-fat cheeses (soy and regular) for toppings on breads, bagels, and crackers.
- Add nuts and seeds to a fruit and yogurt snack.
- Make tofu and tempeh stir-fry.
- Experiment with quick and easy bean recipes such as burritos, casseroles, and salads.
- Make thick soups and stews with beans and lentils.
- Experiment with all the meat replacement soy products on the market such as tofu dogs and burgers.
- Make casseroles, lasagna, and stuffed shell recipes with tofu.

Meal-Planning Tips for Vegetarians

- The health food section of many supermarkets and most health food stores provide a wide selection of vegetarian food choices and convenience items.
- The number of textured vegetable protein products has increased significantly in the past several years. You can now buy products that resemble and taste like hot dogs, burgers, and breakfast sausage; these foods make quick and easy lunches.
- Tofu can be substituted for chicken in most recipes. Seasoned tofu is available, and you can also season the recipe to spice up tofu's milder taste.
- You can substitute vegetable broth when recipes call for beef or chicken stock. Vegetable broth is available in many supermarkets and most health food stores.
- Canned lentils, chickpeas, and beans are a quick and nutritious vegetarian option. When time allows, soak the dried lentil and bean versions. Many bean and lentil recipes can be cooked in batches and frozen for later use.
- If you need assistance, find a vegetarian cookbook with meal ideas suited to athletes.
- Include protein-rich foods at each meal. Because vegetarian options are not as concentrated in protein as animal protein, you need to include adequate portions at most meals and snacks.
- Purchase calcium-fortified soy and rice milks if you drink these products instead of dairy milk.
- Purchase iron-fortified cereals, and consume them with products high in vitamin C such as orange juice.

healthy choices include pasta salad, potato salad, marinated vegetables, cheeses, and bean salads made with oil. Go easy on these items. Try to keep salad dressing portions reasonable, too.

Salad bars have plenty of carbohydrates and fiber, which can help you keep your protein portions low and reasonable. Obviously fresh greens and plain raw vegetables are your best choices. Starches on the salad bar may include chickpeas, kidney beans, green peas, crackers, croutons, and pita bread. Lean protein salad bar choices include plain tuna, cottage cheese, egg, ham, and feta cheese. Try to avoid most cheeses and pepperoni. Keep marinated vegetable portions small, and especially watch out for tuna, chicken, and seafood salad, and macaroni and potato salads that can contain plenty of mayonnaise. High-fat items such as peanuts, sesame seeds, and sunflower seeds, which provide good fats, can be used in small amounts.

PART III

Sport-Specific
Nutrition Guidelines
How to Eat for Your Sport

Each of the five team sports highlighted in this book has its own unique training plan and competition schedule, and therefore its own specific nutritional considerations. Part III focuses on nutrition guidelines for baseball, football, basketball, soccer, and hockey. Sample menus for both male and female competitors are provided for both training days and game day. You can reference the sample menus in various chapters for additional menu ideas.

Topics that are of interest to players in a specific sport are covered—for example, preventing heat cramps in football players and eating on the road for baseball players. However, many of these topics are of interest to all team sport players, so please cross-reference these chapters as needed.

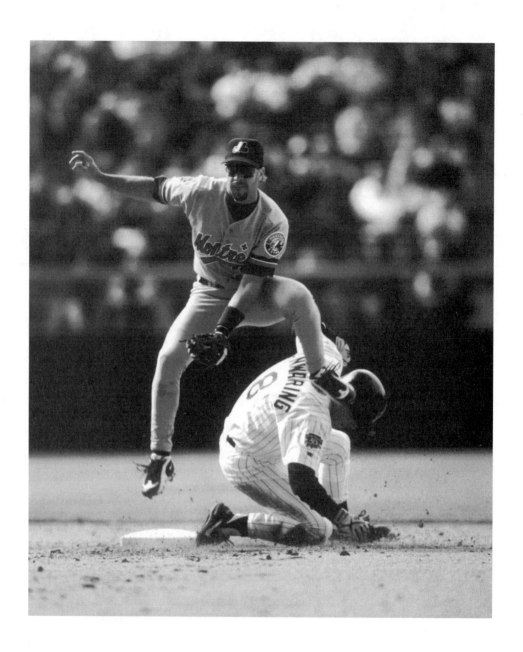

CHAPTER 9

NUTRITION FOR BASEBALL AND SOFTBALL

Baseball is a popular sport at all levels, with over 10 million participants annually. Younger players train and compete in Little League baseball, and they can play at the elementary, middle school, and high school levels. College baseball is also popular, and of course baseball is played in the minor league professional teams, semiprofessional teams, and professional levels. There are women's baseball leagues and amateur clubs, and baseball has been an Olympic sport since 1992.

Many spectators derive much enjoyment from the game, commonly described as one of America's favorite pastimes. Professional baseball talk starts with spring training, when fans are interested in the fitness level of their favorite players, and continues through the fall season with the World Series. In college, baseball is a spring sport, and younger players often participate in their sport through the summer months when out of school.

Softball currently has more than 16 million participants. It was first played in Chicago in 1887 on a cold winter day, when the game of baseball was adapted to be played indoors. It became a national sport in 1933 and was first played in the Olympics in 1996. Softball is a highly popular sport, especially among female participants, and is played on a smaller field than baseball. Equipment includes an oversized ball and smaller bat than those used in baseball. Softball is not a substitute for baseball, but it is a sport that is highly skill-oriented and often very fast-paced as players strategize their way around the smaller dimensions of the playing ground.

DEMANDS OF THE GAME

Baseball is a game between two teams of nine players each, with the objective being to win by scoring more runs than your opponent. Baseball and softball are mainly skill sports in which participants must exhibit fine-motor control, excellent coordination, and swift reaction time. They require both individual and team efforts to win a game. Baseball and softball are distinguished from the more middle-distance and endurance-oriented team sports in that they are not games of continuous activity and they provide opportunities to rest during the game. While players may engage in some general aerobic conditioning, the main training focus is on developing anaerobic power for pitching a fastball, running the bases, batting, and throwing. Baseball practices take place outdoors, often in heat and humidity.

Baseball competition can last several hours and frequently takes place in hot conditions over nine innings. Softball can be played over a number of months, including the hot summer months. During competition, players may stand in the sun for long periods of time (or sit in the dugout) and then require quick bursts of maximum acceleration. Games typically last 2 to 3 hours, and many young softball players can compete in tournaments that require playing in several games in a day and over several days. Baseball and softball are also highly mental games, requiring the ability to make split-second judgments that require good levels of blood glucose. Baseball and softball also demand power and speed that is fueled by phosphocreatine and muscle glycogen stores. A season may entail several games, with players becoming run-down by the end of the season.

Energy Requirements

Development of the skills required for baseball and softball does not necessarily translate to exceptionally high demands for energy. Pitchers likely have higher energy needs than fielders, and many players may engage in various phases of serious resistance training programs to develop muscular strength, which can increase energy needs (see Chapter 6). Because pitchers work harder than other players, they need to eat adequately to maintain muscular power in both their arms and legs. For example, a 170-pound (77-kilogram) pitcher burns 6.7 calories per minute, or 402 calories in 60 minutes of playing time. The same-weight player in the field would burn 5.1 calories per minute, or 306 calories in 60 minutes of playing time. A field player may also have more time of standing and inactivity during that 60 minutes of playing time than a pitcher. In comparison, a soccer player of the same weight would burn almost double the amount of calories in 1 hour at 10.2 calories per minute, for a total of 612 calories per hour. Catchers also work hard during the game and wear heavier equipment. Like pitchers, they also have higher energy requirements than other players.

Body Composition

In recent years, professional baseball players have increased in height and size as there is an intense focus on muscular development to enhance strength and power. Of course, younger baseball players can come in all shapes and sizes. For the more serious players, it would make sense that a healthy level of body fat would improve a player's speed, stamina, and heat tolerance. Because baseball and softball training does not burn a significant amount of calories and optimal body composition improves baseball and softball performance, these athletes should be aware of their energy requirements and practice sensible weight management strategies as outlined in Chapter 6. Baseball and softball players should also focus on specific nutrition strategies for muscle building as described in Chapter 6, when they are focused on that aspect of their training program. Body composition can be monitored at regular intervals to determine the amount of muscle gained and body fat lost.

Diet Composition

The main goals of a baseball and softball player's diet are to provide adequate fuel for training and replace muscle glycogen stores, meet protein requirements for training and resistance training, and keep fat intake to reasonable levels to maintain a healthy weight and good health. Because they rely heavily on muscle glycogen for fuel, baseball players should obtain 50 to 60 percent of their calories from carbohydrates, or 2.5 to 3.0 grams per pound (5.5 to 6.5 grams/kilogram) of body weight to replace liver and muscle glycogen stores depleted from baseball training and/or resistance training. Whole-grain, fruit, and vegetable carbohydrate choices, as described in Chapter 1, should be emphasized. Frequent games and practices can slowly deplete muscle glycogen stores over several days' time if the proper amount of carbohydrate is not consumed. By the end of the week, the baseball or softball player may feel fatigued and not perform at his sharpest.

Protein requirements for aerobic and anaerobic exercise during team training and strength training are easily met with a well-chosen diet and quality protein sources. Protein and carbohydrate intake can be timed properly before and after resistance training for maximizing muscle protein synthesis. Athletes who are trying to lose weight and may be controlling calories should consume protein at the high end of the recommended range. Generally, a protein intake of 15 to 20 percent of calories should meet the protein requirements for baseball and softball training.

Because their calorie needs are not exceptionally high, many baseball and softball players may have too much fat in their diet, pushing out healthy carbohydrate sources and consuming unhealthy fats that increase their risk for cardiovascular disease. Baseball and softball players, competing at many levels, may also eat out frequently due to away game schedules and travel for competition, which can significantly increase fat in the diet. Players can refer to healthy eating out guidelines as described in Chapter 8. The sidebar outlines several calorie levels for a sample for a baseball or softball player's training diet.

Meal Plans for Baseball/Softball Players

Meal Plan for High School Baseball/Softball Players

Morning Conditioning
Afternoon Practice

Breakfast (6:00 a.m.)
Cereal, whole-grain, 1.5 oz. (45 g)
Milk, skim, 8 oz. (240 ml)
Banana, 1 small
Juice, 8 oz. (240 ml)
Egg, 1 whole

Morning Conditioning (60 minutes)
Water at breaks

Postexercise Practice
Milk chug, 12 oz. (360 ml)
Bagel, 4 oz. (120 g)
Nut butter, 4 tsp. (30 ml)
Apple, 1 medium

Lunch (11:30 a.m.)
Peanut butter and jam sandwich
Peanut butter, 4 tsp. (30 ml)
Jam, 2 tbsp. (40 ml)
Bread, 2 slices
Peach, 1 medium
Pretzels, whole-grain, 3/4 oz. (22 g)
Milk, skim, 8 oz. (240 ml)
Assorted raw vegetables, 1 c.

Snack (2:30 p.m.)
Granola bar, 1 medium
Dried fruit, 6 pieces

Practice
Sports drink and water at breaks,
60–90 minutes

Postpractice Snack
Yogurt, 8 oz. (240 ml)
Pear, 1 small
Crackers, whole-grain, 6–8

Dinner (6:30 p.m.)
Poultry, 4 oz. (120 g)
Milk, skim, 8 oz. (240 ml)
Rice, brown, cooked, 2/3 c. (160 ml)
Broccoli, cooked, 1 c.
Bread, 2 slices

Evening Snack (9:00 p.m.)
Toasted cheese
Bread, 2 slices
Cheese, low-fat, 2 oz. (60 g)
Tomato, few slices

3,100 calories
115 g protein (15%)
450 g carbohydrate (58%)
93 g fat (27%)

Meal Plan for College Baseball/Softball Player

Afternoon Practice
Evening Conditioning

Breakfast (7:00 a.m.)
Muesli or granola, 3/4 c. (180 ml)
Apple, 1 medium

Raisins, 3 tbsp. (60 ml)

Soy or dairy milk, 1 c. (240 ml)

Almonds, 6 nuts

Morning Snack (9:30 a.m.)

Energy bar, 1 medium

Juice, 8 oz. (240 ml)

Lunch (12:30 p.m.)

Chicken tacos

Chicken, 3 oz. (90 g)

Beans, 1/2 c. (120 ml)

Rice, 1/2 c. (120 ml)

Tortillas, 2 large

Oil, 2 tsp. (15 ml)

Afternoon Snack (3:00 p.m.)

Banana, 1 large

Crackers, 2 oz. (60 g)

Peanut butter, 2 tbsp. (40 ml)

Dinner (6:00 p.m.)

Stir-fry

Beef, 4 oz. (120 g)

Broccoli, 1 c.

Rice, 2/3 c. cooked (180 ml)

Bread, 2 slices

Oil, 2 tsp. (15 ml)

2,800 calories

430 g carbohydrate (61%)

132 g protein (19%)

69 g fat (22%)

Meal Plan for Little League Baseball Player

Afternoon Practice

Breakfast (6:30 a.m.)

Oatmeal, 1 c. cooked (240 ml)

Strawberries, 1 c.

Juice, 8 oz. (240 ml)

Morning Snack (9:30 a.m.)

Graham crackers, 3

Apple, 1 medium

Lunch (12:30 p.m.)

Chicken, 3 oz. (90 g)

Whole-grain bread, 2 slices

Pretzels, 1.5 oz. (45 g)

Snack (3:00 p.m.)

Bagel, 4 oz. (120 g)

Peanut butter, 2 tsp. (15 ml)

Pear, 1 large

Dinner (6:00 p.m.)

Beef strips, 3 oz. (90 g)

Noodles, 2 c. cooked (480 ml)

Bread, 1 slice

Olive oil, 2 tsp. (15 ml)

Mixed vegetables, 1 c.

2,400 calories

330 g carbohydrate (55%)

122 g protein (20%)

73 g fat (27%)

Important Nutrition Strategies for Baseball and Softball
Hydration, Fluid Replacement, and Carbohydrate Intake

Fluid is likely the most important nutrient for the baseball and softball player. We have all seen our favorite baseball players cooling off in the dugout and pouring water on themselves, as well as drinking ample amounts of rehydrating beverages while coping with heat and high humidity. While baseball is generally played in nine innings and games last less than 4 hours, the game really has no time limit, and players may spend a considerable amount of time coping with the heat. Softball games are often played in the heat, and many players play in tournaments that require a focus on hydration strategies.

Dehydration resulting from sweat losses can negatively affect the performance of baseball and softball players by resulting in overheating and fatigue. Players of all ages should be aware of the signs and symptoms of dehydration such as dark urine, infrequent urination, and headache.

During practice, baseball and softball players should have free access to fluids to replace sweat losses. Studies indicate that optimal fluid consumption is a learned behavior and that players replace fluid losses best by following a schedule or protocol. Younger athletes clearly consume more fluid when given flavored beverages such as a sports drink. Collegiate and professional athletes may drink greater volumes of a flavored sports drink versus water as well. Sports drinks that contain carbohydrate also help the player maintain optimal blood glucose levels, which helps prevent hunger and maintain focus toward the end of the game.

Players should always begin practice or competition fully hydrated. Consuming carbohydrate during games and practice will also help maintain blood glucose levels. During practice, baseball and softball players should follow several fluid and carbohydrate replacement strategies:

- Keep up with daily hydration. Urine is more concentrated and darker in the morning, but it should be clear if you are adequately hydrated.
- The player or athletic trainer should devise an optimal drinking schedule before, during, and after training.
- Consume 16 to 32 ounces (480 to 960 milliliters) fluid in the 60 to 90 minutes before training.
- Drink another 8 to 16 ounces (240 to 480 milliliters) of fluid in the 20 to 30 minutes before training.

- Have or bring your own sports bottle with water or your favorite sports drink on the field during practice. Drink regularly during practice when a break permits.
- Keep fluid replacement beverages cool on the sidelines whenever possible.
- During games, have a sports drink when warming up and between innings.
- Check your weight before and after practice to determine sweat losses and the effectiveness of your drinking strategies. Be aware of how your sweat losses can vary for different types of training sessions and in different environmental conditions.
- Try to have scheduled drink breaks every half hour during training.
- Maintain a regular fluid intake when on the bench during a game.

Precompetition Meal

Precompetition meal timing is important for baseball and softball players who want to have a comfortably digested meal prior to all-out physical efforts at various points in the game. Eating right before the game prevents hunger during the game. An adequate pregame meal can also top off muscle glycogen stores and ensure good blood glucose levels for adequate mental concentration during long games. College and professional players frequently play night games, and younger players may play at various times during the day.

Meal timing should reflect a pregame meal consumed 3 hours or more before the start of the game. Players can aim for 1.0 to 1.5 grams per pound (2 to 3 grams/kilogram) of body weight of carbohydrate food choices that are low in fiber and easy to digest. Moderate amounts of low-fat protein can also be included in this meal to prevent hunger. Fat should be kept to lower levels for easy digestion.

It is also important the players have a plan for the timing of all their meals and snacks for game day. They should not rely on the immediate pregame meal to meet the majority of their food and fluid needs. Baseball and softball players who frequently have night games may arrive for a late-afternoon, pregame practice low on fuel and consume their first substantial meal several hours before the game. This one meal is not likely to adequately replenish body fuel stores, and the player may be running on fumes rather than high-octane fuel by the end of the game. Games are often followed by a large postgame meal.

Baseball and softball players should experiment with their meal timing on game day to fine-tune the timing and portions that work best for them. The sample menu below describes some meal timing and pregame food suggestions for game day. Portions of this sample menu can be trimmed for younger or lower-weight players. The meals emphasize carbohydrates for game day, with moderate amounts of protein and fat to control hunger. Players can also experiment with use of sports nutrition supplements such as gels and sports drinks in the 30 to 60 minutes before the game. These types of products can help maintain blood glucose levels and are easily digested. Blood glucose levels likely start to run low halfway through a game, depending on the position played and the amount of

Sample Competition Day Menu for Baseball/Softball

Game Start 7:00 p.m.

Breakfast (9:00 a.m.)
Cereal, 1.5 oz. (45 g)
Milk, skim, 8 oz. (240 ml)
Banana, 1 small

Lunch (12:30 p.m.)
Turkey sandwich
Pretzels, 1.5 oz. (45 g)
Juice, 8 oz. (240 ml)
Apple, 1 medium
Yogurt, 6 oz. (180 ml)
Almonds, 6

Afternoon Practice
Sports drink, 24 oz. per hour (720 ml)

Pregame Meal (3:30 p.m.)
Fish, 4 oz. (120 g)
Rice, 1.5 c. cooked (360 ml)
Bread, 2 slices
Cooked vegetables, ½ c.
Olive oil, 3 tsp. (20 ml)

Pregame Snack (6:00 p.m.)
Carbohydrate gel, 1 packet
Sports drink, 16–24 oz. (480–720 ml)

During Game
32 oz. sports drink (960 ml)
1–2 gel packets

Postgame Dinner
Beef, lean, 4 oz. (120 g)
Baked potato, 1 medium
Salad, 1–2 c.
Salad dressing, 3 tbsp. (60 ml)
Vegetables, 1 c.
20 oz. (600 ml) of fluid for 1 lb. (2.2 kg)
  weight loss.

3,100 calories
460 g carbohydrate (60%)
125 g protein (165)
83 g fat (24%)

playing time. Consuming a sports drink or gel ensures that blood glucose levels stay within the normal range, fueling your brain to maintain top concentration and focus.

During the off-season, you may need to adjust your nutrition plan for a slightly different training focus. You may emphasize resistance training and complete a moderate aerobic workout for general fitness. The sample menu below provides a menu for off-season training that is focused on weight training. Remember that building muscle requires adequate calories and protein, as well as protein and carbohydrate intake

Game Start 3:00 p.m.

Breakfast (8:00 a.m.)
Oatmeal, cooked, 1 c. (240 ml)
Egg, hard-boiled, 1
Banana, 1 medium
Raisins, 1 tbsp. (20 ml)
Soy or dairy milk, 8 oz. (240 ml)

Lunch (11 a.m.)
Turkey, 4 oz. (120 g)
Bread, 2 slices
Cheese, 1 oz. (30 g)
Juice, 12 oz. (360 ml)
Grapes, 1 c. (240 ml)
Yogurt, 6 oz. (180 ml)

Snack (2:00 p.m.)
Energy bar, 1
Sports drink, 24 oz. (720 ml)

During game
32 oz. sports drink (960 ml)
1–2 gel packets as tolerated

Recovery (6:00 p.m.)
Carbohydrate drink, 24 oz. (720 ml)

Dinner (8:00 p.m.)
Pasta, cooked, 3 c. (720 ml)
Meat sauce, 1 c. (240 ml)
Salad, 2 c. (480 ml)
Dressing, light, 4 tbsp. (80 ml)

3,000 calories
430 g carbohydrate (57%)
110 g protein (15%)
95 g protein (28%)

Off-season Training Menu

Afternoon Weight Training

Breakfast
Bagel, whole-grain, 4 oz. (120 g)
Peanut butter, 2 tbsp. (40 ml)
Jam, 2 tbsp. (40 ml)
Milk, 12 oz. (360 ml)

Snack
Peach, 1 medium

Lunch
Low-fat cheese, 3 oz. (90 g)
Tomato and vegetable slices
Bread, 2 slices
Plum, 2 small
Yogurt with fruit, 6 oz. (180 ml)

Pretraining
Smoothie:
Soy or dairy milk, 8 oz. (240 ml)
Yogurt, 4 oz. (120 ml)
Frozen fruit, 1 c.

Resistance training
Water or sports drink, 16 oz. (480 ml)

Posttraining
Milk, 16 oz. (480 ml)
Banana, 1 large

Dinner
Fish, 6 oz. (180 g)
Sweet potato, 8 oz. (240 ml)
Broccoli, cooked, 1 c.
Salad, 2 c.
Salad dressing, light, 4 tbsp. (80 ml)

3,000 calories
390 g carbohydrate (52%)
135 g protein (18%)
100 g fat (30%)

timed properly after exercise. Light aerobic training also increases your calorie needs, as do any conditioning workouts and plyometrics.

Eating on the Road

Major- and minor-league and collegiate baseball players frequently travel for games, as do softball players who participate in the sport almost year-round. Choosing high-carbohydrate foods and keeping choices low in fat can be challenging when traveling. Chapter 8 reviews healthy eating choices for various types of cuisines and restaurants.

Eating on the Road

Meal	Food Choices
Breakfast	Choose dry and cooked cereals, juices, fresh fruit, waffles, French toast, and pancakes. Keep margarine and butter to a minimum. Order low-fat or skim milk and low-fat yogurt. Bagels and muffins with small amounts of peanut butter and jam are good choices as well. Order omelets made with egg whites and go easy on the cheese, while asking for vegetable fillings.
Lunch	Try to frequent restaurants that have low-fat sandwiches made from poultry or lean meats. Lower-fat tuna salads may be available. Go easy on the cheese, and ask for extra vegetable toppings whenever possible. Choose salads covered with lean protein, baked potatoes, and chili. Choose the regular-sized hamburger or cheeseburger, and split a small French fry serving with a teammate.
Dinner	Choose lean meats, fish, or poultry that is broiled, grilled, baked, or blackened. Ask that potatoes, rice, pasta, or noodles be prepared with less fat. Consume breads and rolls, and go easy on the margarine or butter. Have fruit for dessert whenever possible. Order salad with dressing on the side.
Snacks	Try fresh fruit, dried fruit, granola bars, energy bars. Buy milk chugs and low-fat yogurt whenever possible. Snack on low-fat crackers, instant soups, and pretzels. Drink water and other fluids.

When trying to eat healthfully on the road, it is important to limit hidden fats and fatty foods. Packing your own snacks can also ensure some healthy eating between meals, as can specific restaurant ordering strategies. Some guidelines for eating healthfully on the road include the following:

- Bring your own snacks for travel—for example, fresh fruit, dried fruit, crackers, pretzels, cereals, and energy bars. Try to coordinate items that can be transported in a team cooler such as bagels, yogurt, sandwiches, and milk chugs.

- Drink plenty of liquids from water, juice, and milk to stay hydrated.
- Choose grilled, baked, broiled, and boiled food items rather than fried. Don't hesitate to ask for special requests that reduce fat intake. Pay attention to hidden fats such as high-fat breads and pastries, items cooked with fatty sauces, creamy soups, and mayonnaise-based salad dressings.
- Order individual items à la carte if desired to put together a meal that you would enjoy.
- Have someone with the team call ahead to locate restaurants in the area to which you are traveling that offer menus appropriate for a healthy sports nutrition diet.

Late-night Eating

Because of their travel schedule and evening or night games, baseball and softball players often eat late at night when hunger sets in after a game. Eating foods rich in carbohydrate can replenish muscle glycogen stores, with high-glycemic carbohydrates being the preferred fuel (see Chapter 5). It is important for the baseball and softball player not to overeat at this meal. Chances are that there will be 12 to 16 hours to refuel before the next practice or game. It might also be helpful to have some recovery fluids and fuel on hand after the game, such as a high-carbohydrate drink or smoothie. The player should check body weight and consume 20 ounces (600 milliliters) of fluid for every pound of weight lost. Lean and low-fat choices should be made after this time. Overeating at night could disturb sleep patterns, and caffeine should also be kept to a minimum. Keep portions reasonable so that you can begin the replenishment process again the next day at breakfast. It is important to eat properly in the 4 to 8 hours leading up to the next practice.

Nutrition Supplementation

Creatine Loading for Baseball and Softball

The use of ergogenic aids in baseball received wide attention during the baseball home-run record-setting season of 1998. Because of the increased emphasis on building muscle and developing a more powerful swing, creatine is a much-talked-about supplement in baseball circles. However, data on creatine in baseball players are limited. In theory, creatine loading could help baseball performance by increasing this fuel source in the muscles and raising the rate of resynthesis in the muscle between bouts of exercise. Creatine also supports muscle-building efforts during weight training.

One study measured the effects of creatine loading on female collegiate softball players. Researchers found an increase in strength and endurance with repeated exercise contractions. They speculated that the performance effects of creatine loading were not as pronounced in females as in males.

However, there are several concerns regarding creatine use in baseball and softball players, both male and female. First and foremost, many baseball and softball players are young and in grade school and high school, and there are no short-term safety data regarding creatine and children and adolescents. In addition, we have only limited long-term safety data on creatine use in collegiate athletes and adults. Creatine loading for 5 days in the recommended dose (see Chapter 6) appears safe, but many athletes now consume low doses of creatine every day. This practice raises safety concerns and likely is not necessary for improving performance. It is recommended that young athletes do not take creatine but rather rely on sound training and nutrition strategies for improving performance.

Baseball and softball players should also appreciate that creatine loading produces a weight gain, often as high as 2 to 6 pounds (1 to 2.5 kilograms), depending on the length of supplementation. This weight gain, while mainly fluid held in the muscle from creatine loading, could affect speed and explosiveness.

Anecdotal reports have described cramping and other muscle-related injuries with creatine loading. One study looked at Division I baseball players. Five days of creatine loading and a maintenance creatine dose during the training season did not appear to result in side effects such as cramping or increased incidence of injury. This was a short-term study, however, and does not address possible side effects with long-term use of creatine.

Of course, creatine supplements can be contaminated with banned ingredients if proper quality control is not followed when the raw product is produced or when there is not good quality control at the time of packaging. The NCAA considers creatine nonpermissible and does not encourage use of this supplement.

Recovering from an Injury

At some point in your athletic career, it is possible that you may experience some type of injury from strain, abrasions, bruising, and fractures. The speed at which your injury heals likely is of major concern to you. While you may have a rehabilitation program planned out for yourself, the nutritional guidelines that you should follow while injured may not be as clear. What is clear, however, is that protein, fat, carbohydrates, and vitamins and minerals are essential for timely and complete healing of injuries. Weight management issues may also present themselves at the time of an injury due to a marked decrease in energy expenditure.

Nutritional considerations can vary among specific situations and athletes. But often during rehabilitation a natural fear arises of putting on body fat. Injury often results in significant changes in energy expenditure, owing to a decrease from your usual training program in regard to the types of training and, for a period of time, even its volume and intensity. When you are accustomed to consuming a specific amount of food for your training program, it may be difficult to know how and when to cut back on your caloric intake to achieve the proper caloric balance. Muscle mass may also decrease when you are injured depending on the type of rehabilitation program that you are prescribed.

Depending on the type and extent of the injury, caloric expenditure may decrease by several thousand calories per week. An athlete who decreases training volume by 4 hours a week could experience a weekly 1-pound weight gain if she kept up with her usual eating habits.

However, when recovering from an injury, it is best not to undereat protein and calories. Protein is required for the growth and repair of body tissue, supports healthy immune function, and is required for the synthesis of enzymes and hormones. Undereating can also lead to increased incidence of infection and slower wound healing.

Regardless of the type of injury, it is important to maintain energy balance. Injured athletes can keep a food record and determine their normal caloric intake. They then can trim anywhere from 200 to 500 calories or more daily to prevent weight gain if needed. Sometimes intake of carbohydrate and protein amounts need to be decreased slightly to prevent a gain in body fat. Excess dietary fat that was easily burned off in training should also be shaved down. But avoid drastic dietary restrictions so that you don't miss out on needed nutrients. Often some personalized guidance from a sports nutritionist can be helpful when you are injured.

In many instances, however, a good resistance and rehabilitation program provides a big calorie advantage. Building muscle takes work and energy, allowing you to consume more calories and somewhat offset the decreased caloric expenditure from normal training for your sport. If these weight-training sessions are intense, consuming carbohydrate during training can facilitate recovery and muscle repair.

After an initial period of healing, athletes often engage in rehabilitation programs that are just as demanding as their usual training, though the program may differ in scope and timing. Your usual meal plan may need to be adjusted to support energy levels at specific training times and encourage tissue repair and muscle-building efforts.

Increasing your intake of certain nutrients and perhaps even supplementation may support the healing process. One of the principal functions of vitamin C, for example, is collagen synthesis, a core component of scar tissue. Collagen is also required for the formation and maintenance of connective tissue such as cartilage, tendon, and bone. Vitamin C plays a role in red blood cell synthesis. Load up on some good vitamin C sources, as listed in Chapter 2. Fruits and vegetables are abundant in vitamin C and are also lower-calorie foods. Increasing your intake of fruits and vegetables will also provide antioxidants and bioflavinoids that can protect your muscles against damage during exercise and support the healing process.

Other important vitamins include vitamin A, which supports collagen formation and the immune system. B vitamin requirements can increase if trauma and stress are associated with the injury.

Minerals also play important roles in injury recovery, including iron and zinc. Zinc is an important component of many enzymes involved in energy metabolism and is required for protein synthesis and wound healing. Good sources of zinc include lean red meat, turkey, milk, yogurt, and seafood, especially oysters. Zinc from animal protein is best absorbed. Iron, of course, is needed for oxygen transport and for the formation of hemoglobin and myoglobin so that the athlete can maintain a high level of rehabilitation training. Good sources are listed in Chapter 2.

Your protein and calorie requirements can change at specific phases of the rehabilitation process. However, a nutrient-dense diet is a plus at any time after an injury. A good multivitamin mineral supplement high in antioxidants can also be useful in supporting healthy food choices.

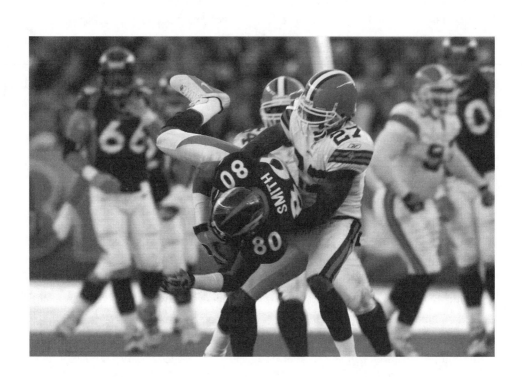

CHAPTER 10
NUTRITION FOR AMERICAN FOOTBALL

Football is a team sport that requires players with speed, agility, tactics, and brute strength, to allow them to push, block, tackle, chase, and outrun each other while trying to force the ball into their opponent's territory. Officially there is 1 hour of game playing time, which often translates into 3 to 4 hours of real time. It can be a very physically demanding sport, with physical contact occurring on every play. Players are getting bigger and stronger, with players in the National Football League often weighing 300 pounds or more.

Of course, professional football is one of the most watched games, but football is played at a number of levels in the United States. Arena football is played indoors, and football is widely played at the high school and college levels. Many recreational players play the less intense versions of flag and touch football. Football is a direct descendent of rugby union football, which descended from soccer. In American football, the player's feet rarely touch the ball, and during the vast majority of the game, the players are holding the ball in their hands.

DEMANDS OF THE GAME

Football is characterized by intermittent activity of short bursts of very intense, often all-out effort, usually not exceeding 15 seconds when the ball is in play, followed by a period of rest between plays. The game requires a high level of anaerobic strength endurance, such as when running with the ball. The more explosive a player's strength, the tougher it is for an opponent to tackle the player. But quickness and agility also benefit a player trying to weave down the field toward a touchdown.

Football is also characterized by the burden of wearing and carrying heavy equipment and by the different characteristics of various positions played. Quarterbacks require speed, agility, and strength; wide receivers, running backs, and defensive backs need quickness; linebackers and tight ends must be fast and strong; and linemen need to be strong and are generally larger in order to block their position.

Regardless of the position played, football is mainly fueled by the creatine phosphate system and muscle glycogen. Football players may also practice twice daily at certain times during the season and are usually participating in a serious weight-training program to build muscle mass and strength.

TRAINING DIET

Energy Requirements

Energy requirements vary from player to player depending on body size and muscle mass, the position played, training program, and body composition goals. Now it is quite normal for offensive linemen in both college and professional ranks to weigh over 300 pounds (136 kilograms), and football players at every level are getting bigger and stronger every year and weigh more for a given height than in previous decades. However, these higher body weights can sometimes translate into a higher rate of injury. Weight loss may also be an issue for lightweight football players, perhaps even leading to unhealthy eating behaviors.

Energy needs clearly can vary greatly from player to player and need to be individualized. Larger players participating in weight training and twice-daily practice can require several thousand calories daily. Recent data presented at the 2004 American College of Sports Medicine meeting indicate that the energy expenditure of linemen during practice may be higher than previously thought, with limited rest periods available to the athletes.

Energy needs of football players can also vary during the season. The most intense time of year is preseason when players participate in twice-a-day practices and weight training. Later in the season, one practice may be a bit lighter or include weight training, with a more demanding second practice later in the day. Calorie needs may dip down from preseason. During the off-season, younger players may participate in other sports during various times during the football off-season, while collegiate and professional players may follow a serious conditioning program and continue weight training when not actively training for football.

Energy expenditure during a game likely is significantly lower, with stops in play and significant rest periods on the sidelines, than during stops in practice. During practice, current estimates place energy expenditure for a 190-pound (86-kilogram) player at 378 calories during 1 hour of play. More data on calorie burning for different positions played and types of activities during football practice are needed. Calorie requirements for the day must be individualized to the player's age, growth and development, training during the season and off-season, and body composition goals.

Body Weight and Body Fat

Regardless of whether a football player is more slightly built and focused on building muscle mass or starts the preseason at a higher body fat than desired, or both, it can be useful to monitor body composition, rather than just body weight. Monitoring body composition, in regard not only to body fat percentages but also to absolute values of fat measurements, can be useful. The athlete and coach or trainer or team nutritionist can determine whether muscle mass is increasing and body fat decreasing. Monitoring weight and body composition can be useful even for the high school football player, as there seems to be a higher rate of obesity among this group of athletes. Often these athletes may attempt to increase calorie and protein intake indiscriminately in an attempt to gain muscle mass, without understanding their energy and protein needs and the proper timing of their nutritional intake (see Chapter 6). Bulking up requires a sound weight-training program, proper nutrition, and realistic expectations as to the rate and amount of muscle gain. Obviously increasing muscle mass and maintaining a healthy level of body fat, not just the body weight on the scale, should be the focus for football players.

One recent study on Division I football players checked body fat levels to determine whether the increase in body mass over the past 10 years has been accompanied by an increase in body fat. It was found that both total body mass and body fat were higher than levels measured in players the two previous decades. Body fat levels varied among positions, with defensive backs, offensive backs, and receivers being the leanest players and offensive linemen and tight ends having the highest levels of body fat. It was also of note that linemen and tight ends on average had body fat levels exceeding 25 percent, an unhealthy and at-risk level in this age group. Much of this excess body fat was concentrated in the abdominal region, which is associated with increased risk for heart disease and stroke. These results underscore the need for nutrition education in this group.

Lighter-weight players may also be focused on maintaining a body weight that allows them to run explosively and swiftly. Their body composition can also be monitored. Energy intake should match their body fat and performance goals. One study found that lightweight college football players may use unhealthy weight control practices such as fasting and using laxatives, diet pills, and diuretics. A large number of these athletes admitted to some type of disordered eating. These reports illustrate, again, the need for appropriate nutrition education and monitoring in this group of athletes.

Diet Composition

Regardless of the position played, adequate carbohydrate stores are critical for the football player, particularly during periods of intense practice and training. Often football players may be under the impression that they require high amounts of protein and may push carbohydrates out of their diet to obtain more of this nutrient. Frequent eating out can also increase the fat content of the diet. Carbohydrate replaces the muscle

Meal Plan for a Football Player

Preseason
Dorm Food Menu

Breakfast (6:30 a.m.)
Pancakes, 4 small
Syrup, 4 tbsp. (80 ml)
Fruit topping, 1 c.
Yogurt, 6 oz. (180 ml)
Milk, 12 oz. (360 ml)

Morning Practice, 60 minutes
Sports drink, 32 oz. (960 ml)

Posttraining Recovery
Smoothie:
    Juice, 12 oz. (360 ml)
    Skim milk powder, 2 tbsp. (40 ml)
    Banana, 1 small
    Wheat germ, 3 tbsp. (60 ml)

Lunch (12:30 p.m.)
Broiled chicken breast, 4 oz. (120 g)
Bun, whole wheat, 1
Pasta salad, 1 c.
Milk, skim, 8 oz. (240 ml)
Orange, 1 medium

Afternoon Practice
Sports drink, 32 oz. (960 ml)

Postpractice
Peanut butter, 2 tbsp. (40 ml)
Jam, 2 tbsp. (40 ml)
Bread, 2 slices
Milk, skim, 8 oz. (240 ml)

Dinner (7:00 p.m.)
Beef, 6 oz. (180 g)
Baked potato, 1 medium
Green beans, 1 c.
Salad, 2 c.
Salad dressing, 4 tbsp. (80 ml)
Fruit salad, 1 c.

Snack (9:30 p.m.)
Cereal, 1.5 oz. (45 g)
Milk, skim, 8 oz. (240 ml)
Raisins, 3 tbsp. (60 ml)

3,600 calories
520 g carbohydrate (58%)
150 g protein (17%)
100 g fat (25%)

glycogen burned for fuel during training. Glycogen can become depleted in specific muscle groups with the repeated high-intensity efforts during practice. Starting practice sessions with replete muscle stores should be the goal of the football player.

Because the majority of football players are involved in intensive weight-training programs, they do have elevated protein requirements. However, these increased protein needs are easily met by consuming a well-balanced diet. The timing of their protein intake

---

Sample Training Menu

Afternoon Practice
Resistance Training

Breakfast (7:00 a.m.)
Egg, 1 whole or egg whites, 3
Whole-grain cereal, 1.5 oz. (45 g)
Dairy or soy milk, 8 oz. (240 ml)
Blueberries, 3/4 c. (180 ml)
Juice, 12 oz. (360 ml)

Lunch (11:30 p.m.)
Bun, whole wheat, 1
Soy burger, 1 medium
Pretzels, 1.5 oz. (45 g)
Milk, skim, 8 oz. (240 ml)
Grapes, 1 c.

Pretraining Snack
Granola bar, 1 medium
Sports shake (with protein), 12 oz.
    (360 ml)
Banana, 1 large

During Training
16–24 oz. sports drink per hour
    (480–960 ml)

Recovery Snack
Peanut butter, 4 tsp. (30 ml)
Jam, 2 tbsp. (30 ml)
Bread, 2 slices

Dinner (7:00 p.m.)
Pork tenderloin, 4 oz. (120 g)
Rice, cooked, 1.5 c. (360 ml)
Corn, 1/2 c. (120 ml)
Bread, whole-grain, 2 slices
Olive oil, 4 tsp. (30 ml)

3,600 calories
470 g carbohydrate (52%)
150 g protein 17%)
120 g fat (31%)

before and after weight training is also essential, as outlined in Chapter 6. Younger athletes should also appreciate that although some protein-containing sports nutrition products may be beneficial, nutritional strategies for weight training can easily be accom-
plished with real food choices that provide vitamins and minerals and are available at
less expense. Overuse of popular protein supplements provides no performance benefits and often results in players exceeding their protein requirements. Excess protein is
burned for fuel, which is not a very efficient process, or simply stored as body fat. Many
protein supplements may contain ingredients or substances not recommended for athletes or developing bodies.

Keeping fat intake to healthy levels can be challenging for the football players.
Younger athletes may frequent fast-food establishments, and frequent eating out and
eating on the run can increase fat intake. (Guidelines for eating out with low-fat options
appear in Chapter 8.) Often, these athletes have limited cooking skills and need assistance in planning and preparing simple meals. (See the sample menus provided.)

Professional football players sometimes hire the services of a chef or a service that
delivers healthy prepared meals. Alcohol intake can also contribute significantly to
caloric intake and is actually metabolized in the body more like fat than carbohydrates,
which is not helpful for an athlete striving for a lean physique. Of course, underage
football players should not be drinking alcohol.

Important Nutrition Strategies for Football
Hydration, Fluid, and Carbohydrate Replacement during Exercise
Football is characterized by repeated high-intensity efforts, which can significantly
deplete both fluid stores and muscle glycogen stores during training. Specific muscle
groups could become depleted of carbohydrate before practice is complete, and players may also need to recover fully after a morning training session to prepare for an
afternoon training session.

Maintaining adequate fluid intake can be a challenge for football players early in the
preseason, when training may occur during hot summer months. The weight of
equipment can also aggravate fluid loss, as can any excess body weight carried by a
player. Younger players or rookies may be less seasoned in proper fluid replacement
practices. Because fluid needs are somewhat based on both body size and sweat rate,
larger players may have very high fluid requirements. Even during practice in cooler
weather later in the season, football players should be on guard against dehydration.

Sports drinks that provide both carbohydrate and fluid are the recommended choice
for football players. Athletes should be encouraged to drink at regular intervals during

practice, with 4 to 8 ounces consumed every 15 to 20 minutes. However, sweat rates can vary greatly from player to player. Athletes should refer to the sidebar, Estimating Fluid Losses in Chapter 7 to calculate their own fluid losses per hour for various types of practices and environmental conditions. The goal is to try to keep up with fluid losses as much as possible and to practice important rehydration strategies after practice. Twenty ounces (600 milliliters) of fluid is recommended for every pound of weight lost.

Carbohydrate replacement is also important to offset decreases in liver and muscle glycogen during training. Carbohydrate will maintain steady blood glucose levels, which supports focus and concentration in a tactical game such as football, and can provide energy for muscle fibers depleted of muscle glycogen from the high-intensity efforts characterized by football. Sports drinks can also be consumed during quarter breaks, when on the sidelines, and at halftime during the game. Trainers should set up protocols during practice and games that encourage fluid intake.

Sodium replacement can also be beneficial for football players who have a higher concentration of sodium in their sweat. Sports drinks high in sodium should be adequate to replace sweat losses. Sodium sweat losses do not have to be replaced completely but adequately to maintain blood sodium levels within the normal range. Fluid replacement with plain water alone does not provide sodium. Having enough salt in the daily diet can also be beneficial. Although guidelines for the average North American encourage decreased sodium intake to prevent hypertension, most athletes have higher sodium needs to replace losses. Clearly sodium recommendations need to be individualized for each athlete based on his medical history, sweat rate, and sodium losses.

Preparing for Competition

Often the pregame meal consists of the foods that the football player likes, feels comfortable consuming, and believes provide a competitive edge. Though carbohydrates are the preferred pregame fuel, players may also like to include some protein in their precompetition meal. Easy-to-digest carbohydrate should be emphasized, as well as lean protein sources in reasonable amounts. Often, players may consume the precompetition meal with the team. The input of a sports nutritionist regarding the menu can be extremely helpful, and players can be advised on their own individualized pregame portions that work for their body weight and tolerances.

During a football game, energy expenditure may not be consistent over the entire 60 minutes, as players are often highly specialized in their position and the skills that they are called on to contribute to a winning game. Players should be encouraged to

Muscle Cramping and Salty Sweaters

Team sport athletes can suffer through muscle cramping during practice or even an important competition. These involuntary and uncontrolled muscle spasms strike quickly and can ruin a key player's performance. What exactly causes muscle cramps remains largely a mystery, and research data in this area are limited. Most likely there are many causes of muscle cramping, such as simple muscular exhaustion, low fuel stores, biomechanical problems, and mineral deficiencies. Each of these requires a variety of treatments specific to each athlete. However, team sport athletes who train and compete in the high temperatures often complain of heat cramps. We may often read or hear about one of our favorite professional players being sidelined by painful heat cramps.

While scientists cannot dive right into the muscle cell to determine precisely what causes heat cramps, data indicate that sodium and fluid imbalances and losses during practice should be considered. There are still more questions than answers regarding heat cramps, but if you suffer from cramping, a few nutritional strategies can help.

Heat cramps do occur in some team sport athletes and are most likely to occur in very hot and humid conditions and when athletes sweat for long periods of time. There is also some emerging data that cramp-prone athletes are "salty sweaters," experiencing significantly higher sodium losses than their non-cramping counterparts.

One recent field study was conducted on college football players who had been identified as having a history of full-body muscle cramping. These cramp-prone players were found to lose 5 to 6 grams of sodium during a 2-hour practice. Players who did not experience muscle cramping, were of similar height, weight, and age, and played the same position lost only 2 grams of sodium during the same 2-hour practice. These cramp-prone athletes increased their salt intake around practice and did not experience cramping that day.

It is possible that for certain football players, and other team sport players, heat cramps are connected to sodium balance. Although well-conditioned athletes generally have lower concentrations of sodium in their sweat, there may be a strong genetic influence as some highly trained athletes do lose large amounts of sodium through sweating. Sodium losses in 1 quart (960 milliliters) of sweat can range from 400 to 1,800 milligrams, or even more in some athletes.

Team sport players prone to heat cramping should ensure that their daily fluid and sodium intake is adequate. While restricting sodium may be appropriate for preventing high blood pressure in sedentary individuals, it could lead to salt depletion problems in team sport athletes who train and compete in hot and humid weather. Salt cravings can be answered by lightly using the salt shaker at the table and by consuming salty foods such as pretzels, soups, and pickles. Cramp-prone team players should start all practices well hydrated. High-sodium sports drinks can also help replace sodium losses during training. Electrolyte tablets that contain sodium are also available if indicated and appropriate for specific players. These products should be consumed appropriately (more is not necessarily better or needed) and taken with plenty of fluid.

There has also been some speculation that other minerals, including potassium, calcium, and magnesium, may be related to muscle cramping. Food sources of these nutrients can also be increased in the diet. Fruits and vegetables provide plenty of potassium. Good sources of calcium include milk, yogurt, dried beans, and green leafy vegetables. Whole grains, almonds, avocados, lentils, wheat germ, and nuts are good sources of magnesium.

Make sure that you test out these strategies for preventing heat cramps carefully during the training season and at practice sessions. It is likely that any nutritional plan for preventing heat cramps has to be personalized to each athlete based on the person's medical history, usual diet, and sweat and sodium losses. If nutritional strategies do not help in solving the mystery of heat cramps, look to resources that can help you determine whether there is a biomechanical cause or problems with stretching or training techniques.

drink water or a sports drink every time they come to the sidelines to maintain adequate hydration. In hot and humid conditions, sports drinks are preferred and should be the first choice for players who receive a lot of playing time. Sports drinks should also be chosen over water if they encourage higher drinking volumes and improved hydration for the football player simply because the taste is preferred. A player who receives a fair amount of playing time could also rapidly deplete specific muscle fibers (fast-twitch) if performing repeated all-out efforts in the game. The carbohydrate in the sports drink would offset this glycogen depletion. See sample competition day menus provided.

Sample Competition Day Menu for Football

Start Time
4:00 p.m. Game Start Time

Breakfast (7:00 a.m.)
Eggs, 2
Bagel, 4 oz. (120 g)
Butter, 2 tsp. (15 ml)
Jam, 2 tbsp. (40 ml)
Juice, 12 oz. (360 ml)
Banana, 1 whole

Snack (10:00 a.m.)
Bread, 2 slices
Jam, 2 tbsp. (40 ml)
Peanut butter, 4 tsp. (30 ml)
Milk, skim, 12 oz. (360 ml)

Pregame Meal (1:00 p.m.)
Broiled chicken breast, 4 oz. (120 g)
Baked potato, 1 medium
Bread, 2 slices

Juice, 12 oz. (360 ml)
Orange, 1 medium

During Game
Water and sports drink
24 oz. (720 ml) or more

Postgame Meal
Beef, lean, 6 oz. (180 g)
Rice, cooked, 1-1/2 c. (360 ml)
Cooked vegetable, 1 c.
Milk, skim, 12 oz. (360 ml)

3,300 calories
450 g carbohydrate (55%)
145 g protein (18%)
100 g fat (27%)

NCAA GUIDELINES FOR ACCLIMATIZING

One of the biggest nutritional risk factors for football players is the prevention of heat illness, which requires appropriate acclimatization. Because of the high risk during early-season workouts in the summer heat, the NCAA has some specific guidelines for college football players. Studies have indicated that football players can lose dangerously high levels of body fluid during two-a-day workouts. Players who are not acclimatized to the heat are also more prone to injury. To prevent heat illness, the NCAA recommends the following practice guidelines in its sports medicine handbook.

Players should complete a health status questionnaire before starting practice along with an initial complete medical history and physical examination. A history of

1:00 p.m. Game Start Time

Breakfast (7:00 a.m.)
Waffles, 3 large or 5 oz. (150 g)
Peach, 1 medium
Syrup, 6 tbsp. (120 ml)
Yogurt, plain, 6 oz. (180 ml)
Juice, 12 oz. (360 ml)
Eggs, scrambled, 3

Pregame Snack (11:00 a.m.)
Energy bar, 1 medium
Sports drink, 24 to 32 oz. (720–960 ml)

During Game
Sports drink 16 to 32 oz. (480–
   960 ml)

Postgame Dinner
Lean steak, 6 oz. (180 g)
Baked potato, 1 large or 10 oz.
   (300 g)
Green beans, 1 c.
Roll, 2 small
Salad, 2 c.
Salad dressing, 4 tbsp. (80 ml)

3,000 calories
435 g carbohydrate (58%)
100 g protein (13%)
96 g fat (31%)

previous heat illness and the athlete's training program the previous month are also important.

Student athletes should gradually increase exposure to hot and/or humid conditions over a period of 7 to 10 days during periods of aerobic conditioning. Intensity and duration of the training should be increased gradually over each training session, until exercise is comparable to competition. If weather conditions are extreme, training should be held at a cooler time of day. Optimal hydration should be maintained during this acclimatization period.

When acclimatizing, use a minimum of protective gear and clothing, and practice in lightweight and light-color clothing because helmets, shoulder pads, and shin guards increase heat stress by interfering with sweat evaporation. Dark clothing also increases the body's absorption of heat. Frequent rest periods are also advised.

Environmental conditions of ambient temperature and humidity should be monitored to prevent heat stress. At high-stress temperature levels, athletic activity should be controlled.

Dehydration should be avoided by having fluid replacement readily available to the athletes, who should be encouraged to drink as much and as frequently as comfort allows. One to 2 cups (240 to 480 milliliters) of fluid should be consumed in the hour before practice, and drinking should continue every 15 to 20 minutes during practice. Weight loss during practice represents fluid loss and should be replaced. Urine volume and color should be used to assess hydration. Carbohydrate–electrolyte drinks (sports drinks) enhance fluid intake and the electrolytes aid in the retention of fluids.

Athletes can record weight before and after practice to monitor body fluid losses and to prevent dehydration. Athletes who lose 5 percent of their body weight or more over several days should be medically evaluated and have their activity restricted until they are rehydrated.

Some student athletes are more susceptible to heat illness. Athletes at greater risk are those who are not acclimatized or aerobically fit, athletes with excess body fat, those with a history of heat illness, and those who regularly push themselves to capacity. Substances that increase the risk of heat illness such as diuretics and stimulants found in over-the-counter drugs and nutritional supplements should not be taken.

Athletes should be monitored for signs of heat illness such as sweating, cramping, weakness and fatigue, rapid and weak pulse, pale and flushed skin, nausea, dizziness, and vision disturbances. Athletes should be under the observation of a coach or athletic trainer.

The NCAA model for football players involves starting off with a 5-day acclimatization period for all players. Coaches can hold one on-field practice per day—the first 2 days, helmets only; the next 2 days, helmets and shoulder pads; and the final or fifth day, one on-field practice with helmets and full pads. Practices are ideally 90 minutes to no more than 3 hours. After the 5-day period, multiple practices should not be conducted on consecutive days in order to promote recovery, not only from heat but from other injuries. During multiple-practice sessions days, three continuous hours of recovery time between practices is required.

Recent data presented at the 2004 American College of Sports Medicine meeting indicate that the new NCAA football acclimatization guidelines have resulted in a decreased incidence of injury rate in the preseason. The preseason traditionally has had a higher incidence of injury rates in college football.

Clearly hydration and acclimatization should be a major focus for coach, trainers, and football players during preseason, hot-weather training.

NUTRITIONAL SUPPLEMENTATION

Several surveys have looked at supplement use in collegiate athletes, including football players. According to one recent survey, vitamin and mineral supplements appear to be the most widely used supplements, followed by calorie replacement drinks. However, use of protein supplements and creatine was also reported to be fairly high.

One study looked specifically at high school football players. The researchers found that 8 percent of athletes used supplements, with the most popular being creatine, HMB, amino acids, DHEA, androstenedione, phosphagen, weight gain products, and tribulus. Another study conducted at a Division I university found that 89 percent of the student athletes took supplements. While females were more likely to take calcium and multivitamins, males had a significant intake for ginseng, amino acids, glutamine, HMB, weight gainers, and whey protein. Energy drinks were the most popular supplements, followed by calorie replacement products, multivitamins, creatine, and vitamin C. Female athletes were more likely to take supplements for health reasons and due to inadequate diet, whereas male athletes wanted to improve speed and agility, develop strength and power, and gain muscle.

Because of the heavy emphasis on increased strength and muscle mass for football, there is often a focus on supplements that promises to make athletes bigger and stronger. One study specifically looked at creatine use in Division I athletes. At least 48 percent of the male athletes reported using creatine, while 4 percent of the female athletes reported using creatine. About one-third of creatine users had started use of this supplement in high school. Friends and teammates were the most common sources of creatine information.

One study has looked at creatine use in collegiate football players. Side effects of creatine use, such as muscle cramping and injury, were studied rather than benefits to performance. Creatine loading took place over 5 days, followed by a maintenance dose taken after workouts, practices, and games. Of course, creatine is now on the NCAA's list of nonpermissible substances. Many creatine users also report an increase in weight with loading. Depending on the field position played, this extra weight may not offer an advantage and could offer a disadvantage in performance. An offensive lineman may derive more benefit from the increased weight than a wide receiver. While creatine use is not advised in both high school and collegiate players, it is important that if taken, this supplement be cycled, not consumed continuously in hopes of ongoing increases in muscle mass.

Players should be educated in the proper dosage, timing, and usage of this supplement to prevent any side effects and health concerns. They should also be familiar with which substances are banned, not permissible, could have potentially harmful side effects, and come with the possibility of product contamination.

CHAPTER 11

NUTRITION FOR BASKETBALL

Basketball is an action-packed game that is exciting to watch. Participation levels at over 36 million players annually make it the number one ranked team sport. It is enjoyed by both female and male players at the high school, college, and professional levels, and it is also an Olympic sport. Five players are on the basketball court during game time, two guards, two forwards, and one center, and they all can play both offense and defense during a game. Because of the combination of team and individual effort in basketball, all the players are highly mobile and cover the whole court when the ball is in play. Players are continually substituted from the bench throughout the game, which is played on the professional level in four 12-minute quarters. The timing clock stops when the ball is not in play, so actual game time is much longer. There is also a break at halftime.

Basketball players possess an admirable combination of power, speed, agility, and finesse to perform intricate and skillful maneuvers throughout the game. Players utilize all three energy systems—the creatine phosphagen system, anaerobic glycolysis, and the aerobic system—as they are both power and endurance athletes. Because of the demands that training and competition place on their bodies, basketball players require a high nutritional intake of energy, fluid, carbohydrates, and proteins to maintain body fuel stores, energy levels, and optimize recovery. Daily practice can easily last 90 minutes. Professionals often practice twice daily, and games may be played frequently during the week. Adequate muscle glycogen stores are essential for these players. Increased strength is clearly an asset to a basketball player, and they may engage in a weight-training program, more likely during off-season training. The pre- or off-season training also includes building a fitness base. Skill work is practiced year-round.

DEMANDS OF THE GAME
Energy Requirements
Energy requirements for basketball players can be quite high, especially when combined with requirements for growth and development. Players at high levels may complete two

intense practices daily. Energy needs can also vary considerably from player to player depending on body size and training schedule. Male professional players practicing twice daily can require over 5,000 calories, whereas a female player in high school may need half this amount at only 2,500 calories daily.

Daily calorie needs are a combination of basic energy expenditure at rest, calories needed for daily activities such as school and work, and the calories expended while training. Training calories per hour of basketball play based on body weight are outlined in Table 5.1. A 180-pound (82-kilogram) male player would burn approximately 710 calories in 1 hour of practice, whereas a 140-pound (64-kilogram) female player would burn about 550 calories in 1 hour of play. Additional and significant calories may also be burned with weight training and aerobic conditioning. Energy requirements can vary from day to day depending on the training schedule and during different periods in the season depending on the training focus at that time of year. For training cycles and days with high energy needs, male basketball players training more than 90 minutes daily may require 23 calories per pound (50 calories/kilogram), with a 180-pound (82-kilogram) player requiring 4,140 calories daily. A female player with similar training time would require 20 to 23 calories per pound (45 to 50 calories/kilogram) and, at 140 pounds, require 2,800 to 3,220 calories daily. Energy needs also change during the off-season, and intake should reflect the calories burned from various components of the off-season program.

Body Composition

While height is often the most notable characteristic in male basketball players, these athletes often have high body weights reflective of their build and large amount of muscle mass. Of course, players at all levels can come in a variety of shapes and builds. Lower body fat levels will offer an advantage to players as this can improve quickness, agility, and jumping ability by decreasing the weight that must be propelled through the air. Body composition of basketball players can be monitored regularly in order to track muscle building and body fat loss. Guidelines for keeping fat in the diet to healthy levels and choosing low-fat options when eating out can also assist athletes in maintaining their optimal level of body fat.

Diet Composition

Basketball players should focus on maintaining adequate carbohydrate in the diet in order to replenish muscle glycogen stores. Carbohydrate requirements are specifically based on the total grams required for the hours of training and the intensity of the workout. Some high-performance players can require anywhere from 3 to 4 grams per pound of weight (7 to 9 grams/kilogram) for the day. Total grams of carbohydrate required should level off at 600 to 700 grams daily for even the highest-weight male players and at 400 to 500 grams daily for female players. Basketball players should appreciate that glycogen is an important fuel supply during practice and that 60 to 90 minutes of moderate- to high-intensity practice can deplete stores significantly. Weight training also depletes this important carbohydrate fuel. Whole-grain, fruit, vegetable, and skim milk carbohydrate sources can be emphasized along with dried peas and beans and soy products to provide the needed grams of carbohydrate. Players with high carbohydrate requirements may require more concentrated supplements and should be aware of carbohydrate amounts per serving size, as outlined in Chapter 8. Carbohydrate amounts required include the daily training diet and carbohydrate intake timed before, during, and after regular training practice.

Basketball players participating in periods of heavy training and cross-training should meet their protein requirements with good food choices providing up to 0.7 gram protein per pound of weight (1.6 grams/kilogram). Adolescent players newer to weight training and also participating in aerobic conditioning may need slightly higher amounts at 0.8 to 0.9 gram per pound (1.8 to 2.0 grams/kilogram). Both carbohydrate and protein intake can be timed properly before and after resistance training to maximize muscle building.

Fat should round out a basketball player's caloric intake, with an emphasis on heart-healthy choices and those high in essential fatty acids, as outlined in Chapter 2. Players with very high energy needs who have met their carbohydrate and protein requirements can intake the rest of their diet from healthy fats. The sidebar provides some sample menus for basketball players. Time and portions can be adjusted as your training schedule, energy needs, and food preferences dictate.

IMPORTANT NUTRITION STRATEGIES FOR BASKETBALL
Hydration, Fluid Replacement, and Carbohydrate Intake

Watching a professional basketball game serves to highlight the high sweat losses of these well-trained athletes. Although sweat rates are highly individual, dehydration is likely to be the most common cause of fatigue during basketball practice and games, long before fuel depletion occurs. Players should monitor their own sweat loss rates by checking weights before and after training as outlined in Chapter 7.

Even body weight losses as little as 1 percent of total body weight, or 1.5 pounds in a 165-pound (0.75 kilogram in a 75-kilogram) player can affecct a player's performance.

Meal Plan for Basketball

Morning Conditioning with Afternoon/Evening Practice

Breakfast (6:30 a.m.)
Waffles, 2 large or 5 oz. (150 g)
Syrup, 4 tbsp. (80 ml)
Fruit topping, 1 c.
Yogurt, 6 oz. (180 ml)
Milk, skim, 8 oz. (240 ml)
Almonds, 12
Egg, 1 or egg whites, 3

Morning Conditioning and Strengthening
Sports drink, 32 oz. (960 ml)

Postrecovery
Toasted cheese sandwich:
    Cheese, low-fat, 2 oz. (60 g)
    Bread, whole-grain, 2 slices
Vegetable salad, 1 c.
Bean soup, 1 c. (240 ml)
Grapes, 30

Lunch (1:00 p.m.)
Tuna salad, low-fat, 4 oz. (120 g)
Bread, whole-grain, 2 slices
Sliced vegetables, 1/2 c.
Yogurt, 6 oz. (180 ml)
Crackers, whole-grain, 8–10

Afternoon Training
Sports drink, 32 oz. (960 ml)

Recovery Snack (5:00 p.m.)
Smoothie:
    Yogurt, 6 oz. (180 ml)
    Milk, skim, 12 oz. (360 ml)
    Frozen berries, 1 c.
Bagel, 4 oz. (120 g)
Nut butter, 4 tsp. (30 ml)

Dinner (7:30 p.m.)
Fish, 6 oz. (180 g)
Rice, cooked, 1-1/2 c.
Cooked vegetables, 1 c.
Salad, 2 c.
Dressing, light, 4 tbsp. (80 ml)
Bread, 2 slices
Spread, 2 tsp. (12 ml)

Dessert (9:00 p.m.)
Sorbet, 1 c. (240 ml)
Yogurt, 4 oz. (120 ml)
Fruit, 1/2 c. (120 ml)

4,400 calories
625 g carbohydrate (57%)
190 g protein (17%)
127 g fat (26%)

Afternoon Practice, 2 hours

Breakfast (7:00 a.m.)
Oatmeal, cooked, 1-1/2 c. (360 ml)
Skim milk, 8 oz. (240 ml)
Bread, 1 slice
Jam, 1 tbsp. (40 ml)
Orange juice, 8 oz. (240 ml)

Lunch (11:00 a.m.)
Chicken, 4 oz. (120 g)
Mayonnaise, light, 2 tbsp. (40 ml)
Rice and bean salad, 1 c. (240 ml)
Grapes, 1 c.

Pretraining Snack (2:30 p.m.)
Energy bar, 1
Banana, 1 small
Yogurt with fruit, 6 oz. (180 ml)

During Practice
32 oz. (960 ml) sports drink

Recovery Snack (5:00 p.m.)
12 oz. (360 ml) high-energy drink

Dinner (7:00 p.m.)
Tofu, 6 oz. (180 g)
Soba noodles, cooked, 2 c. (480 ml)
Vegetables, 2 c.
Sesame seed oil, 3 tsp. (60 ml)

2,800 calories
450 g carbohydrate (64%)
110 g protein (16%)
62 g fat (20%)

Dehydration during practice should easily be prevented with a few useful strategies. Trainers and coaches should ensure that fluids are readily available and provide players plenty of opportunities to drink during breaks. Research indicates that players are more likely to consume fluids and a greater amount of fluid when drinks are flavored. The coaches and trainers should make sure that fluids are close by and easily accessed during practice. Players can also be encouraged to drink on a schedule of 4 to 8 ounces (120 to 240 milliliters) every 10 to 15 minutes. Flavored and cool drinks encourage a greater volume intake, and each player can be assigned his or her own individual hydration bottle. Players can monitor before and after practice weights in relation to the amounts that they consume, and how various fluid amounts and drinking strategies match their sweat losses. High school players can bring frozen bottles of liquid to school to keep cool for after-school practices.

Players can also prehydrate before practice. Urine levels should be clear during the day, though urine tends to be more concentrated in the morning. Players can prehydrate by consuming 16 to 24 ounces (480 to 720 milliliters) 1 hour before practice and 4 to 8 ounces (120 to 240 milliliters) in the 20 minutes beforehand if their schedule allows. Daily hydration strategies should be considered throughout the day, with hydrating fluids consumed at breakfast and lunch and at snacks whenever possible. Most players should aim to consume at least 2 to 3 quarts (approximately 2 to 3 liters) of fluid during the day.

Basketball players can also rehydrate after practice by consuming 20 ounces (600 milliliters) of fluid for every pound of weight loss after exercise. Rehydration should continue after training. Clear urine in the several hours after training is usually a good indicator that an athlete is well hydrated.

Sports drinks not only provide the basketball player with adequate fluid but are an important source of carbohydrate as well. As muscle glycogen and blood glucose levels decrease, power, coordination, speed, and concentration can be affected. Not only is carbohydrate needed to provide muscle for fuel during training, but maintaining blood glucose levels can support the optimal mental focus and stamina needed for making quick decisions and performing a high level of skill. Fatigue can also be a contributing factor to increased susceptibility to injury.

One study looked at the effects of ingesting a sports drink in trained athletes simulating a basketball game, with four 15-minute quarters of stop-and-go running, separated by a halftime. At the end of the experiment, the athletes ran until they were fatigued. A sports drink was consumed before exercise and at the end of each quarter. Researchers found that the carbohydrate ingestion resulted in faster sprinting, a longer run time before fatigue set in, and a beneficial effect on motor skills and mental function.

Carbohydrate replacement can also be achieved with carbohydrate gels consumed with at least 8 ounces (240 milliliters) of water. These products provide an easily digested source of carbohydrate and may be a welcome change from the usual liquid carbohydrates during longer practice breaks.

Some players may also have high sodium losses in their sweat and be "salty sweaters." When combined with a high sweat rate, sodium losses may be substantial. Some basketball players may experience muscle cramping as a reaction to dehydration and sodium loss. At-risk players can consume a high-sodium sports drink and obtain reasonable amounts of sodium in their diet to offset losses.

Nutritional Strategies for Competition
Precompetition Meal

Because the primary fuel for basketball is carbohydrate, the precompetition meal should focus on well-tolerated sources of this fuel. Many players may feel that their protein intake should be maximized before a game and may consume too large an amount at the expense of carbohydrate intake. Players need to fine-tune their optimal competition eating schedule. They may have a light practice the day of an evening game and should also take into consideration their warm-up time. It is important that this meal prevents hunger before and during the game and provides fuel for the game. Of course, basketball players want to know that their food choices are easily digested.

Each basketball player needs to experiment with foods and fluids and meal timing that work best for him or her. If players have to report to the competition area 1 to 2 hours before the game, they may want to pack some light foods and fluids that can be consumed before warm-up and leading up to the start time. Items that are well tolerated include energy bars, liquid sports nutrition supplements that provide mainly carbohydrate and some protein, low-fat smoothies, and sports drinks and gels. Players should focus on prehydrating for the game.

Many basketball players may enjoy having a substantial meal 3 to 4 hours before game time or perhaps even earlier. This meal should include well-tested and well-tolerated carbohydrate foods such as rice, pasta, or potatoes, and moderate amounts of low-fat protein such as poultry or fish, rather than large portions of fatty meats such as steaks. Players can also include some lower-glycemic carbohydrates such as vegetables, fruit, real fruit juice, and skim milk dairy products if that helps to maintain steady blood glucose levels. Having both a substantial meal several hours before the game and a light snack in the 60 to 90 minutes before warm-up may work well for players with very high energy needs. Here are some suggested precompetition meal guidelines:

- Plan your meal ahead of time and make sure that you know your optimal timing.
- Start hydrating immediately, and make sure that any fluid lost during a light practice before the game has been replaced.
- Prepare and pack any needed foods and fluids to be consumed at the game the night before.

- Start your day with a high-carbohydrate breakfast that includes whole grains and fruits.
- Moderate amounts of low-fat protein can be consumed throughout the day to control hunger.
- Keep fat intake to a minimum, with easily digested choices consumed in small amounts as needed to control hunger.
- Have your midday meal consist of a decent portion of low-fat protein, with plenty of carbohydrates.
- Depending on your meal-timing preference, you can adjust your carbohydrate intake according to one of the timing choices listed here. An early pregame meal several hours before the game can also be combined with some easily digested carbohydrate sources in the hour before the game.

  Four hours prior: 2 grams of carbohydrate for every pound of weight (4 grams/kilogram).

  Three hours prior: 1.5 grams/pound (3 grams/kilogram)

  Two hours prior: 1 gram/pound (2 grams/kilogram)

  One hour prior: 0.5 gram/pound (1 gram/kilogram)

- Some basketball players may prefer to eat a fairly nice-sized meal 3 to 4 hours before game time and a light snack within the hour before game time.
- Experiment with various timings and food choices in practice.

Game Time

Players can continue to hydrate prior to game time with sports drinks and consume gels prior to game time for a carbohydrate boost. During the game, some specific strategies can assist the player in maintaining energy levels. Most games are lost when players cannot maintain their intensity and energy levels in the last quarter. Breaks in play should be taken advantage of for refueling and rehydrating. Players should consume a sports drink on the bench, at quarter breaks, and at halftime. They should attempt to consume 30 to 50 grams of carbohydrate at halftime to maintain blood glucose levels. Gels are easily tolerated, as are up to 24 ounces of sports drink, which also provides fluid.

For optimal hydration and blood glucose levels during a game:

- Consume a sports drink during warm-up and up to game time.
- Have 4 to 8 ounces (120 to 240 milliliters) of a sports drink on the bench.
- Drink 4 to 8 ounces (120 to 240 milliliters) of a sports drink at quarter breaks.

• At halftime consume 8 to 16 ounces (240 to 480 milliliters) of a sports drink or a gel with 8 to 16 ounces (240 to 480 milliliters) of water.

The sidebar that follows provides some competition menus for various start times.

Refueling and Replenishing

Basketball is a demanding sport, and a busy season of training and competing can slowly or quickly deplete a player who is not on top of meeting his or her fluid and fuel needs for recovery. Whether after a hard game or a steady practice session, players should refuel with carbohydrate at 0.5 to 0.6 gram per pound (1 to 1.2 grams/kilogram) of body weight. High-glycemic carbohydrates are the best choices to quickly start the replenishment process of fast-twitch muscle fibers. A small amount of high-quality protein, about 10 to 15 grams, can be added to the recovery snack. Often, liquid sports supplements are convenient. Refer to Appendix A for a list of high-glycemic foods.

Your recovery eating and drinking should be in high gear immediately after practice or competition, and your food and fluid choices leading to the next game or practice are also important. A well-balanced carbohydrate-containing meal or snack should be consumed again in 2 hours. For some players, this may include a late after-game meal. Portions should be kept to reasonable amounts late at night. Replenishing should continue the next day at breakfast before the next practice. Athletes who practice in the afternoon should plan ahead to have a healthy lunch and a high-carbohydrate snack in the 90 minutes before practice.

Iron and the Basketball Player

Much of the research on iron status in athletes has been completed on endurance athletes, rather than athletes participating in team sports such as basketball. Both the importance of iron in the diet of athletes and good food sources or iron are reviewed in Chapter 2.

One recent study looked at iron depletion in male and female national basketball team players. Researchers found a high prevalence of iron depletion at 22 percent of subjects, and 25 percent of subjects were found to be anemic. A larger proportion of female basketball players than male players had iron deficiency and anemia. This is mainly attributable to iron losses during menstruation and inadequate dietary intake. Footstrike hemolysis, seen in runners and contributing to iron depletion and anemia, may also be a risk factor in basketball players. Excessive sweating in basketball players with high sweat rates can also be a factor in contributing to iron loss.

Sample Competition Menu

7:30 p.m. Game Start Time

Breakfast (7:00 a.m.)
Waffles, 2 medium or 5 oz. (150 g)
Syrup, 4 tbsp. (80 ml)
Strawberries, 1 c.
Raisins, 1.5 tbsp. (30 ml)
Apple juice, 8 oz. (240 ml)
Nuts, 2 tsp. (15 ml)

Lunch (12:30 p.m.)
Turkey, 6 oz. (180 g)
Bread, 2 slices
Mayonnaise, 4 tsp. (30 ml)
Pasta salad, 1 c. (240 ml)
Oil, 2 tsp. (15 ml)
Orange, 1 medium
Pretzels, 1-1/2 oz. (45 g)
Juice, 12 oz. (360 ml)

Snack (4:00 p.m.)
Cereal, 1-1/2 c. (360 ml)
Milk, 12 oz. (360 ml)
Banana, 1 large

Pre-Game (5:30 p.m.)

Smoothie:
Milk, 12 oz. (360 ml)
Yogurt, 6 oz. (180 ml)
Berries, 1 c.
Granola, 1/4 c. (60 ml)

During Game
Sports drink, 32–40 oz. (960–1,200 ml)
Carbohydrate gel, 1 packet

After Game
Poultry, 4 oz. (120 g)
Rice, cooked, 1-1/2 c. (360 ml)
Vegetable, cooked, 1 c.
Bread, 2 slices

3,500 calories
600 g carbohydrate (68%)
125 g protein (14%)
70 g fat (18%)

Iron stores in both male and female players are easily measured and corrected if needed. Iron stores can be checked preseason on a regular basis and anytime during the season as needed to monitor a dietary increase of high-iron foods or iron supplementation if prescribed by a physician. Iron repletion can improve energy levels and decrease exercise fatigue.

11:00 a.m. Game Start Time

Breakfast (7:00 a.m.)
Pancakes, 4 small
Syrup, 4 tbsp. (80 ml)
Yogurt, 6 oz. (180 ml)
Milk, 12 oz. (360 ml)
Berries, 1 c.

Pre-warm-up
16–24 oz. sports drink (480–720 ml)

During Game
4–8 oz. (120–240 ml) on bench or
between periods
1 gel packet at halftime

Recovery Drink
Recovery sports shake, 12 oz. (360 ml)
(carbohydrate–protein drink)

Dinner (5:00 p.m.)
Linguine, cooked, 3 c. (720 ml)
Vegetables, 1 c.
Seafood mix, 6 oz. (180 g)
Olive oil, 2 tbsp. (40 ml)
Bread, 2 slices
Salad, 2 c.
Dressing, light, 4 tbsp. (80 ml)

3,100 calories
450 g carbohydrate (58%)
100 g protein (13%)
100 g fat (29%)

Ergogenic Aids

Because basketball players are interested in being quick and explosive and in maintaining high power output, they may be interested in supplements that claim to enhance these qualities. Not many studies on ergogenic aids have been conducted on basketball players to consider these claims. One study on creatine did show an improvement in jumping and running performance, which could potentially be applied to basketball. However, product quality continues to be a concern, as do the potential side effects and lack of safety data on creatine use, both short-term and long-term in younger athletes. (See Chapter 6 for more information on ergogenic aids.) Currently it is recommended that basketball players follow sound nutritional practice for building muscle, optimizing energy, and maintaining mental focus during practice.

Eating Well on Campus

Many college food services offer a wide selection of foods for students living in dorms or group home settings such as sororities and fraternities. Campus food courts also provide selections in a variety of locations near classrooms, and of course there is the always-present vending machine. Your challenge is to navigate the selections and find items that support your athletic training, recovery, and good health.

Eating on campus presents several challenges to the collegiate athlete. One is the "all-you-can-eat" setting, with unlimited returns to the table and a wide variety of hot and cold foods that may or may not be prepared with moderate to high amounts of fat. You need to become a savvy consumer at the dorm food service, campus food court, and group-home setting, just as you would at any restaurant and fast-food establishment.

Although typical dorm mealtimes are fairly extensive, it is important that you review your class and practice schedule and have a plan of when and where you will eat for each day of the week. Late nights of studying also may result in evening snacking when hunger hits, so keep a stash of healthy choices in your room. Remember, you are not on a 9-to-5 schedule and you need to be flexible with meal- and snack times, while giving yourself the consistent mealtime structure required for a healthy diet.

While it may be tempting to sleep in, make sure that you always start your day with breakfast. Dorm-style breakfast meals offer a wide variety of choices for ample wholesome carbohydrates and protein. Consider the standard cold and hot cereals and gravitate toward whole-grain, lower-sugar choices. Skim milk and yogurt add more carbohydrates and high-quality protein to the mix. Make sure to include fruit and whole-grain breads as desired. Peanut butter adds some protein, as do eggs—any style. If you do sleep late, try to catch the tail end of breakfast time. You can also keep some simple breakfast items in your room, such as cereal, milk, fruit, and yogurt, so that skipping breakfast is not necessary.

Breakfast choices often go beyond the simple items frequently consumed at home. Food fare that was once limited to weekend brunches such as omelets, waffles, pancakes, sausage, and bacon are now available every day. These items can be part of your breakfast choices, with portions kept to reasonable levels.

Most athletes get hungry every 3 to 4 hours and maybe even sooner after practice. While you should make sure that you sit down to lunch and dinner regularly, it is also important to plan some snacks into your sports diet. Quick items like yogurt and fruit can be purchased on campus, as can granola bars and even a sandwich. Carry snacks with you as needed, and stake out various campus locations close to classrooms for healthy choices.

Try not to arrive for your lunch and dinner meals famished—doing so may tempt you to select overly large portions. Look over the hot menu for that meal and the cold items that are available. Some food services and group homes often post menus ahead of time. Decide on what looks good and best fits your nutritional needs, with an eye out for whole grains, fruits, and vegetables.

The food service can include a salad bar, which can supplement a healthy meal or serve as your main entrée. Choose wisely and adequately from the offerings. Plenty of fresh vegetables such as carrots, mushrooms, cucumbers, and peppers are great, as are leafy greens such as lettuce and spinach. If the salad is to be a main focus of the meal, be sure to include proteins such as cottage cheese, eggs, tuna, cheese, chickpeas, kidney beans, tofu, and turkey. Prepared salads such as pasta salad, potato salad, and marinated vegetable salads also add carbohydrates but

contribute some fat as well, so portion-control these items. Watch out for items loaded with mayonnaise if you are trying not to overdo your fat intake.

Sandwiches remain the mainstay of most lunches. Protein choices include turkey, tuna, peanut butter, and ham. Gravitate toward whole-grain bread, but also vary your choices with pita bread and sandwich wraps. Round out your sandwich with a bowl of soup, fruits, vegetables, and yogurt or a glass of milk. Higher-calorie items would include large bagel or submarine sandwiches, French fries, and milk shakes. Baked potato bars, like sandwich bars, can provide a nice balance of protein and carbohydrate. Spuds can be topped with vegetables, cheese, yogurt, chili, turkey, and sauces.

Hot entrées are available at both lunch and dinner and can run the gamut from healthy stir-fries to fried entrées, though a wider variety of healthy entrée choices seem to be offered at more dorm food services in recent years. Ask questions about how the foods are prepared, and request sauces on the side and specific portions. Veggie and turkey burgers make good low-fat choices, as do pasta plates with red sauces, grilled or broiled fish, and other grilled meats. Regularly offered sides often include steamed rice, baked

Eating Well on Campus (continued)

potatoes, skim milk and yogurt, fresh fruit, and soups.

Desserts are often in abundant supply at the dorm food service. A self-serve frozen yogurt machine and side toppings is a popular choice. Ice cream, cakes, and pies may also be available on a regular basis but are probably highest in calories.

While not every meal needs to end in dessert, some more reasonable choices include fruit bars, yogurt bars, and Popsicles, as well as sorbet and baked or fresh fruit. Set limits on desserts to once daily or several times weekly depending on your energy needs.

CHAPTER 12

NUTRITION FOR SOCCER

Soccer is one of the most popular and widely played team sports in the world. Outside North America, it is commonly referred to as *football*. It is a very old team sport, and its governing body, Fédération International de Football (FIFA), was founded in 1904. American soccer has enjoyed increased popularity since the 1980s, with more than 18 million U.S. participants in the sport. Soccer is enjoyed by men, women, and children participating in recreational leagues and high school and college teams. National and Olympic participants as well as the expanded professional Major League Soccer (MLS) receive plenty of attention from fans. Over one-third of all youth soccer players are girls, and it is one of the most widely played sports for participants under 18 years old.

Soccer is played mainly outdoors, and a team usually consists of 11 players. Positions played include a goalkeeper, defenders, midfielders, and forwards. A regulation game consists of two 45-minute halves, with a 15-minute halftime. This playing time is usually scaled down in youth soccer.

DEMANDS OF THE GAME

Besides being one of the most popular sports in the world, soccer can also be one of the most demanding physically as a high level of conditioning is a requirement just as much as skill. Soccer is characterized by short bursts of high-intensity activity with recovery periods of active rest such as walking or jogging. Most of the energy required to power soccer play is anaerobic, while the recovery process is aerobic. In soccer, the majority of flat-out sprinting involves short bursts lasting 4 to 5 seconds, while rest periods of walking or jogging are about 30 seconds. Soccer players also frequently change pace or direction, about every 5 seconds.

The average distance covered by a top player in a game is 6 miles (10 kilometers), ranging from 3 to 7 miles (5–11 kilometers) per game. Midfielders cover the most distance and are usually the most active players on the field and spend more time jogging than defenders and forwards, as they play both defense and offense. Time at high-intensity levels in a game for a player may range from just under half to two-thirds of total playing time. Goalies spend the least amount of time running and put out many all-out efforts when playing. During the course of a game, soccer players sprint, jog, walk, jump, accelerate, and turn and move sideways and backward.

Much of soccer training is skill oriented, covering techniques and tactics. Good physical conditioning and strength are also essential for top players to develop speed, power, and agility. Drills may be conducted at high intensities with rest periods as seen in a match. Players may also weight train several times weekly. Good strengthening and conditioning can also prevent injury.

Energy Requirements

Soccer players should consume an appropriate amount of calories that supports their body composition goals and training requirements. Most players have high energy needs, and the daily diet should be adequate to replace body fuel stores, particularly muscle glycogen stores. Because soccer players come in a variety of builds and sizes, energy needs can vary from player to player. Energy requirements can also vary depending on the length of practice, percentage of the practice performed at higher intensities, and age and sex of the player. Data indicate that the energy requirement of professional male soccer players can reach 4,000 calories daily during training and slightly less on match days.

While it is important for soccer players to meet and replace the fuel demands of training (Table 5.1), their diet composition is also a key training ingredient because of the fuel demands that soccer places on the body during training and a game. The energy demands of training can also vary considerably throughout the season, depending on the demands and phase of training and competitive schedule. Off-season calorie intake should be adjusted for the player's conditioning program.

Body Composition

Although skill is essential for top performance in soccer, carrying excess body fat can slow down an athlete's speed and affect endurance. Lower body fat levels will reduce the energy demands on a player during training and competition, allowing her to sustain greater efforts. Goalkeepers and defenders are usually taller and heavier than the rest of the team, and goalkeepers usually have a higher level of body fat as their training efforts may not have the same energy demand as other players. Most soccer players are muscular in body type. Body composition can be measured at regular intervals during the season, particularly when the player is actively building muscle. Because of the high energy demands of soccer, excess calorie intake is not a common problem in this sport, though some players can require specific counseling in this area. Conversely, some players may need guidance in choosing adequate calories to cover their training needs.

Diet Composition

The high-intensity, up-and-down physical efforts of a soccer match mean that the player has a heavy reliance on both muscle and liver glycogen stores for fuel. Muscle glycogen concentration will increase in direct proportion to the duration and intensity of the practice or game. The level of muscle glycogen with which the player begins practice or a game depends on the player's fitness level and player's diet. The greater the glycogen content of the muscle, the faster a soccer player can run, sprint, and change direction on the field. High-intensity exercise can deplete muscle glycogen quickly, and significant depletion can be a contributing factor to fatigue in the second half of a game and the latter part of practice. Incomplete glycogen recovery can also occur on a day-to-day basis, compromising training efforts.

Because the amount of carbohydrate consumed in the diet is directly correlated with the amount of glycogen stored in the muscle, soccer players should consume a diet that is at least 60 percent carbohydrate, based on an adequate calorie intake. The total grams of carbohydrate consumed are also important and should range from 3 to 4.5 grams of carbohydrate per pound (6.5 to 10 grams/kilogram) of body weight.

Soccer players do have higher protein needs than sedentary individuals. They require 0.6 to 0.8 gram/pound (1.4 to 1.7 grams/kilogram) daily to meet greater needs for strength. Glycogen depletion during practice or a game can also result in protein oxidation during exercise, contributing to a net loss in protein over time. However, these increased protein requirements are easily met by appropriate food choices and a well-balanced diet. Healthy fats should provide the remainder of calories to meet energy needs in the diet.

IMPORTANT NUTRITION STRATEGIES FOR SOCCER
Hydration, Fluid Replacement, and Carbohydrate Intake

Soccer players practice and compete at high intensities, often in hot temperatures and humid conditions, which contributes to higher sweat losses on the field. Sweat rates can vary considerably from player to player and also depending on the nature of the training session and the weather conditions. Not all practice sessions and games take place in hot and humid conditions, however. The important strategy is for the player to attempt to match fluid losses through sweating with adequate fluid intake. Specific strategies required for keeping up with fluid losses need to be specific to both practices and games, as opportunities to drink vary. One recent study found that sweat losses in male professional soccer players averaged 40 ounces (1,300 milliliters) per hour. Some players in this study also had large losses of sodium in their sweat. Players did not consume enough fluid to replace sweat losses. Higher sweat losses have also been measured in hot training conditions.

Electrolyte losses during practices and games can also vary considerably from player to player and under various playing conditions. Some evidence indicates that exercise-induced muscle cramps can be related to high sodium losses, though this has not been identified specifically in soccer players. However, soccer players with high sweat rates and high-sodium sweat rates should be identified as being at potential risk for losing excess blood sodium during practice and competition.

During training and competition, blood glucose can also be a significant fuel source utilized by the exercising muscles. As training or competition continues, muscle glycogen levels decrease, and blood glucose becomes an even more important fuel source. Low blood glucose, like depleted muscle glycogen, is associated with fatigue during exercise.

To ensure that fluid, electrolyte, and blood glucose levels are maintained during practice and competition, the soccer player should employ some specific fluid intake strategies. A sports drink is the optimal choice for providing the proper balance of fluid, carbohydrate, and sodium, when consumed in adequate volumes. Here are some practice strategies:

- Always begin each training session or competition fully hydrated. This requires rehydrating after the previous training session and maintaining adequate fluid intake throughout the day.
- Check your weight before and after the training session to determine whether fluid intake matches fluid loss. Determine your sweat rate for various types of training sessions and in different environmental conditions. (See the sidebar, Estimating Fluid Losses, in Chapter 7.)
- Drink 16 ounces (480 milliliters) of fluid in the hour before practice or competition and 8 ounces (240 milliliters) in the 30 minutes prior.
- Have your own bottle of fluid available for consumption during practice. Consume anywhere from 4 to 8 ounces (120 to 240 milliliters) during practice

breaks. Ideally, try to consume these volumes every 10 to 20 minutes to match sweat losses.

- At the very least, schedule drinking breaks every 30 minutes.
- Players who have especially high fluid losses as determined by monitoring weight should make sure that they consume adequate volumes of fluid during breaks and know the total volume required to keep up with sweat losses.
- Remember to drink during the warm-up period.
- The recommended fluid intake for male soccer players is 27 to 40 ounces (800 to 1,200 milliliters) per hour, and for female soccer players, 20 to 33 ounces (600 to 1,000 milliliters) per hour. These amounts can be exceeded if the athlete tolerates larger volumes and requires more fluid to replace sweat losses.
- Pay close attention to adequate fluid intake in cooler weather.
- Rehydrate by consuming 20 ounces (600 milliliters) of a sodium-containing beverage for every pound of weight lost.
- Whenever possible, leave a bottle of a sports drink on the perimeter of the field so that you can drink during a small break in play during games.

Opportunities to hydrate and replenish fluid and fuel stores during a game are more limited and challenging than during practice. Maintaining energy stores can enhance performance during the second half of the game. The high-intensity level of the game can also slow the rate at which fluid is emptied from the stomach, so players should be aware of their individual tolerances under game conditions. Here are some guidelines:

- Prehydrate before the game as described earlier for practice. Hydrate in the hours leading up to the game. Clear urine indicates good hydration levels.
- Hydrate whenever you are on the bench.
- Drink a small amount at break in play if your position allows access to fluids. Due to the size of the playing field, quick and easy access to fluids is not always possible.
- Consume 8 to 16 ounces (240 to 480 milliliters) of a sports drink at halftime.
- Consume a carbohydrate gel at halftime to raise blood glucose levels and replenish carbohydrates.

- Rehydrate appropriately after the game for full recovery. Twenty ounces (600 milliliters) is recommended for every pound of weight lost. Fluids with sodium will enhance the rehydration process.

Fluid Intake in Young Soccer Players

Because soccer is such a popular sport for younger players, adequate hydration should be an important consideration in these athletes. Children take longer to acclimatize and produce more heat than adult soccer players, and they often play their sport in the hot summer months. Fluid intake should be encouraged regularly in these young players, as research indicates that they do not usually drink adequate amounts of fluid during

Training Diet Menu for Soccer

Afternoon Practice

Breakfast (7:00 a.m.)
Bread, 2 slices
Peanut butter, 1 tbsp. (20 ml)
Citrus juice, 12 oz. (360 ml)
Banana, 1 whole
Yogurt, plain, 6 oz. (180 ml)

Lunch (12 noon)
Chicken, 4 oz. (120 g)
Bread, 2 slices
Raw vegetable mix, 1 c.
Pudding, 1 c.
Pretzels, 1.5 oz. (45 g)

Snack (3:00 p.m.)
Granola bar, 1 medium
Milk, skim, 8 oz. (240 ml)

During Practice
Sports drink, 24 oz. (720 ml)

Dinner (7:00 p.m.)
Fish, 8 oz. (240 g)
Sweet potato, baked, 8 oz. (240 g)
Broccoli, cooked, 1 c.
Olive oil, 4 tsp. (30 ml)

Snack
Sorbet, 1-1/2 c. (360 ml)
Fig cookies, 2 whole

3,300 calories
500 g carbohydrate (60%)
145 g protein (18%)
80 g fat (22%)

exercise. Flavored sports drinks containing carbohydrate and sodium are generally better accepted by younger athletes and stimulate the desire to drink. Cooler fluids are more likely to be consumed.

Precompetition Nutrition

On rest days before competition, players should consume a high-carbohydrate diet to replenish muscle glycogen stores. Calorie needs may be reduced on these rest days, but a greater percentage of carbohydrate can be consumed to obtain the total grams of carbohydrate provided. The sidebar provides some sample training diet menus for the soccer player.

Another Afternoon Practice

Breakfast (7:00 a.m.)
Orange juice, 1 c. (240 ml)
French toast, 2 slices
Strawberries, 1 c.

Lunch (11:30 a.m.)
Low-fat cheese, 2 oz. (60 g)
Bread, 2 slices
Tomato, 1 whole
Yogurt with fruit, 6 oz.
Pear, 1 whole

Snack (3:00 p.m.)
Crackers, 8 small
Hummus, 4 tbsp. (80 ml)

Carrots, 3
Avocado, 1/4 whole

During Practice
Sports drink, 24 oz. (720 ml)

Dinner (6:30 p.m.)
Rice, cooked, 1.5 c. (360 ml)
Shrimp, 6 oz., cooked (180 g)
Red pepper, 1 whole
Broccoli, 1 c. cooked
Sesame seed oil, 1 tbsp. (20 ml)

2,300 calories
325 g carbohydrate (56%)
100 g protein (17%)
69 g fat (27%)

Meal timing the day of competition depends on the start time. Games are often played in late afternoon or evening but can also be played earlier in the day. Ideally, the player's favorite precompetition meal can be consumed 2.5 to 3 hours before the start time. This meal should provide about 150 to 200 grams of carbohydrate and small amounts of low-fat protein as tolerated. Small amounts of fats may be acceptable as well. For later start times, the athlete may want to eat a fairly large meal earlier in the day and allow plenty of time for digestion. A pregame meal can then be consumed later in the day consisting of the specific foods and portions tolerated by the athlete.

Sample Competition Menu

12:00 p.m. Game Time

Breakfast (7:00 a.m.)
Oatmeal, cooked, 1 c. (240 ml)
Skim milk, 8 oz. (240 ml)
Wheat germ, 2 tbsp. (40 ml)
Bread, 2 slices
Jam, 2 tbsp. (40 ml)
Juice, 12 oz. (360 ml)
Egg, hard-boiled, 1

Pregame Smoothie (10:00 a.m.)
Soy milk, 12 oz. (360 ml)
Frozen berries, 1 c.
Energy bar, 1 medium

During Game
Sports Drink, 32 oz. (960 ml)
Carbohydrate gel, 1 packet

Postgame (3:30 p.m.)
Energy drink, 24 oz. (720 ml)
Energy bar, 1
Carbohydrate recovery drink, 12 oz. (360 ml)
Apple, 1 medium

Dinner (5:00 p.m.)
Chicken fajitas:
   Chicken, 6 oz. (180 g)
   Tortilla, 4 small
   Salsa, 1 c. (240 ml)
   Peppers, 1 c. (240 ml)

Snack
Frozen yogurt, 1 c. (240 ml)
Frozen berries, 1 c.

3,400 calories
560 g carbohydrate (65%)
110 g protein (13%)
83 g fat (22%)

Players can also consume easily digested sports bars and gels in the 90 minutes leading up to a game.

Soccer games can be scheduled close together, and travel may be required to go to a game. Players should pack some of their favorite travel snacks and fluids. They should appreciate the importance of adequate nutritional recovery between games and consume high-glycemic carbohydrates shortly after the game and again in 2 hours. Carbohydrate amounts of 50 to 75 grams are recommended. Small amounts of protein can be added to these recovery snacks. Meal and snack times can be adjusted as needed for game times and energy needs.

Light Practice Day before Competition High-carbohydrate Menu

Breakfast (7:30 a.m.)
Raisin Bran, 1.5 c. (45 g)

Milk, skim, 8 oz. (240 ml)

Grapefruit, 1 whole

Bagel, 3 oz. (90 g)

Cheese, low-fat, 2 oz. (60 g)

During Practice
16 oz. (480 ml) sports drink

Postpractice
Recovery drink, 16 oz. (480 ml)

Banana, 1 large

Lunch (12:00 p.m.)
Peanut butter, 4 tsp. (30 ml)

Jam, 2 tbsp. (40 ml)

Bread, 2 slices

Orange, 1 medium

Yogurt with fruit, 6 oz. (200 ml)

Dinner (5:00 p.m.)
Grilled chicken, 6 oz. (180 g)

Sweet potatoes, 8 oz. (240 g)

Peas, cooked, 1 c.

Bread, 2 slices

Olive oil, 5 tsp. (40 ml)

Fruit salad, 1 c.

3,200 calories

520 g carbohydrate (65%)

110 g protein (14%)

75 g fat (21%)

Do Nutritional Needs Differ for Male and Female Athletes?

Despite the well-established physiological differences between female and male athletes, female athletes are routinely prescribed sports nutrition recommendations based on male-subject-derived scientific data. Fortunately, the past decade has seen increased scientific focus and study of nutritional requirements unique to female athletes. While much of this research has focused on endurance exercise, rather than the type of training programs practiced in team sport, a few key points can be considered by female athletes.

A full body of research utilizing solely female athletes that can be compared to the existing data on men is lacking, but emerging data do provide some practical gender-specific considerations for carbohydrate loading, nutritional intake during training, and recovery strategies, as well as gender-specific topics for future consideration.

Consuming adequate carbohydrate to optimize body glycogen fuel stores when resting or decreasing training prior to competition is an important nutritional strategy for female athletes, just as it is for their male counterparts. To load glycogen effectively, women need to consume an adequate number of grams of carbohydrate, but they appear to glycogen load only to about 50 percent of the magnitude of men. Female athletes competing on soccer, basketball, and hockey teams should not pass up the performance benefits of tapering and eating a high-carbohydrate diet, but they can appreciate that the benefit may be less than conventionally ascribed to this nutritional strategy.

Researchers have also studied gender difference regarding carbohydrate consumption during exercise with useful results. Because female athletes do not respond as robustly as men to carbohydrate loading, the consumption of a sports drink appears to be one place they can make up this difference. Subjects cycled at 60 percent VO_2max for 90 minutes while consuming an 8 percent carbohydrate beverage (1 gram carbohydrate per kilogram body weight). This study demonstrated that when female athletes performing endurance exercise were provided with sports drinks during exercise, they oxidized or burned more of the sports drink than males. Overall, though, women still burn more fat than carbohydrate during exercise when compared to men. Carbohydrate consumption during higher training intensities would also be expected to benefit female athletes. Future research is needed to determine whether the benefits hold up during the high-intensity, intermittent training seen in team sports.

Consuming carbohydrate immediately after training improves muscle glycogen resynthesis and recovery. Female athletes benefit from this strategy as much as their male counterparts. Research indicates that males and females appear to store glycogen at similar rates when carbohydrate is given immediately after endurance exercise. Future research can determine how this nutritional recovery strategy affects training programs specific to team sports.

Another recent study also points to the need for more data to fine-tune the unique daily nutritional requirements of female athletes and the effect of diet manipulations on performance, particularly for carbohydrate intake. Researchers had well-trained female triathletes and cyclists consume a low-carbohydrate diet of 1.4 grams per pound (3 grams/kilogram), a moderate-carbohydrate diet of 2.25 grams/per pound (5 grams per kilogram), and a high-carbohydrate diet of 3.5 grams per pound (8 grams/kilograms). Subjects cycled to exhaustion. Interestingly, subjects had difficulty consuming the prescribed amount of carbohydrate on the high-carbohydrate diet.

When completing a time trial after cycling at 70 percent VO_2max, no significant performance differences were found among the diets. More research and performance testing on various carbohydrate dietary levels in female athletes participating in team sports is needed. Past studies have demonstrated a difference in fuel metabolism between men and women. In the future, it is expected that nutritional recommendations are to be more sex-specific.

Women have a greater increase in core temperature given similar heat exposure when compared to men. Onset of sweating may occur at higher body temperatures, and sweat rates may be lower. However, there are likely more differences in sweat rates among individual women athletes than between men and women. Female athletes should consume fluid during exercise to attempt to match their fluid losses, while staying within their gastrointestinal tolerances. One study indicated that replacing body fluid after exercise is not affected by the phase of the menstrual cycle.

Although protein needs of female team sport athletes are higher than the general population, there appear to be no significant differences between men and women at this time. Recommendations are based on body weight and specific training programs, and they can vary with the amount of calories and carbohydrate consumed. Of course, adequate caloric intake allows for more optimal utilization of the protein consumed.

Do Nutritional Needs Differ? (continued)

With a greater number of female athletes reaching lower body fat levels, and women having to work harder to achieve the same level of leanness as men, health could be compromised. When a female athlete's caloric intake is inadequate, her body may be more prone to defend or maintain the current weight than would a man's. Recent data indicate that inadequate caloric intake is the main trigger for hormonal imbalances, absence of menstruation, and, subsequently, compromised bone health.

While more specific nutritional training recommendations for women need to be tested and formulated, women athletes should practice some focused strategies to ensure optimal performance. For example, they should consistently practice optimal recovery nutrition following hard training, glycogen load in combination with adequate caloric intake, and make sure to consume enough carbohydrate during training and competition.

CHAPTER 13

NUTRITION FOR HOCKEY

Ice hockey is enjoyed by players of all levels across North America and is extremely popular, with over 2 million participants, respectively, in the United States and Canada. Participation can begin at an early age for both boys and girls, at the club, amateur, high school, and collegiate levels. The National Hockey League was formed in Canada in 1920 and now consists of 30 professional teams in the both the United States and Canada.

Hockey is played almost year-round at some level, and the professional hockey season is one of the most physically demanding in regard to training and the competitive schedule. Training for ice hockey takes place both on and off the ice.

DEMANDS OF THE GAME

Ice hockey is a demanding sport both aerobically and anaerobically. During a game, hockey is characterized by repeated high-intensity efforts interspersed with periods of moderate activity and rest during play stoppage. While most of the effort during a game is powered by the anaerobic system, using creatine phosphate and muscle glycogen as a fuel, the aerobic system is also crucial for hockey players. The aerobic system fuels a small part of the energy required for intense hockey play, and most of the energy at moderate activity levels. Most important, in ice hockey, a well-trained aerobic system is crucial for recovery between plays and during time on the bench. Top players who have more ice time have even less time on the bench, making the aerobic system even more important for recovery.

Hockey players move on the ice at speeds that may reach 30 to 40 miles per hour (48 to 64 kilometers per hour), and their goal shots may send the puck flying at up to 100 miles per hour (160 kilometers per hour). Hockey players must possess muscular strength, muscular endurance, and general aerobic fitness. Of course, they also need a high level of skating skill, superior strength endurance, and the ability to move explosively, turn quickly, and maneuver while fending off an opponent's body checks. Hockey can be a very exciting game to watch because of its fast pace and frequent change in action.

During a game, hockey is unique in that player substitutions can be made during play. Except for the goalie, players are usually on the ice for 45 to 90 seconds per shift, with top players perhaps playing a total of 30 cumulative minutes. Players may have 4 to 5 minutes of recovery between shifts, and games lasts for three 20-minute periods. These high-speed efforts receive fuel from the phosphocreatine and anaerobic glycolysis system, making muscle glycogen an important fuel source.

Hockey training is also very intense and demanding, working both the high-intensity anaerobic systems and the aerobic system. Between bouts of all-out efforts, a well-trained aerobic system improves the player's recovery between shifts and between games. Players may build aerobic fitness through bike riding, stair climbing, and a strength-training program. Other components of a training program consist of drills, plyometrics, and on-ice skills.

Energy Requirements

Hockey players have high-energy needs during the season, and they should adjust their caloric intake accordingly for their off-season training. Hockey players are large and more muscular than in past decades and may have high-calorie needs due to their high body weight. A 180-pound (82-kilogram) hockey player may burn 12 calories per minute during an intense practice, or burn 600 calories in 50 minutes. These calories would be required in addition to basic calorie requirements of 2,300 calories. The player may also participate in other training sessions, requiring anywhere from another 500 to 1,000 calories daily. Depending on the playing level of the athlete and the time of season, male hockey players may require over 4,000 calories daily. Female hockey players also need a high amount of calories per pound or kilogram of body weight based on their training program and level of play.

Body Composition

Body composition and body weight goals need to be individualized to the player, his or her training and competition schedule, and level of play. Often, high-level hockey players have trouble maintaining weight during the season due to the high energy demands of training and competing. They can play several games per week and experience frequent travel, which takes a toll on their body and can result in unwanted weight loss that diminishes their power and performance.

Young hockey players often desire to gain muscle mass and should follow the nutritional requirements outlined for weight training in Chapter 6. These young hockey players will have higher daily protein and calorie needs, and they need to time meals and snacks appropriately around their weight-training and other training sessions. Supplements targeted for muscle building are generally not advised for this age group.

Appropriate body composition is also advised for hockey players, as moving excess body fat during play requires more effort and energy. Hockey players should reach body composition goals gradually, as rapid weight loss can decrease power and compromise fuel stores. Players should avoid excess body fat gain in the off-season and begin body fat loss efforts preseason, reaching goals before the competition season. During the season, efforts should focus on maintenance and maintaining muscle mass.

Diet Composition

Carbohydrate is the preferred fuel for hockey practice and competition, and players should focus on maintaining adequate carbohydrate in their diet. Carbohydrate depletion can become a significant factor in the quality of workouts and during competition, particularly in the third period when fuel stores run low. As occurs in many team sport competitions, the winning team often consists of the players with the most fuel reserves and energy to score.

One study measured muscle glycogen in elite hockey players in Sweden. Researchers determined that a high-carbohydrate diet, with about 60 percent carbohydrate calories, resulted in a higher level of muscle glycogen before competition than a diet that was lower in carbohydrate and that may typically be followed by hockey players. The higher muscle glycogen levels also translated into improved performance. Players consuming the high-carbohydrate diet had greater skating speed, skated more shifts and longer shifts, and skated a greater distance. The differences between the players on the high-carbohydrate diet and those on the mixed diet (40 percent carbohydrate) were most evident during the third period of the game. Researchers noted that the low pregame muscle glycogen stores could be due not only to insufficient diet but also to inadequate recovery between games.

Training between games also depletes muscle glycogen stores, and players should pay close attention to their carbohydrate intake when their schedule is filled with practice sessions and competition. One study found that muscle glycogen stores were depleted by 60 percent in varsity players in a single game. Combined with inadequate carbohydrate intake, intense training can result in low muscle glycogen stores that could compromise performance.

Hockey players also have the highest protein requirements of team sport and strength athletes. The required daily amount of 0.6 to 0.8 gram per pound (1.4 to 1.7 grams/kilogram) is easily met in a well-planned diet. Glycogen depletion during practice or a game can also result in protein oxidation during exercise, contributing to a net loss in protein over time. However, a well-planned diet that includes appropriate carbohydrate intake should prevent this from happening. Healthy fats should provide the remainder of calories to meet energy needs in the diet.

IMPORTANT NUTRITION STRATEGIES FOR HOCKEY
Hydration, Fluid Replacement, and Carbohydrate Intake

Despite being played on the ice in relatively cooler temperatures, hockey players can incur high sweat losses during practice and a game. During their high-intensify training, an increase in body temperature is seen, and the result is a high sweat rate. The amount of equipment and pads that hockey players wear also increase their risk for dehydration. Goalies are even more susceptible to dehydration because of the weight of the heavy equipment that they wear. Dehydration compromises performance long before fuel depletion, and hockey players should monitor their sweat losses during various types of practice sessions and training intensities. Significant weight loss during a training session indicates that players are not drinking adequately and not keeping up with their sweat losses.

Hockey players need to drink fluids on a schedule before, during, and after practice to maintain adequate hydration levels. Strategies can be individualized to sweat rates during on-ice practices, weight-training sessions, general aerobic conditioning, and off-ice anaerobic training. Various types of training sessions offer different opportunities to drink during training. Players should appreciate that these opportunities to drink should be maximized in an effort to maximize performance and recovery.

Training and games place a high demand on muscle glycogen for fuel, and the fluids consumed should contain carbohydrate. Sports drinks provide a good balance of fluid and carbohydrate for the hockey player and should be the beverage of choice during intense training sessions. Sports drinks also help players maintain adequate blood glucose levels during intense training and games, which is important for concentration and maximizing the rapid reaction times during play. Players should be aware that maintaining optimal hydration allows fluids to more quickly empty from the stomach and can prevent delayed stomach emptying and the feeling of fluid sloshing in the stomach during intense efforts.

During games and intense practices, hockey players can also consume high-carbohydrate gels. These supplements offer a concentrated source of carbohydrate that quickly raises blood glucose levels and provides fuel between periods. One gel packet should be consumed with at least 8 ounces (240 milliliters) of water.

Despite maximizing opportunities to drink during practice and games, hockey players should make an effort to rehydrate after games, especially if they have lost more than 1 percent of their body weight, or about 2 pounds for a 180-pound player (1 kilogram for an 82-kilogram player). Rehydration choices should include a drink that contains some sodium. Players should drink 20 ounces (600 milliliters) for every pound (0.5 kilogram) of weight lost. Concentrated carbohydrate drinks provide carbohydrate for glycogen replenishment, fluid for rehydration, and sodium to enhance the rehydration process.

Some hydration and carbohydrate replacement strategies specific to the hockey player include the following:

- Check morning weight several times weekly to determine if daily hydration is adequate.
- Drink 14 to 20 ounces (400 to 600 milliliters) of fluid in the 2 hours before practice or a game. Stop drinking 30 to 60 minutes before a game to empty your bladder.
- Take small sips of fluid during the game when you are on the bench, about 4 to 6 ounces (120 to 180 milliliters) whenever possible.
- Consume 8 ounces (240 milliliters) or more of a sports drink between periods, or consume one carbohydrate gel and 8 ounces (240 milliliters) of water.
- Rehydrate with at least 40 ounces (1,200 milliliters) of a carbohydrate drink after practice or competition.

The sidebar provides some training diet menus that provide guidelines for meals, snacks, and fluid intake around exercise.

Fluid Intake in Young Players

Young hockey players also need to keep up with their fluid losses during practice. Players can become dehydrated during practice sessions lasting under 1 hour. Sports drinks are still the preferred choices during these practice sessions and games, because research indicates that a sports drink can enhance intermittent, high-intensity exercise lasting only 60 minutes. Flavored drinks also improve hydration efforts among young athletes.

Precompetition

Hockey players can time their eating before practice and particularly competition to maximize their fuel stores, particularly body carbohydrate stores, and minimize any unwanted gastrointestinal side effects. A high-carbohydrate pregame meal can top off

Sample Menu for Hockey Players

Afternoon Practice

Breakfast (6:30 a.m.)
Breakfast, cereal, 2 c. or 3 oz.
  (90 g)
Milk, skim, 12 oz. (360 ml)
Orange juice, 8 oz. (240 ml)
Banana, 1 small
Toast, 2 slices
Margarine, 2 tsp. (15 ml)
Jam, 2 tbsp. (40 ml)

Conditioning (7:30 a.m.)
Water to maintain hydration

Snack (8:30 a.m.)
Yogurt, 6 oz. (180 ml)
Peach, 1 medium

Lunch (12:00 p.m.)
Turkey sub:
Turkey, 6 oz. (180 g)
Bread, 2 slices
Mayo, 2 tsp. (15 ml)

Juice, 12 oz. (360 ml)
Yogurt, 6 oz. (180 ml)

Snack (3:00 p.m.)
Granola bar, 1
Apple, 1 medium

During Practice
Sports drink, 24 oz. (720 ml)

Dinner (7:00 p.m.)
Lean beef, 4 oz. (120 g)
Baked potato, 1 large or 10 oz. (300 g)
Mixed vegetables, 1 c.
Garden salad, 2 c.
Dressing, light, 4 tbsp. (60 ml)

Snack
Milk, 8 oz. (240 ml)
Crackers, whole-grain, 8 small

3,500 calories
500 g carbohydrate (57%)
135 g protein (15%)
109 g fat (28%)

muscle glycogen and fill liver glycogen stores. Meal timing is essential, and most players should be comfortable consuming 150 to 200 grams of carbohydrates about 2 to 3 hours beforehand. Small amounts of easily digested protein such as skim milk, soy milk, and poultry can be consumed. Other protein choices that are often well tolerated before competition include peanut butter and low-fat cheeses in small amounts. Fats such as oils and spreads should be kept to reasonable amounts for easy digestion.

Hard Evening Practice

Breakfast (7:30 a.m.)
Grits, cooked, 1 c. (240 ml)
Raisins, 2 tbsp. (40 ml)
Yogurt, nonfat, plain, 6 oz.
  (180 ml)
Cashews, 2 tsp. (12 ml)

Lunch (11:30 a.m.)
Tuna, 4 oz. (120 g)
Pita bread, 1 round or 2 oz. (60 g)
Celery, pepper, carrots, 2 c.
Apple juice, 12 oz. (360 ml)

Snack (3:00 p.m.)
Bagel, 4 oz. (120 g)
Nut butter, 2 tbsp. (40 ml)
Apple, 1 large

During Practice
Sports drink, 40 oz. (1,200 ml)

Recovery (6:30 p.m.)
Smoothie:
    Milk, 12 oz. (360 ml)
    Yogurt, 6 oz. (180 ml)
    Frozen berries, 1 c.

Dinner (8:00 p.m.)
Pork tenderloin, 4 oz. (120 g)
Rice, cooked, 1.5 c. (360 ml)
Corn, 1/2 c. (120 ml)
Mushrooms, 1/4 c. (60 ml)
Bread, 2 slices
Olive oil, 4 tsp. (30 ml)
Sherbet, 1 c. (240 ml)
Raspberries, 1 c.

3,300 calories
520 g carbohydrate (63%)
110 g protein (13%)
88 g fat (24%)

Meal timing should reflect personal tolerances and game timing. Players may want to have a larger midday meal the day of an evening game and a light easily digested meal or large snack 2 to 3 hours beforehand. While meal and snack timing should reflect game time and tolerances, players should appreciate that their carbohydrate intake for the day should be adequate to ensure recovery from the last practice session and fill glycogen stores prior to the game. Players can experiment with use and intake of various sports nutrition products such as liquid meal replacements, gels, and high-carbohydrate drink in the 2 to 3 hours prior to the game. Products should be tested in practice and never on game day.

Postgame Recovery

Because hockey players may play several games in a week, participate in weekend tournaments, or have a busy schedule of both practices and games, postgame recovery

Hockey Game Day Plan

7:00 p.m. Game Start Time

Breakfast (8:30 a.m.)
Oatmeal, cooked, 1 c. (240 ml)
Egg, 1
Toast, 1 slice
Margarine, 2 tsp. (15 ml)
Juice, 8 oz. (240 ml)

Lunch (1:00 p.m.)
Baked chicken, 6 oz. (180 g)
Rice, cooked, 2 c. (480 ml)
Vegetables, cooked, 1 c.
Milk, 12 oz. (360 ml)
Frozen yogurt, 12 oz. (360 ml)
Fruit, 1 c.

Snack (4:00 p.m.)
Bread, 2 slices
Honey, 2 tbsp. (40 ml)
Peanut butter, 4 tsp. (30 ml)
Water, 16 oz. (480 ml)

Game
Sports drink every shift, 4–6 oz.
  (120–180 ml)
Sports drink between periods, 16 oz.
  (480 ml)

Postgame
High-carbohydrate recovery drink, 16 oz.
(480 ml)

Dinner (10:00 p.m.)
Pasta, cooked, 3 c. (720 ml)
Meat sauce, 1-1/2 c. (360 ml)
Salad
Dressing, light, 4 tbsp. (80 ml)
Bread, 2 slices

4,100 calories
600 g carbohydrate (60%)
130 g protein (13%)
120 g fat (27%)

should be optimized to replenish muscle glycogen stores prior to the next training session or game. Within 30 minutes of a game, the athlete should consume 0.5 gram of carbohydrate per pound of body weight (1 gram/kilogram). This recovery snack can also include 15 to 20 grams of protein. These carbohydrate and protein amounts can be repeated with a meal or snack in 2 hours to continue the muscle glycogen replenishment process. The sidebar provides some sample menus for various game start times, including fluids to be consumed during competition and recovery meals and snacks.

3:00 p.m. Game Start Time

Breakfast (8:00 a.m.)
Cereal, 1.5 oz. (45 g)
Milk, skim, 8 oz. (240 ml)
Strawberries, 1 c.
Juice, 12 oz. (360 ml)
Eggs, scrambled, 2
Toast, 2 slices
Peanut butter, 4 tsp.

Lunch (12 noon)
Roast turkey, 4 oz.
Bread, 2 slices
Mayo, light, 2 tbsp.
Pretzel, 1.5 oz.
Orange, 1 medium
Juice, 12 oz.

Snack
Gel, 1 packet
Sports drink, 24 oz. (360 ml)

During Game
4–6 oz. (120 to 180 ml) on the bench
8 oz. (240 ml) between periods

Postgame
Carbohydrate recovery drink, 12 oz. (360 ml)

Dinner (7:00 p.m.)
Chicken and bean burrito, 1 large
Chicken, beans, rice, cheese

3,200 calories
530 g carbohydrate (66%)
120 g protein (15%)
67 g fat (19%)

Nutrition and Your Immune System

Periods of heavy training are associated with a depressed immune function, and compromised immune function can be further aggravated by inadequate nutrition. Combining training with school and/or work can overtax an athlete's resources, stress your body, and compromise your ability to fight infection. A strong immune system should result in fewer colds or viruses, and if the athlete does get sick, recovery should be quicker. Dedicated team sport athletes don't want to encounter an unwanted halt to their training program due to illness. Specific foods can strengthen your immune system.

One of the nutrients most commonly associated with preventing colds is vitamin C, which has a widespread reputation as an immune system booster. A daily multivitamin and mineral supplement may contain the Daily Value of vitamin C, but don't underestimate the importance of ample food sources of this nutrient. Athletes can consume over three servings of fresh fruit daily and up to 2 cups of cooked vegetables daily for ample amounts of dietary vitamin C. High doses of vitamin C have not been shown to protect the immune system, and 250 milligrams is adequate to saturate body stores.

Fruits and vegetables also contain hundreds of phytochemicals that provide many preventative health benefits and are also excellent sources of carotenoids that boost the activity of white blood cells called lymphocytes. Beta-carotene can also be con-

verted to vitamin A, an important nutrient for the immune system.

Other nutrients important for a strong immune system include adequate intakes of zinc, iron, and vitamins B6 and B12. A good daily multivitamin and mineral supplement providing 100 percent of the Daily Values ensures adequate nutrient intake. Megadosing with vitamins and minerals can compromise the immune system, and excessive intakes of iron, zinc, and vitamin E are not advised.

Consuming adequate calories is not only beneficial for an athlete's recovery and energy levels but also important to maintaining a healthy immune system. Falling short of your calorie requirements can compromise your immune system. Poorly planned and low-calorie diets can also be low in protein, which can compromise your immune system. Diets too low in energy can result in inadequate intake of vitamins and minerals, which also decreases immunity.

Training with optimal stores of carbohydrate not only provides fuel for your workouts but boosts your immune system. Athletes who train in the carbohydrate-depleted state experience greater increases in the stress hormones that go up during exercise. Consuming carbohydrate during exercise also seems to diminish some of the immunosuppressive effects of intense training. Overall, good carbohydrate replacement supports your immune system.

CREATINE AND HOCKEY PLAYERS

Creatine is often a popular ergogenic aid with hockey players who want to build muscle and improve strength. One study of elite ice hockey players looked at the performance effects of creatine loading for 5 days, followed by a 10-week maintenance dose. Over the 10-week period, an improvement was seen in on-ice sprint performance. Further studies specific to ice hockey training and performance are needed.

One of the side effects of creatine loading is an immediate weight gain, most likely fluid gain. Hockey players may not like training with this additional weight. Concerns with creatine use in young athletes and possible harmful side effects persist. There is also concern that the use of such supplements in young athletes may encourage the use of more harmful and illegal supplements. Young hockey players should follow the proper nutritional guidelines for muscle building and strength as outlined in Chapter 6.

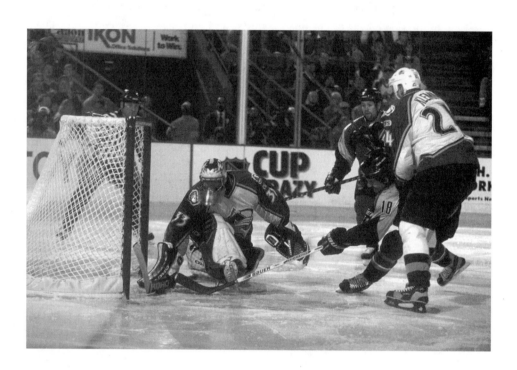

GLYCEMIC INDEX OF FOODS

GLYCEMIC INDEX OF FOODS			
Food, portion	**Grams of carbohydrate per serving**	**Glycemic load per serving**	**Glycemic index for 50 g**
High-Glycemic Foods (GI > 70)			
Glucose (test dose)	50		100
Potato, instant, mashed, 5 oz. (150 g)	22.8	22.1	97
Baguette, 1 oz. (30 g)	15.9	15.1	95
Potato, baked, 6.5 oz. (200 g)	29	27.3	94
Rice, instant, 5 oz. (200 g)	42	36.5	87
Corn Flakes, 1 oz. (30 g)	25	21.5	86
Pretzels, 2 oz. (60 g)	39	32.2	83
Rice Krispies, 1 oz. (30 g)	29	24	82
Waffles, 2 oz. (60 g)	24.7	19.2	76
Doughnut, 1.6 oz. (47 g)	19	14.3	76
Total cereal, 1 oz. (30 g)	25	19	76
Waffle, 2 oz. (60 g)	25	19.3	76
Soda crackers, 0.8 oz. (25 g)	17.8	13.1	74
Cheerios, 1 oz. (30 g)	25	18.5	74
Watermelon, 8 oz. (240 g)	12	8.6	72
Bagel, white, 2.25 oz. (70 g)	35.5	25.5	72
Millet, 5 oz. (150 g)	34.8	24.7	71
Bread, white, 2 oz. (60 g)	26.8	18.8	70
Pancakes, from mix, 2.7 oz. (80 g)	32.5	21.8	67
Moderate-Glycemic Foods (GI 55–70)			
Croissant, 1.9 oz. (57 g)	14.7	22	67
Shredded Wheat, 1 oz. (30 g)	21.7	14.6	67
Cream of Wheat, 1 oz. (30 g)	20	13.2	66
Pineapple, 4 oz. (120 g)	9.6	6.3	66
Oat kernel bread, 2 oz. (60 g)	25.6	16.6	65
Raisins, 2 oz. (60 g)	42.7	27.3	64
Rye crispbread, 1 oz. (30 g)	16	10.1	63
Muffin 1.9 oz. (57 g)	27.7	17.2	62
Corn, sweet, 2.6 oz. (80 g)	16	9.5	62
Ice cream, 1.6 oz. (50 g)	9.9	6.1	62

GLYCEMIC INDEX OF FOODS, *CONTINUED*

Couscous, 5 oz. (150 g)	14.3	8.7	61
Bran muffin, 1.9 oz. (57 g)	20.9	12.5	60
Spaghetti, white, durum wheat, 6 oz. (180 g)	44.3	25.6	58
Pita bread, 1 oz. (30 g)	16	9.2	57
Orange juice, 9 oz. (264 g)	21	12	57
Muesli, 2 oz. (60 g)	32	17.9	56
Oat Bran, raw, 2 oz. (60 g)	30	16.5	55
Popcorn, 2 oz. (60 g)	19	10.5	55
Pumpernickel bread 1 oz. (30 g)	13.4	7.4	55

Low-Glycemic Foods (GI <55)

Pound cake, 1.75 oz. (53 g)	25	13.4	54
Buckwheat, 5 oz. (150 g)	28.8	14.6	51
Bread, whole-grain, 2 oz. (30 g)	23	12	51
Banana, ripe, 4 oz. (120 g)	23.9	12.1	50
All-Bran, 2 oz. (60 g)	36.8	18.4	50
Rice, brown, 5 oz. (150 g)	47.7	23.9	49
Porridge oatmeal, 8 oz. (250 g)	20.3	9.9	48
Sweet potato, 5 oz. (150 g)	26	12.5	48
Bulgur, 5 oz. (150 g)	26	11.9	46
Lactose	50	21.5	43
Chickpeas, 5 oz. (150 g)	21	8.6	42
Grapefruit juice, 8 oz. (260 g)	15.7	7.5	41
Pear, Bartlett, 4 oz. (120 g)	11.3	4.6	40
Apple juice, 8 oz. (243 g)	26	10.4	40
Apple, 4 oz. (120 g)	14.6	5.9	33
Apricots, dried, 2 oz. (60 g)	25	8	32
Fettuccine, 4 oz. (120 g)	30	9.6	32
Yogurt, fruited, 6.5 oz. (200 gm)	33	10.9	32
Milk, skim, 8 oz. (259 g)	13	4.1	32
Spaghetti, whole-meal, 4 oz. (120 g)	30	9.6	28
Peach, 8 oz. (240 g)	15	4.2	28
Lentils, 5 oz. (150 g)	14.9	4.1	28
Kidney beans, 5 oz. (150 g)	24	5.5	23
Fructose (test portion)	50	10	20

Values are based on a glucose rating of 100. Source: *The GI Factor,* Dr. Jennie Brand-Miller, and www.glycemicindex.com.

APPENDIX B

FACTS ABOUT VITAMINS AND MINERALS

FACTS ABOUT VITAMINS AND MINERALS			
Vitamins	**DRIs**	**Major Sources**	**Major Functions**
Thiamin (vitamin B1)	**Males** 14–70 yrs: 1.2 mg **Females** 14–70 yrs: 1.1 mg	Wheat germ, whole-grain breads and cereals, organ meats, lean meats, legumes	Energy production from carbohydrate, essential for healthy nervous system
Riboflavin (vitamin B2)	**Male** 14–70 yrs: 1.3 mg **Females** 14–18 yrs: 1.0 mg 18–70 yrs: 1.1 mg	Milk and dairy products, green leafy vegetables, lean meats, beans	Energy production from carbohydrates and fats, healthy skin
Niacin (nicotinamide, nicotinic acid)	**Males** 14–70 yrs: 16 mg **Females** 14–70 yrs: 14 mg	Lean meats, fish, poultry, whole grains, peanuts	Energy production from carbohydrate, synthesis fat, blocks release FFA
Vitamin B6 (pyridoxine)	**Males** 14–50 yrs: 1.3 mg 51–>70 yrs: 1.7 mg **Females** 14–18 yrs: 1.2 mg 19–50 yrs: 1.3 mg 50–>70 yrs: 1.5 mg	Liver, lean meats, fish, poultry, legumes, bran cereal	Role in protein metabolism, necessary for formation of hemoglobin and red blood cells, synthesis essential fatty acids, required for glycogen breakdown
Vitamin B12 (cobalamin)	**Males** 14–>70 yrs: 2.4 µg **Females** 14–>70 yrs: 2.4 µg	Lean meats, poultry, dairy products, eggs	Formation of red blood cells, metabolism nervous tissue, involved folate metabolism, formation DNA

FACTS ABOUT VITAMINS AND MINERALS, *CONTINUED*

Vitamins	DRIs	Major Sources	Major Functions
Folic acid (folate)	**Males** 14–>70 yrs: 400 µg **Females** 14–>70 yrs: 400 µg	Green leafy vegetables, legumes	Role in red blood cell and DNA formation
Biotin	**Males** 14–18 yrs: 25 µg 19–>70 yrs: 30 µg **Females** 14–18 yrs: 25 µg 19–>70 yrs: 30 µg	Meats, legumes, milk, egg yolk, whole grains	Role in metabolism of carbohydrate, protein, fat
Pantothenic acid	**Males** 14–>70 yrs: 5 mg **Females** 14–>70 yrs: 5 mg	Liver, lean meats, eggs, salmon, all animal and plant foods	Role in metabolism of carbohydrate, protein, fat
Vitamin C	**Males** 14–18 yrs: 75 mg 19–>70 yrs: 90 mg **Females** 14–18 yrs: 65 mg 19–>70 yrs: 75 mg	Citrus fruits, green leafy vegetables, broccoli, peppers, strawberries, potatoes	Essential for connective tissue development, role in iron absorption, antioxidant, role wound healing
Fat-Soluble			
Vitamin A (retinol, provitamin carotenoids)	**Males** 14–>70 yrs: 900 µg **Females** 14–>70 yrs: 700 µg	Liver, milk, cheese, fortified margarine, carotenoids in plant foods (orange, red, deep green in color)	Maintains healthy tissue in skin and mucous membranes, essential night vision, role in bone development
Vitamin D (cholecalciferol)	**Males** 14–50 yrs: 5 µg 50–70 yrs: 10 µg >70 yrs: 15 µg **Females** 14–50 yrs: 5 µg 51–70 yrs: 10 µg >70 yrs: 15 µg	Vitamin D–fortified milk and margarine, fish oil, action of sunlight on skin	Increase intestinal absorption of calcium, promotes bone and tooth formation
Vitamin E (tocopherol)	**Males** 14–>70 yrs: 15 mg **Females** 14–>70 yrs: 15 mg	Vegetable oils, margarine, green leafy vegetables, wheat germ, whole-grain products	Formation red blood cells, antioxidant
Vitamin K (phylloquinone)	**Males** 14–18 yrs: 75 µg 19–>70 yrs: 120 µg **Females** 14–18 yrs: 75 µg 19–>70 yrs: 90 µg	Liver, soybean oil, spinach, cauliflower, green leafy vegetables	Essential normal blood clotting

FACTS ABOUT VITAMINS AND MINERALS, *CONTINUED*

Vitamins	DRIs	Major Sources	Major Functions
Major Minerals			
Calcium	**Males** 14–18 yrs: 1,300 mg 19–50 yrs: 1,000 mg 50–>70 yrs: 1,200 mg **Females** 14–18 yrs: 1,300 mg 19–50 yrs: 1,000 mg 51–>70 yrs: 1,200 mg	Milk, cheese, yogurt, ice cream, dried peas and beans, dark-green leafy vegetables	Bone formation, enzyme activation, nerve impulse transmission, muscle contraction
Phosphorus	**Males** 14–18 yrs: 1,250 mg 19–>70 yrs: 700 mg **Females** 14–18 yrs: 1,250 mg 19–>70 yrs: 700 mg	Protein foods: meat, poultry, fish, eggs, milk, cheese, dried peas and beans, whole grains	Bone formation, cell membrane structure, B vitamin activation, component of ATP-CP, and other important organic compounds
Magnesium	**Males** 14–18 yrs: 410 mg 19–>70 yrs: 420 mg **Females** 14–18 yrs: 360 mg 19–30 yrs: 310 mg 31–>70 yrs: 320 mg	Milk, yogurt, dried beans, nuts, whole grains, tofu, green vegetables, chocolate	Roles in protein synthesis, glucose metabolism, muscle contraction
Trace Minerals			
Iron	**Males** 14–18 yrs: 11 mg 19–>70 yrs: 8 mg **Females** 14–18 yrs: 15 mg 19–50 mg.: 18 mg 50–>70 yrs: 8 mg	Organ meats, lean meats, poultry, shellfish, dried peas and beans, whole-grain products, green leafy vegetables	Hemoglobin formation, oxygen transport
Zinc	**Males** 14–>70 yrs: 11 mg **Females** 14–18 yrs: 9 mg 19–>70 yrs: 8 mg	Organ meats, meat, fish, poultry, shellfish, nuts, whole-grain products	Part of enzymes involved in energy metabolism, immune function
Copper	**Males** 14–18 yrs: 890 mg 19–>70 yrs: 900 mg **Females** 14–18 yrs: 890 mg 19–>70 yrs: 900 mg	Organ meats, meat, fish, poultry, shellfish, nuts, bran cereal	Role in use of iron and hemoglobin by body, involved in connective tissue formation and oxidation

FACTS ABOUT VITAMINS AND MINERALS, *CONTINUED*

Vitamins	DRIs	Major Sources	Major Functions
Fluoride	**Adequate intake** **Males** 14–18 yrs: 3 mg 19–>70 yrs: 4 mg **Females** 14–>70 yrs: 3 mg	Milk, egg yolks, drinking water, seafood	Helps form teeth and bones
Selenium	**Males** 14–>70 yrs: 55 µg **Females** 14–>70 yrs: 55 µg	Meat, fish, poultry, organ meats, seafood, whole grains and nuts from selenium-rich soil	Part of antioxidant enzyme
Chromium	**Adequate intake** **Males** 14–50 yrs: 35 µg 50–>70 yrs: 30 µg **Females** 14–18 yrs: 24 µg 19–50 yrs: 25 µg 50–>70 yrs: 20 µg	Organ meats, meats, oysters, cheese, whole-grain products, beer	Enhances insulin function as glucose tolerance factor
Iodine	**Males** 14–>70 yrs: 150 µg **Females** 14–>70 yrs: 150 µg	Iodized table salt, seafood, water	Part of thyroxine that plays role in reactions involving cellular energy
Manganese	**Adequate Intake** **Males** 14–18 yrs: 2.2 mg 19–>70 yrs: 2.3 mg **Females** 14–18 yrs: 1.6 mg 19–>70 yrs: 1.8 mg	Beet greens, whole grains, nuts, legumes	Part of essential enzyme systems
Molybdenum	**Males** 14–18 yrs: 43 µg 19–>70 yrs: 45 µg **Females** 14–18 yrs: 43 µg 19–>70 yrs: 45 µg	Legumes, cereal grains, dark-green leafy vegetables	Part of essential enzymes involved in carbohydrate and fat metabolism

COMPARISON OF SPORTS NUTRITION PRODUCTS

COMMERCIAL SPORTS DRINKS (8-OZ. SERVING)					
Product	Type of Carbohydrate	Carbohydrate Concentration (%)	Calories	Carbohydrate (g)	Sodium (mg)
Accelrade	Sucrose, fructose, maltodextrin (also contains small amounts branched-chain amino acids)	7.75	93	17	127
All Sport	Fructose, sucrose	7	70	19	55
Body Fuel	Maltodextrin, fructose	7	70	17	70
Cytomax	Fructose, maltodextrin, polylactate, glucose	8	83	19	70
Endura	Glucose polymers, fructose	6	60	15	92
Exceed	Glucose polymer, fructose	7	70	17	50
Gatorade	Sucrose, glucose	6	50	14	110
Gatorade Endurance Drink	Sucrose, glucose	6	60	15	200
Gookinaid	Glucose, fructose	5	43	10	69
GU$_2$O	Maltodextrin, fructose	5.5	52	13	120
Hydra Fuel	Glucose polymer, fructose, glucose	7	66	16	25
Met-Rx ORS	Rice syrup solids, glucose	8	70	19	125
Perform	Glucose, fructose, maltodextrins	7	60	16	110

COMMERCIAL SPORTS DRINKS (8-OZ. SERVING), *CONTINUED*

Product	Type of Carbohydrate	Carbohydrate Concentration (%)	Calories	Carbohydrate (g)	Sodium (mg)
Performance	Maltodextrin, fructose	10	100	25	115
PR Solution	Maltodextrin, fructose	12.5	120	30	50
Power Ade	Fructose, sucrose	6	55	14	50
PowerBar Endurance Sports Drink	Maltodextrin, dextrose, fructose	7	70	17	160
Red Bull	Sucrose, glucose	12	112	28	215
Revenge	Maltodextrin, amylopectin starch	9	90	23	100
Warp Aide	Fructose, maltodextrin	8	70	19	80
Coca-Cola	High fructose corn syrup, sucrose	12	108	29	9
Orange juice	Fructose, sucrose	11–15	112	26	2.7
Water		0	0	0	0

RECOVERY DRINKS

Product	Serving Size	Calories	Carbohydrate (g)	Protein (g)	Fat (g)
Boost	8-oz. can	240	33	15	6
EndoroxR4	2 scoops	280	53	14	1.5
Ensure	8-oz. can	250	40	9	6
Gatorade Energy Drink	12 oz.	310	78	0	0
Gatorade Nutrition Shake	11-oz. can	370	54	20	8
Metabolol	2 scoops	200	24	14	5
Metabolol II	2 scoops	260	40	18	3
Met-Rx	1 packet	260	24	37	2
Optimizer	2 scoops	280	58	11	0
Physique	4 scoops	210	38	14	0
UltraFuel	16 oz.	400	100	0	0

CARBOHYDRATE GELS

Product	Serving	Calories	Carbohydrate (g)	Sodium (mg)
Accel Gel	41-g packet	90	20 (plus 5 g protein)	95
Carb BOOM	41-g packet (1.4 oz.)	110	27	50
Clif Shot	32-g packet (1.1 oz.)	100	37	50
Gu	32-g packet (1.1 oz.)	100	30	20
Power Gel	41-g packet (1.1 oz.)	110	33	50

GLYCEMIC INDEX OF CARBOHYDRATE SOURCES AND SELECTED SPORTS NUTRITION PRODUCTS

Drink	Glycemic Index
Gatorade	89
XLR8	68
Poweraid	65
Cytomax	62
Allsport	53

Carbohydrate Source	Glycemic Index
Frustose	22–24
Galactose	22–24
Honey	55
Sucrose	65
Glucose	100
Maltodextrin	105

SAMPLE MENUS

Sample menus of varying calorie and carbohydrate levels are provided here. You can adjust portions and make substitutions as desired to raise or lower calorie and carbohydrate intake. The vegetarian menus can be used by animal protein eaters to obtain additional meal ideas. Vegetarians can use the animal protein–containing menus by making plant protein substitutions. Use the food lists provided in Chapter 8 to make substitutions for ingredients that are not available.

SAMPLE MENUS

2,200 calories
290 g carbohydrate (51%)
143 g protein (25%)
60 g fat (24%)

Cooked grain cereal, 1 c.
  (240 ml)
Banana, 1 small
Cottage cheese, 1/2 c.
  or egg, 1
Nuts, 1 tbsp. (15 ml)

Recovery smoothie:
12 oz. dairy milk (360 ml)
Frozen fruit, 1 c. (240 ml)

Low-fat tuna salad, 3 oz.
  (100 g)
Bread, 2 slices
Lentil salad or pasta salad,
  1/2 c. (120 ml)

Salmon, 6 oz. (180 g)
Buckwheat or rice, 1 c.
  cooked
Asparagus, 1 c.
Salad, 2 c.
Olive oil, 2 tsp. (20 ml)
Salad dressing, 2 tbsp.
  (30 ml)

Sorbet or frozen yogurt, 1/2 c.
  (120 ml)
Peach, 1 medium

2,500 calories
415 g carbohydrate (64%)
110 g protein (17%)
53 g fat (19%)

Oatmeal, 1 c. cooked
  (240 ml)
Apple, 1 medium
Juice, 8 oz. (240 ml)

Yogurt, 6 oz. (180 ml)
Strawberries, 1 c. (240 ml)

Chicken, 3 oz. (100 g)
Whole-grain bread, 2 slices
Pretzels, 3/4 oz. (22 g)
Pear, 1 large

Bagel, 3 oz. (90 g)
Peanut butter, 1 tsp. (8 ml)

Beef strips, 3 oz. (100 g)
Noodles, 2 c. cooked
  (480 ml)
Bread, 1 slice
Olive oil, 2 tsp. (15 ml)
Mixed vegetables, 1 c.

2,600 calories
335 g carbohydrate (50%)
139 g protein (21%)
83 g fat (28%)

Muesli, 3/4 c. (180 ml)
Apple, 1 medium
Raisins, 2 tbsp. (30 ml)
Soy or dairy milk, 1 c.
  (240 ml)
Almonds, 2 tsp. (15 ml)

Granola bar, 1 medium
Peach, 1 medium

Chicken tacos:
Chicken, 3 oz. (100 g)
Kidney or pinto beans,
  1/2 c. (120 ml)
Rice, 1 c. (240 ml)
Tortillas, corn, 2
Oil, 2 tsp. (30 ml)

Papaya, 1 whole
Crackers, 2 oz. (60 g)
Cream cheese, 2 tbsp.
  (40 ml)

Risotto:
Beef, 4 oz. (120 g)
Broccoli, 1 c.
Rice, 1-1/2 c. cooked
Bread, 2 slices
Oil, 2 tsp. (15 ml)

SAMPLE MENUS, *CONTINUED*

3,200 calories	3,200 calories	4,300 calories
480 g carbohydrate (59%)	488 g carbohydrate (59%)	610 g carbohydrate (56%)
147 g protein (18%)	146 g protein (18%)	168 g protein (15%)
90 g fat (24%)	87 g fat (24%)	137 g fat (28%)

Column 1 (3,200 calories)

Waffles, 4 squares
Syrup, 1/2 c. (120 ml)
Berries, 1 c.
Hard-boiled egg, 1
Soy or dairy milk, 12 oz.
  (360 ml)

Roast turkey, 3 oz. (100 g)
Avocado or hummus, 2 tbsp.
  (30 ml)
Toasted pita, 1 round
Plums, 3 medium
Soy or dairy milk, 8 oz.
  (240 ml)
Nonfat yogurt, 6 oz. (180 g)

Pasta, 3 c. cooked
Marinara sauce, 1 1/2 c.
  (360 ml)
Lean beef, 3 oz. (100 g)
Bread, 2 slices
Salad, 2 c.
Olive oil, 3 tsp. (20 ml)
Salad dressing, 2 tbsp.
  (30 ml)

Column 2 (3,200 calories)

Raisin bran, 1 1/2 c.
Milk, 8 oz. (240 ml)
Grapefruit, 1 whole
Bagel, 3 oz. (100 g)
Low-fat cheese, 2 oz. (60 g)

Recovery smoothie:
Milk, skim, 16 oz. (480 ml)
Granola, 1/2 c.
Banana, 1 large

Peanut butter, 1 tbsp.
  (15 ml)
Jam, 2 tbsp. (30 ml)
Bread, 2 slices

Orange, 1 medium
Yogurt with fruit, 8 oz.
  (240 ml)

Grilled chicken, 6 oz.
  (180 g)
Sweet potatoes, 10 oz.
  (300 g)
Peas, 1 c. cooked
Bread, 2 slices
Olive oil, 5 tsp. (50 ml)
Fruit salad, 1 c. (240 ml)

Sorbet, 1 c. (240 ml)
Strawberries, 1 c.

Column 3 (4,300 calories)

Bran flakes, 1 c.
Milk, 1 c. (240 ml)
English muffin, 2
Melted low-fat cheese,
  2 oz. (60 g)
Smoothie:
Soy milk, 12 oz. (360 ml)
Banana, 1
Wheat germ, 1 tbsp.
  (15 ml)
Sports drink, 40 oz.
  (1,200 ml)

Beef and bean burritos:
Beef, 8 oz. (240 g)
Rice, 1/2 c. cooked
Beans, 1 c.
Tortillas, 2 large
Salsa, 1 c. (240 ml)
Canola oil, 4 tsp. (30 ml)

Gingersnaps, 6
Juice, 8 oz. (240 ml)

Tofu stir-fry:
Tofu, 4 oz. (120 g)
Brown rice, 1 1/2 c. cooked
Sweet peppers, broccoli,
  1 c. cooked (240 ml)
Sesame seed oil, 1 tbsp.
  (15 ml)
Granola bar, 1
Ice cream, 1 c. (240 ml)
Chocolate syrup, 2 tbsp.
  (30 ml)
Nuts, 2 tsp. (15 ml)

SAMPLE MENUS, *CONTINUED*

2,200 calories
340 g carbohydrate (60%)
99 g protein (18%)
56 g fat (22%)

Orange juice, 1 c. (240 ml)
French toast, 2 slices
Syrup, 1/2 c. (120 ml)
Strawberries, 1 c.

Low-fat cheese, 2 oz. (60 g)
Bread, 2 slices
Tomato, 1 whole
Yogurt with fruit, 1 c.
   (240 ml)
Pear, 1 whole

Crackers, 8 small
Hummus, 1/2 c.
Milk, skim, 8 oz. (240 ml)

Rice, cooked, 1-1/2 c.
   (360 ml)
Shrimp, 6 oz. cooked
   (180 g)
Red pepper, 1 whole
Broccoli, 1 c. cooked
Sesame seed oil, 1 tbsp.
   (15 ml)

Frozen yogurt, 1 c. (240 ml)
Fruit slices, 1/2 c.

2,400 calories
346 g carbohydrate (58%)
99 g protein (17%)
68 g fat (26%)

English muffin, 1 whole
Cream cheese, 2 tbsp.
   (30 ml)
Jam, 2 tbsp. (30 ml)
Grapefruit juice, 12 oz.
   (360 ml)
Egg, 1 whole

Pinto beans, 1/2 c.
Rice, cooked, 1 c.
Tortilla, 1 whole
Salsa, 4 tbsp. (60 ml)
Cheese, 1 oz. (30 g)
Avocado, 1/4 whole

Granola bar, 1
Peaches, 2
Almonds, 1 tbsp. (15 ml)

Pasta, cooked, 2 c.
Lean beef, 3 oz. (100 g)
Marinara sauce, 1 c.
   (240 ml)
Green salad, 2 c.
Salad dressing, 2 tbsp.
   (30 ml)

Frozen yogurt, 1 c. (240 ml)
Blueberries, 1/2 c.

2,700 calories
380 g carbohydrate (55%)
130 g protein (19%)
86 g fat (27%)

Oatmeal, cooked, 1 1/2 c.
   (360 ml)
Skim milk, 8 oz. (240 ml)
Wheat germ, 4 tbsp. (60 ml)
Bread, 2 slices
Jam, 2 tbsp. (30 ml)
Orange juice, 8 oz.
   (240 ml)

Chicken, 4 oz. (120 g)
Bread, whole-grain, 2 slices
Mayonnaise, light, 2 tbsp.
   (30 ml)
Rice and bean salad, 1/2 c.
Grapes, 1 c.

Energy bar, 1
Banana, 1
Yogurt with fruit, 8 oz.
   (240 ml)

Tofu, 6 oz. (180 g)
Asian noodles, cooked, 2 c.
   (480 ml)
Vegetables, 2 c.
Sesame seed oil, 2 tbsp.
   (30 ml)

SAMPLE MENUS, *CONTINUED*

3,000 calories	3,700 calories	4,500 calories
430 g carbohydrate (58%)	630 g carbohydrate (68%)	775 g carbohydrate (67%)
176 g protein (23%)	130 g protein (14%)	140 g protein (12%)
63 g fat (19%)	75 g fat (18%)	105 g fat (21%)

3,000 calories

Bagel, 4 oz. (120 g)
Peanut butter, 2 tbsp.
  (30 ml)
Citrus juice, 12 oz. (360 ml)
Banana, 1 whole
Yogurt, plain, 1 c. (240 ml)

Tuna, 4 oz. (120 g)
Mayonnaise, 1 tbsp. (15 ml)
Pita bread, 1 round
Pretzels, 1.5 oz. (45 g)
Raw vegetable salad, 1 c.
Soy or dairy milk, 12 oz.
  (360 ml)
Peach slices, 1 c.
Granola, low-fat, 1/4 c.
  (60 ml)

Halibut, 8 oz. (240 g)
Buckwheat, cooked, 1 1/2 c.
Asparagus, 1 c. (360 ml)
Canola oil, 2 tsp. (15 ml)

Sorbet, 1 c. (240 ml)
Fig cookies, 3 small

3,700 calories

Grits, cooked, 1 c. (240 ml)
Raisins, 2 tbsp. (30 ml)
Yogurt, nonfat, plain, 1 c.
  (240 ml)
Dried cherries, 10
Cashews, 1 tbsp. (15 ml)

Hummus, 1/2 c.
Pita bread, 2 rounds
Celery, pepper, carrots, 2 c.
  (480 ml)
Apple juice, 12 oz. (360 ml)

Bagel, 2 oz. (60 g)
Nut butter, 2 tbsp. (30 ml)
Apple, 1 large

Pork tenderloin, 8 oz. (240 g)
Rice, cooked, 1-1/2 c.
  (360 ml)
Corn, 1/2 c. (120 ml)
Mushrooms, 1/4 c. (60 ml)
Bread, 2 slices
Olive oil, 4 tsp. (15 ml)

Sherbet, 1 c. (240 ml)
Raspberries, 1 c. (240 ml)

4,500 calories

Pancakes, 4 small
Maple syrup, 3/4 c. (180 ml)
Banana, 1 large
Raisins, 2 tbsp. (30 ml)
Nuts, 1 tbsp.
Soy milk, 12 oz. (360 ml)

Sports drink, 40 oz.
  (1,200 ml)

Burrito:
Chicken, 5 oz. (150 g)
Rice, cooked, 2 c.
Pinto beans, 1 c.
Avocado, 1/4 whole
Salsa, 1/2 c. (120 ml)

Linguine, cooked, 3 c.
Mixed vegetables, 1 c.
  (240 ml)
Bread, 2 slices
Olive oil, 2 tbsp. (30 ml)
Salad, 2 c.
Salad dressing, 2 tbsp.
  (30 ml)

Frozen yogurt, 2 c. (480 ml)
Cookies, 2
Strawberries, 1 c.

Vegetarian Menus

2,200 calories
348 g carbohydrate (62%)
95 g protein (17%)
53 g fat (21%)

Farina, cooked, 1 c.
(240 ml)
Skim milk, 8 oz. (240 ml)
Nuts, 1 tbsp. (15 ml)
Apple, 1
Orange juice, 12 oz.
(360 ml)

Soy burger, 1 patty
Bun, 1 whole
Cheese, low-fat, 1 oz. (30 g)
Lentil or bean salad, 1/2 c.
(120 ml)
Vegetables, raw, 1 c.
(240 ml)
Avocado, 1/4 whole

Kidney beans, 1 c.
Rice, cooked, 1 c.
Tortilla, 1 whole
Green salad, 1 c.
Salad dressing, 2 tbsp.
(30 ml)

Granola bar, 1 whole
Peach, 1 whole
Yogurt with fruit, 8 oz.
(240 ml)

2,400 calories
390 g carbohydrate (63%)
105 g protein (17%)
56 g fat (20%)

Muesli, 3/4 c. (180 ml)
Soy or dairy yogurt, 8 oz.
(240 ml)
Blueberries, 1 c. (240 ml)

Garbanzo beans, 1/3 c.
Salad greens/vegetables, 3 c.
Pita, 1 large
Cheese, low-fat, 2 oz. (60 g)
Grapefruit juice, 8 oz.
(240 ml)

Energy bar, 1 medium
Apple, 1

Tempeh, 3/4 c. (180 ml)
Rice, 1-1/2 c. cooked
Broccoli, cooked, 1 c.
Sesame seed oil, 1 tbsp.
(15 ml)

Orange, 1 medium
Almond, 2 tsp. (15 ml)

3,000 calories
475 g carbohydrate (67%)
102 g protein (14%)
60 g fat (19%)

Waffles, 2 small
Maple syrup, 4 oz. (120 ml)
Raspberries, 1 c.
Skim milk, 1 c. (240 ml)

Hummus, 1/2 c.
Rice, cooked, 1/2 c.
Lentil salad, 1/2 c.
Pita bread, 1 round
Carrots and celery, 2 c.

Bagel, 4 oz. (120 g)
Cheese, low-fat, 2 oz. (60 g)
Apple, 1

Tofu, 4 oz. (120 g)
Soba noodles, cooked, 2 c.
(480 ml)
Greens, cooked, 1 c.
Sesame seed oil, 1 tbsp.
(15 ml)

Pear, 1 large

SAMPLE MENUS, *CONTINUED*

2,900 calories
470 g carbohydrate (62%)
113 g protein (15%)
78 g fat (23%)

Pancakes, 4 small
Syrup, 6 tbsp. (90 g)
Raisins, 2 tbsp. (30 ml)
Apple juice, 8 oz. (240 ml)
Eggs, 2 whole

Soy or dairy yogurt with fruit,
    8 oz. (240 ml)
Almonds, 2 tbsp. (30 ml)

Bean soup, 1-1/2 c. (360 ml)
Rye crackers, 4
Vegetable salad, 1 c.
Soy milk, 12 oz. (360 ml)

Potato, 1 large
Kidney beans, 1 c.
Cheese, low-fat, 1 oz. (30 g)
Green salad, 2 c.
Salad dressing, 3 tbsp. (45 g)

Frozen yogurt, 1 c. (240 ml)
Banana, 1 large

3,600 calories
635 g carbohydrate (68%)
134 g protein (14%)
73 g fat (18%)

Bran flakes, 1-1/2 c.
    (360 ml)
Wheat germ, 2 tbsp. (30 ml)
Soy or dairy milk, 8 oz.
    (240 ml)
Peach, 1 medium

Recovery Drink:
Juice, 12 oz. (360 ml)
Yogurt, 1 c. (240 ml)
Banana, 1 whole

Nut butter, 2 tbsp. (30 ml)
Bread, 2 slices
Bean soup, 1 c. (240 ml)
Raw vegetables, 1 c.

Tofu, 8 oz. (240 g)
Peas, 1 c.
Noodles, 2 c. (480 ml)
Rolls, 2
Vegetable oil, 2 tbsp.
    (30 ml)
Green salad, 2 c.
Salad dressing, 2 tbsp.
    (30 ml)

Sports drink, 40 oz.
    (1,200 ml)

3,300 calories
550 g carbohydrate (65%)
120 g protein (14%)
77 g fat (21%)

Oatmeal, cooked, 1-1/2 c.
    (360 ml)
Skim milk, 1 c. (240 ml)
Wheat germ, 2 tbsp. (30 ml)
Orange juice, 12 oz.
    (360 ml)
Yogurt, 1 c. (240 ml)
Apple, 1 large

Sports drink, 40 oz.
    (1,200 ml)

Thin-crust pizza, easy
    cheese, 3 slices
Green salad, 2 c.
Salad dressing, 2 tbsp.
    (30 ml)
Soy milk, 8 oz. (240 ml)

Pretzels, 2 oz. (60 g)
Hummus, 1/2 c.
Raw vegetables, 1 c.

Spaghetti, cooked, 3 c.
    (720 ml)
Marinara sauce, 2 c.
    (480 ml)
Parmesan cheese, 3 tbsp.
    (45 ml)
Italian bread, 2 slices
Olive oil, 1 tbsp. (15 ml)

Sorbet, 1-1/2 c. (360 ml)
Fig bars, 2

SELECTED BIBLIOGRAPHY

Åkermark, C, et al. 1996. Diet and muscle glycogen concentration in relation to physical performance in Swedish elite ice hockey players. *International Journal of Sport Nutrition* 6 (3): 272–284.

Armstrong, LE. Caffeine, body fluid-electrolyte balance, and exercise performance. *International Journal of Nutrition and Exercise Metabolism* 12 (2): 189–206.

Balsom, PD, et al. 1999. Carbohydrate intake and multiple sprint sports: with special reference to football (soccer). *International Journal of Sports Medicine* 20 (1): 48–52.

Bangsbo, JL, et al. 1992. The effect of carbohydrate diet on intermittent exercise performance. *International Journal of Sports Medicine* 13: 152–157.

Beals, K. 2004. *Disordered Eating among Athletes*. Human Kinetics, Champaign, IL.

Børsheim, E, et al. 2004. Effect of amino acid, protein, and carbohydrate mixture on net muscle protein balance after resistance exercise. *International Journal of Sport Nutrition and Exercise Metabolism* 14 (3): 255–271.

Bosco, C, et al. 1997. Effect of oral creatine supplementation on jumping and running performance. *International Journal of Sports Medicine* 18 (5): 369–372.

Broad, EM, et al. 1996. Body weight changes and voluntary fluid intakes during training and competition sessions in team sports. *International Journal of Sport Nutrition* 6 (3): 307–320.

Burke, L, and Deakin, V. 2000. *Clinical Sports Nutrition*. McGraw-Hill, Sydney.

Burke, LM, et al. 1993. Muscle glycogen storage after prolonged exercise: Effect of the glycemic index of carbohydrate feedings. *Journal of Applied Physiology* 75: 1019–1023.

Burke, LM, et al. 1996. Muscle glycogen storage after prolonged exercise: effect of frequency of carbohydrate feedings. *American Journal of Clinical Nutrition* 64: 115–119.

Burns, RD, et al. 2004. Intercollegiate student athlete use of nutritional supplements and the role of the athletic trainers and dietitian in nutrition counseling. *Journal of the American Dietetic Association* 104 (2): 246–249.

Casa, DJ, et al. 2004. Heat acclimatization of football players during initial summer practice sessions. *Medicine and Science in Sport and Exercise* 36:S49 (abstract).

Catlin, D, et al. 2000. Trace contamination of over-the-counter androstendione and positive urine test results for a nandrolone metabolite. *Journal of the American Medical Association* 284: 2618–2621.

Criswell, D, et al. 1991. Influence of a carbohydrate-electrolyte beverage on performance and blood homeostasis during recovery from football. *International Journal of Sport Nutrition* 1 (2): 178–191.

Crowe, MJ, et al. 2003. The effects of B-hydoxy-B-methylbutarate (HMB) and HMB/creatine supplementation on indices of health in highly trained athletes. *International Journal of Nutrition and Exercise Metabolism* 13 (2): 184–197.

Davis, JM, et al. 1997. Carbohydrate drinks delay fatigue during intermittent, high-intensity cycling in active men and women. *International Journal of Sports Nutrition* 7 (4): 261–273.

DePalma, MT, et al. 1993. Weight control practices of lightweight football players. *Medicine and Science in Sport and Exercise* 25 (6): 694–701.

Dubnov, G, and Constantini, NW. 2004. Prevalence of iron depletion and anemia in top-level basketball players. *International Journal of Nutrition and Exercise Metabolism* 14 (1): 30–37.

Febbraio, MA, et al. 1996. Carbohydrate feedings before prolonged exercise: effect of glycemic index on muscle glycogenolysis and exercise performance. *Journal of Applied Physiology* 81: 1115–1120.

Gomez, JE, et al. 1998. Body fatness and increased injury rates in high school football linemen. *Clinical Journal of Sports Medicine* 8 (2): 115–120.

Hawley, JA, et al. 1994. Carbohydrate, fluid, and electrolyte requirements of the soccer player: a review. *International Journal of Sport Nutrition* 4 (3): 221–236.

Herbold, NH, et al. 2004. Traditional and nontraditional supplement use by collegiate female varsity athletes. *International Journal of Sport Nutrition and Exercise Metabolism* 14 (5): 586–593.

Heyward, VH, and Stolarczyk, LM. 1996. *Applied Body Composition Assessment*. Human Kinetics, Champaign, IL.

Ivy, JL, et al. 1988. Muscle glycogen storage after different amounts of carbohydrate ingestion. *Journal of Applied Physiology* 64 (5): 2018–2023.

Ivy, JL, et al. 1988. Muscle glycogen synthesis after exercise: effect of time of carbohydrate ingestion. *Journal of Applied Physiology* 64 (4): 1480–1485.

Izquierdo, M, et al. 2002. Effects of creatine, supplementation on muscle power, endurance, and sprint performance. *Medicine and Science in Sports and Exercise* 34 (2): 332–343.

Kaplan, TA, et al. 1995. Effect of obesity on injury risk in high school football players. *Clinical Journal of Sports Medicine* 5 (1): 43–47.

Kirwan, JP, et al. 1988. Carbohydrate balance in competitive runners during successive days of intense training 65 (6): 2601–2606.

Kovacs, EMR, et al. 2002. Effect of high and low fluid intake on post-exercise rehydration. *International Journal of Sport Nutrition and Exercise Metabolism* 12: 14–23.

Kreider, RB, et al. 1998. Effects of creatine supplementation on body composition, strength, and sprint performance. *Medicine and Science in Sport and Exercise* 30 (1): 73–82.

Leiper, JB, et al. 2001. Gastric emptying of a carbohydrate-electrolyte drink during a soccer match. *Medicine and Science in Sports and Exercise* 33 (11): 1932–1938.

Lemon, P, et al. 1992. Protein requirements and muscle mass/strength changes during intensive training in novice bodybuilders. *Journal of Applied Physiology* 73: 767–775.

Maughan, RJ, et al. 2004. Fluid and electrolyte intake and loss in elite soccer players during training. *International Journal of Sport Nutrition and Exercise Metabolism* 14 (3): 333–346.

Miller, SL, et al. 2003. Independent and combined effects of amino acids and glucose after resistance exercise. *Medicine and Science in Sports and Exercise* 35 (3): 449–455.

Minehan, M, et al. 2002. Effect of flavor and awareness of kilojoule content of drinks on preference and fluid balance in team sports. *International Journal of Sport Nutrition and Exercise Metabolism* 12 (1): 81–92.

Nicholas, CW, et al. 1995. Influence of ingesting a carbohydrate-electrolyte solution on endurance capacity during intermittent, high-intensity shuttle running. *Journal of Sports Science* 13 (4): 283–290.

NCAA. 2002. *Out of Season Football Conditioning: Educational Initiatives*. 1–8. NCAA, Indianapolis.

Nicholas, C, et al. 1997. Carbohydrate intake and recovery of intermittent running capacity. *International Journal of Sport Nutrition* 7 (4): 251–260.

Nowak, RK, et al. 1988. Body composition and nutrient intakes of college men and women basketball players. *Journal of the American Dietetic Association* 88 (5): 575–578.

Palumbo, C, and Clark, N. 2000. Case problem: nutrition concerns related to the performance of a baseball team. *Journal of the American Dietetic Association* 100 (6): 704–707.

Parkin, J, et al. 1997. Muscle glycogen storage following prolonged exercise: effect of timing of ingestion of high glycemic index food. *Medicine and Science in Sport and Exercise* 29: 220–224.

Rico-Sanz, J. 1998. Body composition and nutritional assessment in soccer. *International Journal of Sport Nutrition* 8 (2): 113–123.

Rico-Sanz, J, et al. 1998. Dietary and performance assessment of elite soccer players during a period of intense training. *International Journal of Sport Nutrition* 8 (3): 230–240.

Rico-Sanz, J, et al. 1999. Muscle glycogen degradation during simulation of a fatiguing soccer match in elite soccer players examined noninvasively by 13-c-MRS. *Medicine and Science in Sports and Exercise* 31 (11): 1587–1593.

Rosenbloom, CA, ed. 2000. *Sports Nutrition: A Guide for the Professional Working with Active People*. American Dietetic Association, Chicago.

Roy, B, Tarnopolsky, M, et al. 1998. Influence of differing macronutrient intakes on muscle glycogen resynthesis after resistance exercise. *Journal of Applied Physiology* 84 (3): 890–896.

Roy, R, et al. 1997. Effect of glucose supplement timing on protein metabolism after resistance training. *Journal of Applied Physiology* 82 (6): 1882–1888.

Sherman, WM, et al. 1989. Effects of 4 h preexercise carbohydrate feedings on cycling performance. *Medicine and Science in Sports and Exercise* 21 (5): 598–604.

Sherman, WM, et al. 1991. Carbohydrate feedings 1 h before exercise improves cycling performance. *American Journal of Clinical Nutrition* 54: 866–870.

Shirreffs, S, et al. 1996. Post-exercise rehydration in man: effect of volume consumed and drink sodium content. *Medicine and Science in Sports and Exercise* 28 (10): 1260–1271.

Simard, C, et al. 1988. Effects of carbohydrate intake before and during an ice hockey game on blood and muscle energy substrates. *Research Quarterly for Exercise and Sport* 59: 144–147.

Slater, G, et al. 2001. B-hydoxy-B-methylbutarate (HMB) supplementation does not affect changes in strength or body composition during resistance training in trained men. *International Journal of Nutrition and Exercise Metabolism* 11 (3): 384–396.

Smith Rockwell, M, et al. 2001. Nutrition knowledge, opinions, and practices of coaches and athletic trainers at Division I University. *International Journal of Nutrition and Exercise Metabolism* 11 (2): 174–185.

Stofan, JR, et al. 2003. Sweat and sodium losses in NCAA Division I football players with a history of whole body muscle cramping. *Medicine and Science in Sports and Exercise* 35:S48 (abstract).

Stover, EA, et al. 2004. Drinking strategy for improving hydration status in high school football players. *Medicine and Science in Sports and Exercise* 36:S49 (abstract).

Tarnopolsky, MA, and MacLennan, DP. 2000. Creatine monohydrate supplementation enhances high intensity exercise performance in males and females. *International Journal of Sport Nutrition and Exercise Metabolism* 10 (4): 452–463.

Tarnopolsky, MA, et al. 1997. Postexercise protein-carbohydrate and carbohydrate supplements increase muscle glycogen in men and women. *Journal of Applied Physiology* 83 (6): 1877.

Tarnopolsky, MA, et al. 2001. Gender differences in carbohydrate loading are related to energy intake. *Journal of Applied Physiology* 91: 225–230.

Tipton, KD, and Wolfe, RR. 2004. Protein and amino acids for athletes. *Journal of Sports Science* 22 (1): 65–79.

Welsh, RS, et al. 2002. Carbohydrates and physical/mental performance during intermittent exercise. *Medicine and Science in Sports and Exercise* 34 (4): 723–731.

Yaspelkis, B, et al. 1993. Carbohydrate supplementation spares muscle glycogen during variable-intensity exercise. *Journal of Applied Physiology* 75: 1477–1485.

Yoshida, T, et al. 1995. Effect of aerobic capacity on sweat rate and fluid intake during outdoor exercise in the heat. *European Journal of Applied Physiology* 71: 235–239.

INDEX

ABOUT THE AUTHOR

Monique Ryan, MS, RD, LDN is a nationally recognized nutritionist with over twenty years of experience. She is founder of Personal Nutrition Designs, a nutrition consulting company based in the Chicago area. Started in 1992, Personal Nutrition Designs provides nutrition programs for diverse groups of people with an emphasis on long-term follow-up and support programming. Ryan has developed thousands of nutrition plans for clients in the areas of sports nutrition, weight management, women's health, eating disorder recovery, various medical and health concerns, and disease prevention and wellness. Her clients are provided with practical, cutting-edge nutrition information based on current scientific research.

Ryan is a nationally recognized sports nutritionist and was a member of the Performance Enhancement Team for USA Triathlon, USA Cycling (Women's Road Team), and Synchro Swimming USA up until the 2004 Athens Olympic Games. She has worked with the Timex Multisport Team, and was the nutritionist for the Saturn Cycling Team from 1994 to 2000. Ryan has consulted with many professional endurance triathletes and mountain bike teams. She has also lectured extensively on sports nutrition to coaches, trainers, and amateur athletes who train at all levels.

Ryan has also written *Sports Nutrition for Endurance Athletes*. She is the author of over 150 published articles. For the past fourteen years, she has written sports nutrition articles for *VeloNews*, and has written regularly for *Inside Triathlon* since 1994.

Monique Ryan has a Bachelor of Science degree in Nutrition and Dietetics and a Master of Science Degree in Nutrition. She completed her clinical training at Northwestern Memorial Hospital Medical Center in Chicago. She is a registered dietitian (RD) and licensed in the state of Illinois (LDN). Ryan is a member of the American College of Sports Medicine (ACSM) and is an ACSM Health Fitness Instructor. Ryan has competed in the sports of road cycling and mountain biking.